UROLOGICAL NURSING

Second edition

Edited by

Sharon Fillingham and Jean Douglas

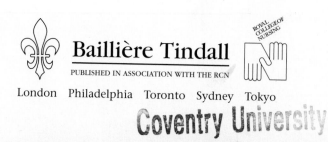

Baillière Tindall

PUBLISHED IN ASSOCIATION WITH THE RCN

London Philadelphia Toronto Sydney Tokyo

Baillière Tindall

An imprint of Harcourt Publishers Limited

© 1997 Baillière Tindall
© Harcourt Publishers Limited 2000

First published in 1994 by Scutari Press

❀ is a registered trademark of Harcourt Publishers Limited

This book is printed on acid-free paper

A catalogue record for this book is available from the British Library

ISBN 0-7020-2303-5

Typeset by J&L Composition Ltd, Filey, North Yorkshire
Printed in China
EPC/02

UROLOGICAL NURSING

5

UROLOGICAL NURSING

second edition

CONTENTS

CONTRIBUTORS

Rachel Anson RGN Dip. N(Lond), ENB 134, 998, 978, Senior Staff Nurse, Haemodialysis Unit, Royal Sussex County Hospital, Brighton
Chapter 6: Urinary Tract Stones

Louisa Ashford BSc(Hons), RGN, ENB 998, Clinical Practitioner, UCLH NHS Trust, London
Chapter 17: Developments in Urological Nursing – Expanding Nursing Roles in Urology

Martin Beynon BSc(Hons), RGN, ENB 134, 978, 998, Lecturer Practitioner Urology Nursing, UCLH NHS Trust, London
Chapter 1: Anatomy and Physiology of the Urinary Tract
Chapter 2: Urological Investigations

Jane Champion BSc(Hons), RGN, ENB 978, 998, 225, Senior Nurse Manager, Uro-Nephrology, UCLH NHS Trust, London
Chapter 6: Urinary Tract Stones

Daphne Colpman BSc(Hons), RGN ENB 134, 978, 998, PgDip Health Promotion, Continence Advisor, UCLH NHS Trust, London
Chapter 4: Conservative Management of Urological Problems
Chapter 7: Reconstructive Surgery for Urinary Tract Defects

Jean Douglas RGN, SCM, Dip. N(Lond), FETC, ENB 134, 978, Formerly Clinical Nurse Facilitator, UCLH NHS Trust, London
Chapter 14: Reassignment Surgery

Sue Fell RGN, ENB 941, 998, 980, 134, 216, HDQC Physiology, Clinical Nurse Specialist Stoma Care/Continent Diversions, UCLH NHS Trust, London
Chapter 13: Scrotal Disorders

Elizabeth Fenwick RGN, ENB 134, 998, Cert. Couns., Clinical Nurse Specialist, Chemotherapy, UCLH NHS Trust, London
Chapter 10: Urological Cancers

Sharon Fillingham BSc(Hons), RGN, Dip. Couns., ENB 978, 980, 216, 998, 870, HA Colorectal Nursing, Clinical Nurse Specialist Stoma Care, UCLH NHS Trust London
Chapter 11: Urological Stomas
Chapter 12: Penile Disorders

Helen Forristal RGN, ENB 134, 998, 237, MacMillan Urology Nurse Specialist, Joyce Green, Dartford
Chapter 9: Prostatic Problems

Helen Harvey RGN, ENB 998, 980, 134, Ward Sister, UCLH NHS Trust, London
Chapter 11: Urological Stomas

Sue Keeble RSCN, RGN, ENB 138, 978, 998, Clinical Nurse Specialist/ Continence Advisor Paediatric Urology, The Portland Hospital for Women and Children, London
Chapter 15: Paediatric Urology

Caroline Leach BSc(Hons), RGN, DipCouns, Clinical Practitioner, UCLH NHS Trust, London
Chapter 16: Psychological Effects of Urological Problems – Adults

Rachel Busuttil-Leaver BSc(Hons), RGN, ENB 998, 134, 978, 980, 870, Clinical Nurse Specialist Continent Diversion, UCLH NHS Trust, London
Chapter 8: Reconstructive Surgery for the Promotion of Continence

Alison Lungley RSCN, RGN, ENB 134, 998, Senior Nurse Specialist, Healthcare at Home, Brentford, Middlesex
Chapter 15: Paediatric Urology

Margaret Macaulay RGN, ENB 134, 978, 998, DN, Continence Advisor, Wandsworth Community Health Trust, London
Chapter 5: Urinary Drainage Systems

Jane Maxfield RGN, ENB 998, 134, 978, 941, N37, Clinical Nurse Practitioner, UCLH NHS Trust, London
Chapter 9: Prostatic Problems

Claire Nicholls RGN, ENB 134, 998, 978, Ward Sister, UCLH NHS Trust, London
Chapter 1: Anatomy and Physiology of the Urinary Tract
Chapter 2: Urological Investigations

Sharon Rainsbury RGN, BSc(Hons), ENB 134, 978, 998, Formerly Ward Sister, UCLH NHS Trust, London
Chapter 6: Urinary Tract Stones

Maryam Sokootifar BSc(Hons) HV (Health Visitor), RGN, RSCN, ENB 138, 998, Senior Staff Nurse Paediatrics, UCLH NHS Trust, London
Chapter 16: Psychological Effects of Urological Problems – Adolescents

Judith Susser RGN, ENB 980, 978, 134, Research Sister, Clinical Trials and Research Unit, Institute of Urology and Nephrology, UCLH NHS Trust, London
Chapter 17: Developments in Urological Nursing – Research Nursing in Urology

Kate Welford RGN, ENB 134, 978, 998, 870, Continence Advisor, UCLH NHS Trust, London
Chapter 3: Urodynamics
Chapter 4: Conservative Management of Urological Problems

Patricia de Winter RGN, ENB 138, 998, Research Sister, Clinical Trials and Research Unit, Institute of Urology and Nephrology, UCLH NHS Trust, London
Chapter 17: Developments in Urological Nursing – Research Nursing in Urology

PREFACE

The second edition of this textbook has been prepared in response to the many recent innovations and treatments in the field of urology.

All the contributors to this textbook have been employed within St Peter's Hospital/Institute of Urology and Nephrology which is now part of the University College London Hospitals (UCLH) NHS Trust.

St Peter's is an amalgamation of four smaller hospitals which were originally situated around the Covent Garden area of London and relocated with UCLH in 1992. Considerable experience in the field of uro-nephrology has been established within the unit which continues to be responsive to urological research and education needs of both nursing and medical staff.

As with the first edition, the contributors have not been constrained by a particular framework of presentation; neither a universal nursing model nor a standard chapter layout has been adopted. It is hoped that such an approach will make the text more accessible, providing the reader with a resource which is both readable and user-friendly, and it is our aim to provide a book which will appeal to all individuals involved in the field of urology.

It is hoped that after the success of the first edition, the second edition, with its updated material and additional chapters, will continue the trend.

The contributors acknowledge the many colleagues from St Peter's who have assisted them during the preparation of this book. Brenda Roe is thanked for her assistance with the chapter on urinary drainage systems. We would also like to thank Rosemary Clark and Robin Douglas for their untiring secretarial support.

Finally, we would particularly like to thank and acknowledge Clive Laker, whose original idea to produce such a textbook has given us the opportunity to be involved in this exciting project.

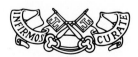

In acknowledgement of the staff at the Institute of Urology and Nephrology, St Peter's Hospital, The University College London Hospitals NHS Trust

PUBLISHER'S ACKNOWLEDGEMENTS

We wish to thank the following companies for their generous contributions towards the production costs of this book:

ConvaTec

 Osbon Medical UK

Yamanouchi Pharma Ltd

ANATOMY AND PHYSIOLOGY OF THE URINARY TRACT

1

Contents

This chapter outlines the structure and function of the adult upper and lower urinary system. The embryological development of the urinary system is discussed in Chapter 15.

The urinary tract comprises kidneys, ureters, urinary bladder and urethra (Figure 1.1). The function of the urinary tract is to remove the waste products of metabolism, to regulate fluid and electrolyte balance, to regulate acid–base balance, and to transport and store urine; it thus plays a vital role in maintaining homeostasis.

ANATOMY OF THE KIDNEY

The kidneys are a pair of bean-shaped organs which lie posterior to the parietal peritoneum within the retroperitoneal space. They are situated high in the abdominal cavity and, relative to the spinal vertebrae, occupy a position between the twelfth thoracic and fourth lumbar vertebrae, though the right kidney is slightly lower owing to the anatomical position of the liver. The kidneys are partially protected by the eleventh and twelfth rib pairs: other key anatomical relationships are shown in Figure 1.2. The adult kidneys are similar in both shape and size, measuring about 10–12 cm in length, 5–7 cm in width and 2–5 cm in thickness. Each weighs approximately 150 g.

The lateral surface of the kidney is convex and its medial surface is concave; there is a cleft in this medial portion known as the renal hilum. There are

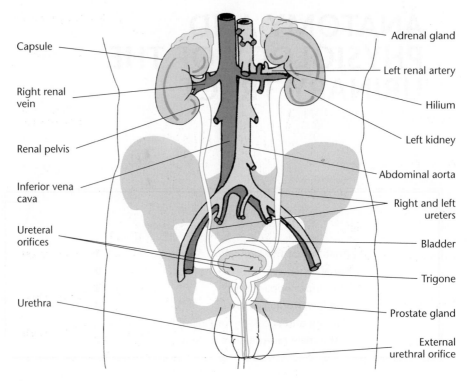

Figure 1.1 *Anatomy of the urinary tract*

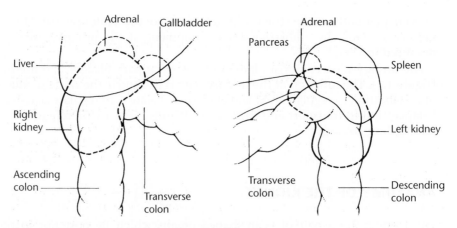

Figure 1.2 *Key anatomical relationships of the kidney*

several structures that enter or exit the kidney at this point, e.g. the renal pelvis (ureter), blood vessels, lymphatics and nerves.

Each kidney is surrounded by three layers of supportive tissue. The first of these layers (closest to the kidney) is the smooth, fibrous renal capsule which is continuous with the outer layer of the ureter at the renal hilum; its purpose is as a barrier against infection and direct trauma. The middle protective layer is the adipose capsule (perinephric fat) which holds the kidney in place within the abdominal cavity and cushions it from direct trauma. Should

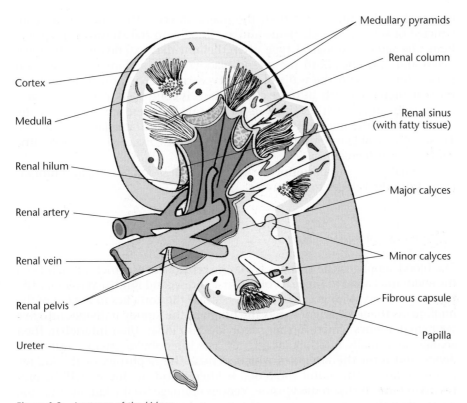

Figure 1.3   Anatomy of the kidney

the amount of fatty tissue diminish rapidly the kidneys drop down from their normal anatomical position causing kinking of the ureter and hydronephrosis – an event known as 'ptosis'. The outer protective layer is a dense fibrous connective tissue called the renal fascia, which anchors the kidney to its surrounding structures and the posterior abdominal wall.

A longitudinal coronal section through the kidney reveals several macroscopic structures (Figure 1.3). The kidney is divided into an outer darker area, the cortex, and an inner lighter-coloured area, the medulla. The nephrons (functional units of the kidney) extend throughout both the cortical and medullary regions.

Within the medulla there are 10–18 triangular structures known as the renal pyramids. They are striated (striped) in appearance as a result of the presence of straight renal tubules (from the nephrons) and coexistent blood vessels. The pyramids direct urine down into the initial part of the collecting system (calyces). It can be seen in Figure 1.3 that the cortex of the kidney extends from the outer boundary down to the bases of the renal pyramids, as renal columns. Further, the cortex subdivides into an outer zone and an inner juxtamedullary zone. This is an important anatomical distinction, as those nephrons responsible for water balance extend deeply into the juxtamedullary zone.

The renal cortex, in association with the pyramids, constitute the renal parenchyma. In the average adult kidney the renal parenchyma consists of approximately 1 million nephrons. Urine draining from the renal pyramids is

collected in the minor and then the major calyces. The calcyces are constructed of smooth muscle tissue and are lined with transitional cell epithelium, the same histological type of epithelium that extends into the renal
pelvis and also lines both ureter and bladder. Contractions of the smooth
muscle fibres within the walls of the calyces and pelvis propel urine down
into the ureter. The rate of these contractions is controlled by intrinsic pace-
maker cells situated within the walls of the calyces (these are not neuronally
innervated, as the mechanism remains intact within transplanted kidneys).
These cells are able to monitor urinary flow: as the calyces distend peristaltic
contraction is increased.

The renal pelvis lies posterior to the main renal blood vessels, and funnels
urine from the calyces to the ureter.

Renal circulation

The blood supply to the kidneys is via the renal arteries which branch from
the abdominal aorta at the level of the first and second lumbar vertebrae. The
right renal artery is longer than the left because the aorta lies to the left of the
midline. As the renal artery enters the hilum of the kidney it divides into five
segmental arteries which further subdivide into lobar, then interlobar, then
arcuate, and finally interlobular arteries. The interlobular arteries ultimately
divide and form the arterioles which perfuse the nephrons of the kidney
(Figure 1.4a). At this point the blood is filtered and the filtrate will be pro-
cessed to form the byproduct, urine. Venous drainage for the kidney is via the
renal veins; this runs a course roughly parallel to that of the arterial supply,
but there are no lobar or segmental veins. The renal veins empty into the
inferior vena cava. The left renal vein is longer than the right, as the inferior
vena cava lies to the right of the vertebral column.

The kidneys receive approximately 25% of the total cardiac output under
resting conditions.

Innervation of the kidney

The nerve supply to the kidneys is from the sympathetic (autonomic) nervous
system via the renal plexus. These are vasomotor nerves and accompany the
renal arteries and their branches throughout the renal parenchyma, regulating renal blood flow by altering the diameter of the arterioles.

Microscopic structure of the kidney

The functional unit of the kidney is the nephron (Figure 1.4b). Each nephron
consists of two principal structures, first a 'tuft' of capillaries known as the
glomerulus (approximately six to eight capillary loops in total); and secondly
a renal tubule approximately 6 cm long and lined throughout by a modified
columnar epithelium. Each part of the renal tubule has a unique cellular
anatomy which reflects its specific function (Figures 1.5 and 1.6).

The proximal end of the renal tubule (Bowman's capsule) is cup-shaped

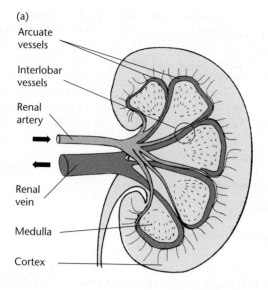

(a)

Arcuate vessels

Interlobar vessels

Renal artery

Renal vein

Medulla

Cortex

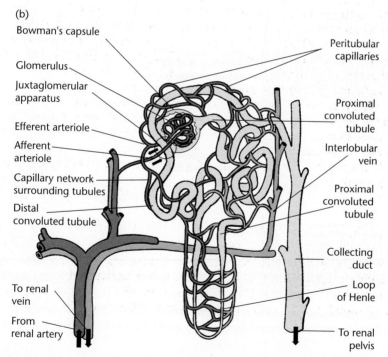

(b)

Bowman's capsule

Glomerulus

Juxtaglomerular apparatus

Efferent arteriole

Afferent arteriole

Capillary network surrounding tubules

Distal convoluted tubule

To renal vein

From renal artery

Peritubular capillaries

Proximal convoluted tubule

Interlobular vein

Proximal convoluted tubule

Collecting duct

Loop of Henle

To renal pelvis

Figure 1.4 *Cross-section of the kidney (a), showing the anatomy of the juxtaglomerular nephron and associated blood vessels (b)*

and invaginates the glomerulus; filtration is achieved within this first portion of the nephron. The capillaries within the glomerulus are more permeable to water and solutes than the extrarenal capillaries, owing to the size of the fenestrations (pores) in the single layer glomerular endothelium. Solute-rich filtrate from the glomerulus contains large proteins but not cells. The

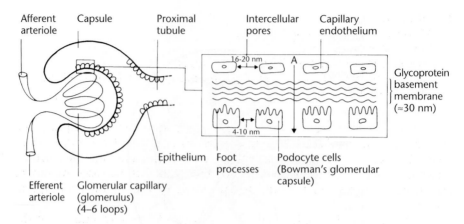

Figure 1.5 *Fine structure of Bowman's capsule*

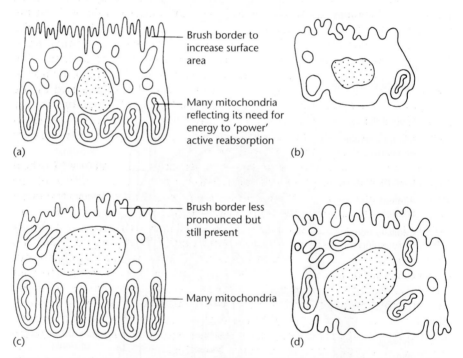

Figure 1.6 *Histological appearance of cells within different functional areas of the nephron: (a) proximal tubular cell; (b) thin loop of Henle cell; (c) distal tubular cell; (d) collecting duct cell*

glomerular endothelium rests upon a basement membrane, this inhibits the filtration of large protein molecules. The capsular epithelium is lined with podocytes. These cells possess foot-like structures called pedicles which, except for filtration pores, cover the basement membrane. Small molecule proteins cannot pass through the capsular epithelium; the resulting filtrate comprises water, electrolytes, urea, glucose, polypeptides and amino acids.

The other key functional areas of the nephron can be divided into the following stages:

1. Filtration.
2. Mass salvage of essential substances.
3. Water balance.
4. Fine control of water, sodium and hydrogen.
5. Facultative water reabsorption under hormonal control (via the influence of antidiuretic hormone).

The proximal convoluted tubule follows from the Bowman's capsule and extends for a length of 12–24 mm through the cortex of the kidney. This region is lined by large columnar epithelial cells which are modified on the internal surface to form a brush border of microvilli: this increases the surface area inside the proximal tubule where much of the solute reabsorption occurs.

The thin-walled descending limb of the loop of Henle extends from the proximal convoluted tubule. It passes into the medulla and forms a U shape, moving back into the cortex via a thicker-walled ascending limb. In both limbs the columnar cells are flatter and they contain fewer microvilli on the internal surfaces. The ascending limb of the loop of Henle leads into the distal convoluted tubule, the first part of which folds back in proximity to the afferent arteriole, where it forms a region known as the macula densa. The specialized epithelial cells of the macula densa monitor the sodium chloride concentration of fluid flowing through this area and comprise part of the juxtaglomerular apparatus. The distal convoluted tubule is comparatively short (4–8 mm) and leads into the collecting ducts which join together as they move through the medulla, finally opening at the tips of the medullary papillae into the calyces of the renal pelvis.

Nephrons are categorized as either 'cortical' or 'juxtamedullary'. Cortical nephrons (85%) have glomeruli located towards the outer surface of the cortex and short loops of Henle, some of which extend down to the outer medulla. The juxtamedullary nephrons (15%) are located close to the corticomedullary junction and have long loops of Henle which extend deeply into the medulla. In addition these nephrons possess a larger glomerulus and the efferent arteriole forms not only a peritubular network of capillaries, but also a series of vascular loops known collectively as the vasa recta. The vasa recta descend into the medulla and form a collective network of capillaries that surround the collecting ducts and ascending limbs of the loops of Henle. Essential nutrients are supplied to the renal medulla and blood then returns to the cortex via the ascending vasa recta. These juxtamedullary nephrons are crucial for the production of concentrated urine.

Figure 1.7 illustrates the main regional specialization of reabsorption and secretion within the nephron (McLaren, 1996).

Microcirculation

Nephrons are associated with two capillary beds: the glomerulus and the peritubular capillary bed. The glomerulus is unique as it is fed and drained by arterioles – the afferent and efferent arterioles. The afferent arterioles are supplied by the interlobular arteries. The blood pressure within the glomerulus is higher than in other capillary beds as the afferent arteriole is larger in diameter than the efferent arteriole, also they are both high-resistance vessels.

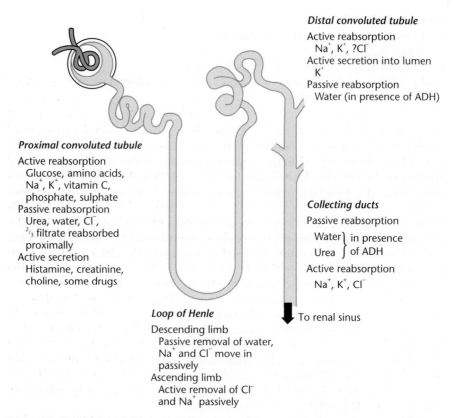

Distal convoluted tubule

Active reabsorption
Na$^+$, K$^+$, ?Cl$^-$
Active secretion into lumen
K$^+$
Passive reabsorption
Water (in presence of ADH)

Proximal convoluted tubule

Active reabsorption
Glucose, amino acids,
Na$^+$, K$^+$, vitamin C,
phosphate, sulphate
Passive reabsorption
Urea, water, Cl$^-$,
$^2/_3$ filtrate reabsorbed
proximally
Active secretion
Histamine, creatinine,
choline, some drugs

Collecting ducts

Passive reabsorption
Water ⎱ in presence
Urea ⎰ of ADH
Active reabsorption
Na$^+$, K$^+$, Cl$^-$

Loop of Henle

Descending limb
Passive removal of water,
Na$^+$ and Cl$^-$ move in
passively
Ascending limb
Active removal of Cl$^-$
and Na$^+$ passively

To renal sinus

Figure 1.7 *Regional specialization in reabsorption and secretion in the nephron*

Renal blood pressure falls from approximately 95 mmHg in the renal arteries to approximately 8 mmHg in the renal veins (Marieb, 1995), but pressure within the glomerulus will normally remain unaffected by fluctuations in systemic blood pressure. The high pressure therefore enables fluid and solutes to be filtered through the glomerular capsule. The volume of plasma filtered through the glomeruli per minute is known as the glomerular filtration rate (GFR) and it provides a reliable measure of renal function; normal GFR approximates 120 ml per minute. In instances where there may be poor renal perfusion (e.g. hypovolaemic shock), the GFR falls sharply.

The majority of the filtrate is selectively reabsorbed by the cells throughout the length of the renal tubule, and returned to the circulation via the peritubular capillary beds. The peritubular capillary beds arise from the efferent arterioles that drain the glomerulus. They follow the route of the renal tubules and drain into venules of the renal venous system. These low-pressure capillaries are adapted to absorb solutes and water from the renal tubular cells.

In addition to filtration and selective reabsorption the kidney performs other specialist functions that maintain the body's internal homeostatic environment.

RENAL FUNCTION

Autoregulation of renal blood pressure

Owing to the high perfusion requirement of the adult kidney, the kidney possesses an intrinsic ability to autoregulate (i.e. to maintain its own blood flow) over a range of systemic arterial pressures. As volume decreases, the homeostatic response attempts to maintain sufficient blood flow to retain renal viability, and also to reduce filtration capacity in the short term (as the GFR falls) until normal levels of perfusion are restored. This pressure range is approximately 80–180 mmHg, which allows the kidney to cope with a wide fluctuation in perfusion input from the aorta. Further, the GFR remains constant over this range, primarily owing to the ability of the kidney to alter its vascular tone within the efferent and afferent arterioles. These arterioles are smooth muscle structures, innervated with sympathetic nerve fibres, which primarily cause vasoconstriction. Thus, if afferent constriction occurs the GFR will decrease as blood flow decreases. If the efferent vessels constrict the GFR will increase, as effective filtration pressure will be increased. This mechanism is not solely innervated neuronally, however, as transplanted kidneys still display the ability to autoregulate; it is thought likely to be under hormonal control via adrenergic receptors on the smooth muscle cells of the arterioles. Sympathetic nervous system activity, via the influence of adrenaline, decreases the renal blood flow (vasoconstriction) and thus the GFR. Blood is then transferred to the vital organs and results in the production of small volumes of concentrated urine (oliguria), e.g. in patients suffering from hypovolaemia.

Normal postural adjustments also require the sympathetic nervous system to adjust the level of arterial blood pressure, by constriction of vessels within the skin and viscera. In these circumstances the GFR remains stable, since autoregulation occurs via the afferent or efferent arterioles, thus maintaining perfusion and therefore function.

Renin–angiotensin mechanism

A further potent homeostatic mechanism which aims to conserve blood flow in the kidney is that of the renin–angiotensin system (Figure 1.8), which also directly influences systemic blood pressure. Angiotensinogen is an alpha-2 globulin produced by the liver. It provides the substrate for renin (therefore acting as an enzyme) to cleave the angiotensinogen molecule. Renin itself is produced by the polar cuff cells of the afferent arterioles (Figure 1.9). The macula densa cells (in the distal tubule) are primarily sodium sensitive; however, as a result of the close anatomical arrangement between the juxtaglomerular apparatus and the macula densa, renin release can be stimulated in response to three separate stimuli:

1. Low blood pressure: within the walls of the afferent arterioles there are pressure sensors (baroreceptors) which respond when the arteriole is stretched or constricted. Thus dilation of the arterioles, i.e. increased blood flow, stretches the afferent arteriolar wall, causing a decrease in

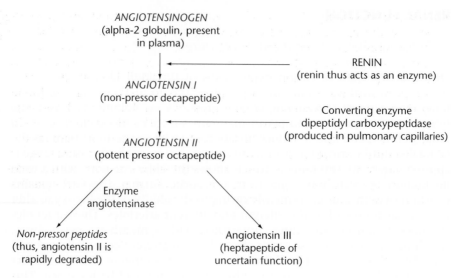

Figure 1.8 *The renin–angiotensin mechanism*

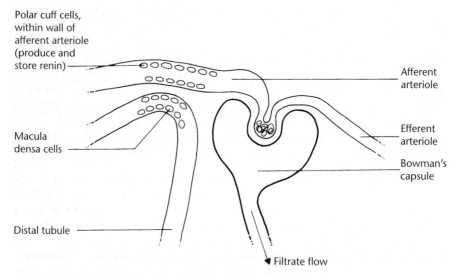

Figure 1.9 *Renin and its site of production*

renin secretion. In conditions of low blood flow stretch is reduced and renin production therefore increases, in an attempt to compensate.

2. Sodium signal: renal secretion would also seem to be controlled by the amount of sodium chloride within the glomerular filtrate, passing through the macula densa cells of the distal tubule. In circumstances of low blood volume (i.e. haemorrhage), the urine becomes more concentrated, and this stimulates the macula densa cells which transfer information to the polar cuff cells, thus initiating renin release. The sodium 'signal' allows the kidney to respond to changes in sodium concentration as well as to blood volume – reflecting a tubular mechanism of regulation rather than a vascular one.

3. Adrenergic system: this stimulus occurs via the sympathetic nervous system during stress situations (e.g. haemorrhage or hypotension). It constitutes a neuronal signal which causes renin release. Additionally, the presence of adrenaline and noradrenaline also leads to renin release. From Figure 1.8 it can be seen that angiotensin II is a potent pressor substance, increasing the total peripheral resistance and therefore blood pressure. Its second major function is its direct influence on the adrenal cortex, initiating the release of aldosterone – this process takes 45–60 minutes. Aldosterone is then 'renally' active, causing an increase in tubular sodium reabsorption which in turn increases the rate of passive water reabsorption. Thus water is absorbed from the tubules with sodium and the net effect is one of increasing the effective plasma volume (rather than plasma sodium in isolation).

Antidiuretic hormone

Antidiuretic hormone (ADH) exerts a crucial effect upon the renal tubules by increasing water reabsorption in the terminal portion of the distal tubule and within the individual collecting ducts. It would appear to do this by initiating the formation of specific channels which are highly permeable to water (within the distal tubule and collecting duct cells) (Guyton, 1991). Water will therefore move from the tubule owing to the high osmotic potential of the renal interstitium, and is taken up by the vasa recta. From these vessels it passes to the systemic circulation. In the absence of ADH virtually no water is absorbed at all from the distal tubule and collecting duct cells, and huge amounts of very dilute urine are produced (as in diabetes insipidus).

The renin–angiotensin system would be unable to exert its mechanism of increasing systemic volume via the effect of aldosterone, without the influence of the neurosecretion ADH, produced from the posterior pituitary gland. As plasma sodium concentration increases, this is sensed in the hypothalamus (as well as in peripheral chemoreceptors) and ADH is released: ADH targets the cells of the collecting duct and changes their permeability to water, so increasing the intracellular pore size and facilitating increased water reabsorption owing to the high osmotic potential of the renal interstitium. The water reabsorbed passes via the vasa recta to the systemic circulation.

Acid–base balance

Acid–base balance is achieved by:

1. The active reabsorption of virtually all filtered bicarbonate.
2. The regeneration of new bicarbonate, to replace that used in plasma buffering.
3. The formation of titratable acid salts which can be excreted in the urine.

The process of urinary acidification provides the only means of removing non-volatile acid from the circulation. Metabolic acidosis is a key problem in patients with renal failure. The urinary pH is normally between 4 and 8, which reflects the urinary route for acid excretion.

Some bacteria (e.g. *Proteus* sp.) have the capacity to split the urea within urine via the enzyme urease, so releasing ammonia and making the urine more alkaline. The alkalinity then causes the precipitation of key ionic species such as calcium and phosphate and may lead to the formation of stones if prolonged.

Production of erythropoietin

Erythropoietin is a hormone that forms the primary stimulus to bone marrow tissue, resulting in the production of new red blood cells. Such erythropoietic activity is stimulated by relative hypoxia, which then causes the release of renal erythropoietic factor from the kidney and liver, although the kidney produces by far a greater percentage – probably over 80%. Once in the plasma, renal erythropoietic factor acts as a specific plasma protein, and is converted to the hormone erythropoietin which then stimulates red blood cell production. Without this mechanism chronic refractory anaemia results.

A significant advance for patients suffering from chronic renal failure who experience such anaemia has been the successful production of human erythropoietin using recombinant DNA technology. This can be given intravenously at the end of haemodialysis or subcutaneously two or three times weekly, depending on the patient's haemoglobin results. It produces a dramatic increase in the quality of life.

It is not known at present exactly where in the kidney erythropoietin is produced, though several sites are currently implicated. These include the mesangial cells of the glomerulus, which extend into the tuft of glomerular capillaries, and the renal tubular epithelial cells (Guyton, 1991). In conditions of low oxygen tension, erythropoietin production begins within minutes or hours and reaches maximum production within 24 hours. If there is no renal function at all anaemia is inevitable, as the 20% of erythropoietin formed in other tissues is only adequate to sustain between 30% and 50% of required red blood cell production.

Vitamin D activation

The kidney is also responsible for the activation of vitamin D. The term 'vitamin D' refers to a group of compounds which are synthesized within the skin from a precursor molecule already present. This process of synthesis is reliant upon the presence of ultraviolet radiation from direct sunlight. The precursor substance is called 7-dehydrocholesterol, and sunlight converts this to cholecalciferol (vitamin D_3). The liver then converts vitamin D_3 to 25-hydroxycholecalciferol, i.e. adds an hydroxyl group. It is this substance that the kidney then further changes to 1,25-dihydroxycholecalciferol (calcitriol), which is the most active form of vitamin D and acts as a hormone to stimulate calcium and phosphate absorption from the gut. This conversion process occurs in the proximal tubular cells of the nephrons.

Calcitriol is up to a thousand times more active than any of its precursor

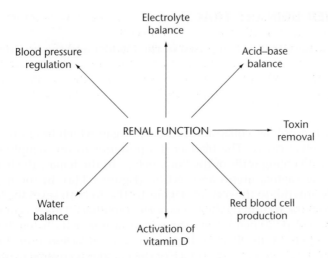

Figure 1.10 *Summary of renal function*

substances and therefore in the absence of kidney function, vitamin D loses almost all of its ability to induce calcium absorption (Guyton, 1991).

A summary of renal function is given in Figure 1.10.

THE UPPER URINARY TRACT

The upper urinary tract is made up of the renal pelves and the ureters. The renal pelvis funnels urine from the calyces down into the ureter. The ureter is a slender tube approximately 25–30 cm in length and 6 mm in diameter. Each ureter begins at the level of the second lumbar vertebra and is a continuation of the renal pelvis (pelviureteric junction, PUJ). The ureter then passes behind the peritoneum and descends to the posterior surface of the bladder.

The ureters enter the bladder wall at an oblique angle (vesicoureteric junction) creating a functional valve that will prevent reflux of urine back into the kidneys; during the filling phase and the voiding phase of the bladder the ureters will be compressed.

The wall of the ureter comprises three layers: the inner mucosa is transitional epithelium, the middle layer is composed of two muscle sheets (the inner is longitudinal in arrangement and the outer is circular; the proximal third of the ureter does, however, contain outer longitudinal muscle fibres), and the outer layer or adventitia is comprised of fibrous connective tissue which anchors the ureter within the retroperitoneal cavity. Peristaltic waves initiated in the renal pelvis propel urine into the ureter. The ureter in turn becomes distended which stimulates contraction of the muscle layer forcing urine along its length and into the bladder.

THE LOWER URINARY TRACT

The lower urinary tract is comprised of the bladder and the urethra.

The urinary bladder

The bladder is a hollow, collapsible muscular organ which lies in the anterior part of the pelvic cavity. The bladder lies posterior to the symphysis pubis, lateral to the diverging walls of the bony pelvis. In the female the bladder lies anterior to the vagina, uterus and rectum (Figure 1.11a). In the male it lies immediately anterior to the rectum (Figure 1.11b). In both sexes the bladder is separated from the rectum by the fascia of Denonvilliers. This is a combination of fused layers of peritoneum from the retrovesical pouch. Its tough, impenetrable nature acts as an effective barrier to rectal invasion from bladder or prostatic tumours. The superior surface of the bladder is covered by the peritoneum, which is reflected upwards onto the anterior abdominal wall, and which peels upward and backward as the bladder rises out of the pelvic cavity on filling. It is therefore possible surgically to approach the anterior aspect of the bladder via the retropubic space, effectively bypassing the peritoneal cavity.

In males the vas deferens and the seminal vesicles lie adjacent to the base of the bladder. Beneath the bladder and attached to the bladder base is the prostate gland, through which the urethra passes.

At the base of the bladder is a small triangular area known as the trigone. The trigone represents the area between the two ureteric orifices and the internal urethral meatus. The trigone during the filling phase of the bladder changes little in size. It is highly sensitive to stretch, and is the area irritated by the presence of foreign bodies, e.g. indwelling urinary catheters.

The bladder is described as having four layers (Bullock *et al.*, 1991).

1. The innermost layer is composed of a mucus-secreting transitional cell epithelium which facilitates stretch. When the bladder is empty this urothelium is six to eight cells deep and is thrown into folds (rugae). As the bladder distends the urothelium stretches and thins to a thickness of two or three cells, and the rugae disappear.
2. The second or submucosal layer is known as the lamina propria and is constructed of connective tissue. It is present above the urothelium in the distensible part of the bladder but absent in the trigonal area.
3. The third muscular layer is collectively known as the detrusor. The detrusor muscle contains both longitudinal and circular fibres and there is controversy over the exact nature of their arrangement. It has been suggested that the detrusor is made up of three layers – an inner longitudinal layer, a middle circumferential layer and an outer longitudinal layer. However, a more complex meshwork of layers is more likely. Stretch receptors within the detrusor play a vital role in bladder filling and emptying.
4. The fourth outer layer (known as the serosa or adventitia) is not a distinct continuation of bladder tissue as such, as it is formed by the peritoneum. It provides separation from adjacent structures and only covers the superior surface of the bladder.

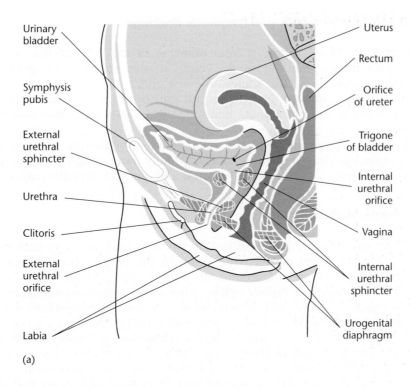

(a)

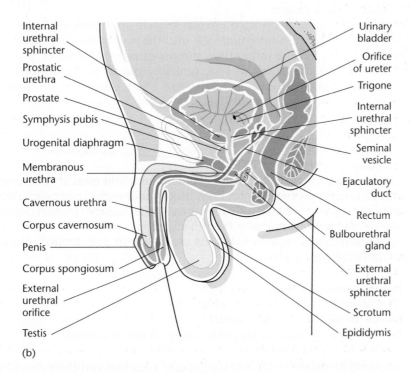

(b)

Figure 1.11 Anatomy of the lower urinary tract in (a) the female and (b) the male

Blood supply, venous and lymphatic drainage

The bladder's blood supply is from branches of the internal iliac artery: principally the superior and inferior vesical arteries. Venous drainage of the bladder is achieved via two routes. The first utilizes the internal iliac veins to the inferior vena cava, and the second runs from the internal iliac veins to the veins of the innominate bones, femoral heads and lower vertebral bodies.

There is a widespread lymphatic drainage system within the deep muscle layer of the bladder, via the internal iliac and obturator groups of nodes, and also via the lymphatics of the bony pelvis and upper ends of the femur.

Bladder neck structure

The anatomical nature of the bladder neck is at present an area of urological controversy. It differs between the sexes. In the male, a circular layer of smooth muscle is present around the bladder neck, which then passes down into the prostatic capsule below, along with longitudinal muscle fibres. These muscle fibres are richly innervated with adrenergic sympathetic nerves sensitive to noradrenaline, and are responsible for bladder neck contraction upon orgasm, thus preventing retrograde ejaculation of semen up into the bladder. The exact role of these muscle fibres in maintaining urinary continence is unclear and it would seem likely that other mechanisms (e.g. circular elastic muscle fibres) may be more important in keeping this area of the bladder neck closed.

In the female, there is no such circular muscle arrangement. Rather, the smooth muscle fibres run longitudinally into the wall of the urethra and are innervated via cholinergic rather than adrenergic nerves. However, the bladder neck still remains closed at rest, probably owing to the influence of circular elastic fibres and also the valve-like effect caused by the urethral mucosa which is highly vascular.

The male urethra

The urethra is a tube that starts at the bladder neck and ends at the external meatus. Its function is to transport both urine and semen. Apart from a small region of squamous epithelium close to the external urethral meatus the male urethra is lined by transitional cell epithelium.

The male urethra is approximately 23 cm in length and divided into four distinct areas (Figure 1.12):

1. Prostatic urethra (3–4 cm in length).
2. Membranous urethra (2–3 cm in length).
3. Bulbar urethra (1.5 cm in length).
4. Penile or spongy urethra (approximately 15 cm in length).

The prostatic urethra originates at the bladder neck and vertically pierces the prostate gland through its anterior aspect. Secretory ducts from within the prostate, which contribute to ejaculatory volume, open onto the posterior

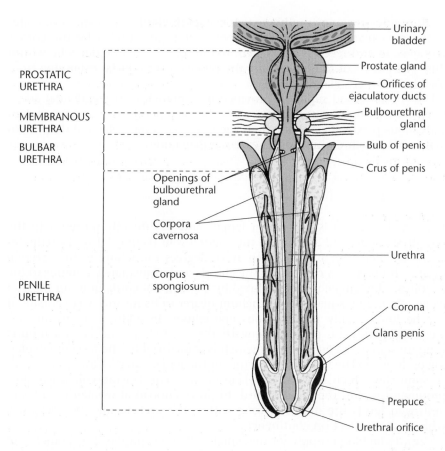

Figure 1.12 The male urethra

aspect (at the utriculus). This part of the urethra also contains a pyramid-shaped structure known as the verumontanum, which is anatomically above the level of the external sphincter. The verumontanum acts as a 'surgical landmark', enabling surgeons to avoid damage to the external sphincter during transurethral surgery. The ejaculatory ducts which bring sperm from the vas deferens and secretions from the seminal vesicles open on either side of the verumontanum.

The membranous urethra extends from the base of the prostate to the bulbar area of the urethra and pierces the pelvic floor musculature (the levator ani/urogenital diaphragm). It is thin-walled, non-distensible and highly susceptible to stricture formation and rupture. The ligaments supporting the prostatic urethra attach it to the symphysis pubis, while the bulbar and penile urethra are supported by dense attachments to the corpus cavernosa, held in turn by the ischial tuberosities. Thus any fracture that displaces the bones of the pelvis is likely to tear the membranous urethra.

The bulbar urethra or urethral bulb is surrounded by the bulbospongiosus muscle. Contraction of this muscle assists in urethral emptying at the termination of voiding, and also aids the expulsion of semen during orgasm and ejaculation.

The penile or spongy urethra extends from the bulbar area and terminates at the navicular fossa of the glans penis. It is surrounded by the corpus spongiosum and receives many periurethral glands, whose ducts lie within this. The largest of these ducts are the two Cowper's ducts, extending from the four Cowper's glands.

The arterial blood supply is provided by a branch of the pudendal artery (urethral artery). Venous drainage is via the deep penile vein and the pudendal venous plexus. Lymphatic drainage is via the superficial and deep inguinal nodes which drain into the external iliac nodes.

The female urethra

The female urethra is 4–5 cm in length and lies directly posterior to the symphysis pubis and anterior to the vaginal wall (Figure 1.13). It originates at the bladder neck and is angled at 16 degrees tunnelling to the external meatus. It opens 2–3 cm behind the clitoris and immediately anterior to the introitus. The female urethra is lined by transitional epithelium for most of its length and by squamous epithelium nearer to its meatus. Occasionally it can be lined totally by squamous epithelium. In addition many mucus-secreting glands are present. Beneath the epithelium the lamina propria supports a rich vascular network which is influenced by the level of circulating oestrogens. The muscular structure of the female urethra forms an intrinsic sphincter, which allows urethral closure to occur. The musculature is most prominent within the middle third. In postmenopausal women with lower oestrogen levels the muscular tone within the urethra may be decreased, which has an effect on continence.

The arterial blood supply for the female urethra is provided by branches of the vaginal artery. Venous drainage is via the pelvic venous plexus. Lymphatic drainage is provided mainly by the internal iliac nodes: additional drainage is via the external iliac nodes.

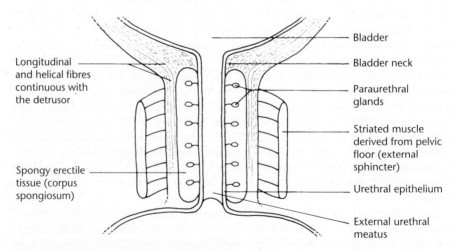

Longitudinal and helical fibres continuous with the detrusor

Spongy erectile tissue (corpus spongiosum)

Bladder

Bladder neck

Paraurethral glands

Striated muscle derived from pelvic floor (external sphincter)

Urethral epithelium

External urethral meatus

Figure 1.13 Structure of the female urethra

External sphincter mechanism

The external sphincter is constructed of an inner longitudinal smooth-muscle layer and an outer circular striated-muscle layer.

The action of the male external sphincter has been traditionally explained as arising from fibres of the levator ani muscle, which surrounds the membranous urethra. However, more recent anatomical studies have shown that these fibres do not constitute a complete muscle ring, but rather only form an arrangement comparable to a 'urethral sling' providing support as opposed to prolonged contraction (Bullock *et al.*, 1991). These are 'fast-twitch fibres' which appear to contract during sudden rises in intra-abdominal pressure caused by such events as coughing, laughing and running.

The main contribution to the external sphincter appears to come from the urethral wall itself. At this point the urethral musculature within the area of the membranous urethra contains an outer circular layer of striated muscle fibres which are designed for prolonged contraction (slow-twitch fibres). These fibres receive innervation via somatic (voluntary) nerves from the level of sacral vertebrae 2 and 3. In the male the external sphincter mechanism exerts a higher closure pressure than the bladder neck mechanism.

In the female the external sphincter extends throughout the whole length of the urethra, but as mentioned above is more pronounced in the middle third. As in the male, the 'urethral sling' comprises fast-twitch fibres arising from the levator ani fibres, and serves to raise urethral closure pressure during episodes of raised intra-abdominal pressure. It is the external voluntary sphincter, however, that is responsible for the maintenance of urinary continence.

Innervation of the bladder and physiology of micturition

The innervation of the bladder and the sphincters comprises a complex system of intrinsic and extrinsic nerve pathways. For effective bladder function, autonomic plus somatic nerve fibres from the bladder and urethra pass to the spinal cord at the level of S2–S4 via the pelvic parasympathetic nerves. This area of the cord is known as the 'spinal micturition centre' which co-ordinates incoming sensory impulses and outgoing parasympathetic motor impulses, to and from the detrusor muscle and the sphincters. Until the age of approximately 2–4 years the bladder is emptied by a simple spinal reflex arc. As the bladder fills, stretch receptors in the detrusor send sensory impulses to the spinal micturition centre. When the initial urge to void occurs, the micturition centre responds by sending motor impulses to the detrusor to contract and the sphincters to relax. The process is completed when the bladder is empty and the filling phase will begin again.

Voluntary control of the micturition cycle occurs when the central nervous system matures and the child develops the ability to appreciate bladder filling and the social advantages of continence. From the spinal micturition centre nerve fibres ascend to the 'higher' micturition centres within the brain, i.e. the pons and the cerebral cortex. These centres allow the inhibition of the simple spinal reflex arc: sensory impulses from the detrusor pass into and through the spinal cord, and are co-ordinated in the pons. The pons is controlled by the cortex which can send either inhibitory or facilitative impulses back to the spinal cord, and thus will block or allow micturition.

Detrusor contraction occurs via impulses from parasympathetic, cholinergic nerves which pass to the detrusor along parasympathetic pelvic fibres. Sympathetic nerves also provide bladder innervation via the hypogastric nerves, and are mainly motor contractile fibres. The sphincter mechanism is innervated by both somatic voluntary nerves (from S2 to S3) and autonomic fibres, the autonomic innervation provides control for the smooth, slow-twitch inner muscle layer of the urethra. The fast-twitch periurethral sling is innervated by somatic voluntary nerves. Figure 1.14 gives an overview of bladder innervation and Figure 1.15 illustrates the normal bladder cycle as described below.

The filling phase

During the filling phase the bladder volume increases with very little change in intravesical pressure as the bladder is highly compliant and there is little cholinergic activity (Berne and Levy, 1990). The bladder is inhibited from emptying by the process described above. The stretch receptors within the detrusor continue to send impulses to the higher centres, and at a 'critical'

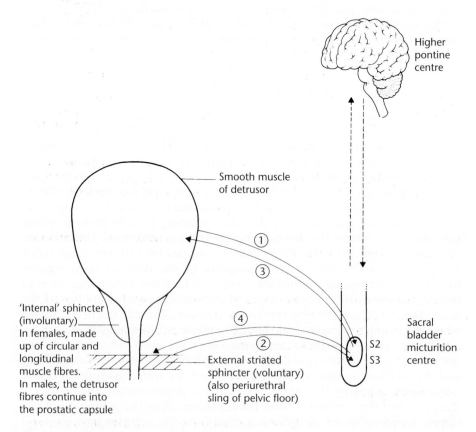

Figure 1.14 Innervation of the bladder

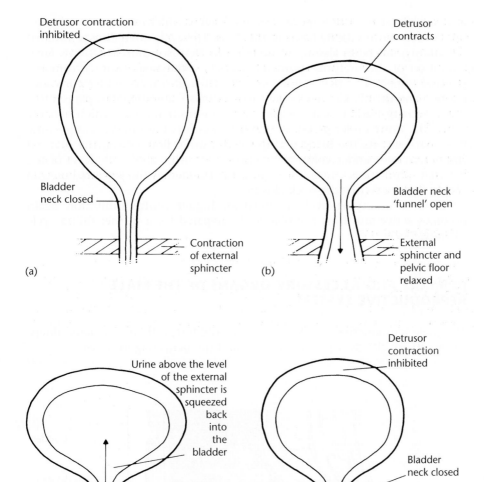

Figure 1.15   *Normal bladder cycle: (a) resting or storage phase; (b) voiding phase; (c) voiding begins to terminate; (d) termination of voiding*

bladder pressure (when the volume reaches about 200 ml) the first sensation to void is experienced. This desire can be suppressed until it is convenient and socially acceptable to void. Contraction of the external sphincter and the bladder neck prevents leakage during the filling phase.

The voiding phase

Voiding involves the co-ordinated relaxation of the external sphincter, relaxation of the bladder neck and contraction of the detrusor muscle. This is achieved via the 'spino-pontine-spinal' reflex which involves the higher micturition centres located within the pons. The cycle of voiding is initiated voluntarily, but relies also upon involuntary detrusor muscle activity. First, relaxation of the urethral sphincter leads to a fall in pressure within the urethral lumen. The pelvic floor muscles then also relax under conscious control, and the bladder neck opens (or 'funnels'). Simultaneous parasympathetic activity leads to contraction of the detrusor muscle, which actively expels the urine under pressure. When this occurs the intravesical pressure rises markedly. As the bladder empties and urine flow ceases, the urethral sphincter closes under voluntary control. Any urine above the level of the external sphincter is 'milked' back into the bladder, as the proximal urethra contracts prior to bladder neck closure.

Once the emptying cycle is finished, higher centre inhibition again becomes active and thus the bladder is prepared for a further filling cycle (Blandy, 1992).

PRIMARY AND ACCESSORY ORGANS OF THE MALE REPRODUCTIVE SYSTEM

The male reproductive system consists of the testes, their associated ducts, the accessory glands (e.g. the prostate) and the penis (Figure 1.16).

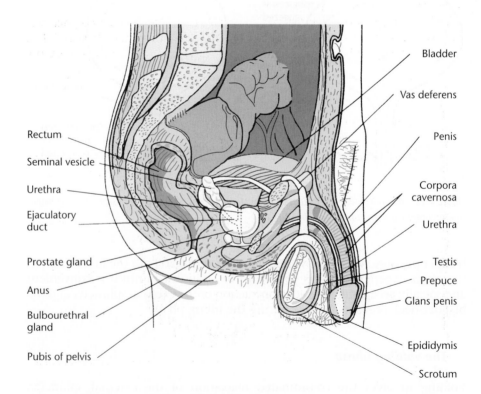

Figure 1.16 *Anatomy of the male reproductive system*

The testes and scrotum

The testicles are the primary sex organs of the male. They are responsible for the production of androgens and spermatozoa; these functions are performed by two distinct cell groups, the Leydig (interstitial) cells and the Sertoli cells.

The paired oval testicles are situated within the scrotum. A midline septum divides the scrotum, providing a compartment for each testis. The testicles are suspended from the external inguinal ring by the spermatic cord, which houses nerve fibres (autonomic), blood vessels and lymphatics.

The testes need to be at a constant temperature of approximately 35°C to enable sperm production. Muscle fibres within the spermatic cord (cremaster muscles) enable it to shorten, thus the testes will be moved upwards towards the body if the external temperature falls. The dartos muscle situated within the superficial fascia of the scrotal skin also assists with temperature control: when it is cold the skin is heavily wrinkled to reduce heat loss, and when it is warm the scrotal skin is flaccid and loose to aid cooling.

The blood supply to the testicles is from the testicular arteries. These arteries leave the aorta at the level of the renal arteries, pass via the retropubic space into the groin, then along the inguinal canal and down the spermatic cord via the inguinal ring (a slit-like opening in the transversus abdominis muscle). The venous drainage also occurs through the spermatic cord and from there passes to the left renal vein and then the vena cava. Drainage is facilitated by the pampiniform plexus which surrounds the testis and epididymis, and is also thought to act as a heat exchanger, to assist in keeping the testes at their optimum temperature.

Each testicle is surrounded by two layers, the fibrous tunica albuginea and the double-layered outer tissue known as the tunica vaginalis (Figure 1.17). The tunica vaginalis is derived from the peritoneum; it helps protect the

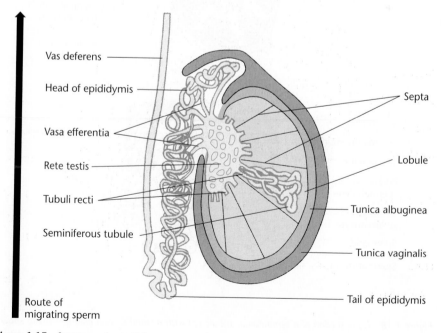

Figure 1.17 Structure of a testicle

testicle from injury and sheathes the testis during intrauterine life. Between the layers of the tunica vaginalis lies a small amount of lubricating fluid which further helps protect the testes from sudden movement. This potential cavity can expand and fill with fluid, in which case a hydrocele results. The tunica albuginea covers the testis and projects into the testicular tissue, dividing it into 200–300 wedge-shaped compartments containing the seminiferous tubules, which are the functional part of the organ (Figure 1.18). Each compartment contains one to four coiled seminiferous tubules and they converge to form a short, straight tubule – the tubulus rectus – which conveys sperm into the rete testis. The rete testis is a network of tubules found on the posterior aspect of the testis. Sperm are transported from here via the efferent ductules to the epididymis.

The soft connective tissue around the seminiferous tubules contains the interstitial cells (Leydig cells). These cells are responsible for the production of androgens such as testosterone, which is secreted into the interstitial fluid.

The epididymis

The epididymis is a long, highly convoluted tube, packed tightly within each testis and lined with secretory columnar epithelium. If uncoiled the epididy-

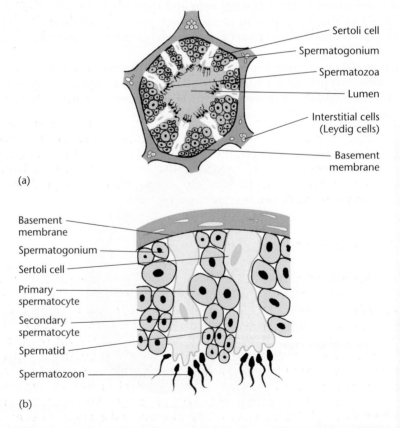

(a)

(b)

Figure 1.18 Cross-section of a seminiferous tubule (a) with a small section enlarged (b) to show microscopic structure of testes

mis would measure approximately 6 metres in length. By palpation the epididymis can be felt on the posterior testicular aspect, as a rough, 'string-like' mass.

The epididymis is divided into three sections: head, body and tail. The head receives sperm from the efferent ductules and the body and tail regions provide storage. The tail of the epididymis then drains into the vas deferens. Storage of sperm is necessary because, although production of mature sperm is a continuous process, ejaculation may only occur irregularly. If no ejaculation occurs within 40–50 days, the sperm stored within the epididymis degenerate, via a process of liquefaction, and are removed by phagocytosis.

The vas deferens

The vas deferens (ductus deferens) is approximately 45 cm in length. It passes upwards from the epididymis into the pelvic cavity via the inguinal canal as part of the spermatic cord. It passes anterior to the symphysis pubis and then arches over the ureter, before descending posterior to the bladder. The distal region of the vas deferens connects with the duct of the seminal vesicle which forms the ejaculatory duct. The ejaculatory duct enters the prostate gland and in turn empties into the urethra.

The wall of the vas deferens contains three layers of smooth muscle, held together with connective tissue and innervated via the autonomic nerve supply. This allows the vas deferens to contract rapidly during ejaculation which propels the sperm forward into the urethra.

The seminal vesicles

The seminal vesicles lie on the posterior region of the bladder and are approximately 5–7 cm in length. They are secretory glands and produce about 60% of semen volume. The seminal fluid produced is yellow, viscous and alkaline, comprising fructose, ascorbic acid, prostaglandins and a coagulating enzyme. Sperm and seminal fluid mix together in the ejaculatory duct and enter the prostatic urethra on ejaculation.

The prostate gland

The prostate gland is situated around the bladder neck, and the portion of the urethra which emerges from the bladder at this point. It lies behind the symphysis pubis, to which it is attached by a tough layer of fascia. On either side the pubis and ischial tuberosities curve around it. The size of the prostate varies according to age; it increases rapidly in size at the age of puberty. A normal gland is approximately 15 g in weight and 3 cm in diameter, the size remaining constant until approximately the age of 45–50 years. The shape of the prostate is likened to that of a chestnut, which reflects its non-uniform nature. Around 1 in 10 men over the age of 55 years will require surgery to relieve urinary obstruction caused by prostatic enlargement (Figure 1.19). Benign prostatic hyperplasia and carcinoma of the prostate are discussed in Chapter 9.

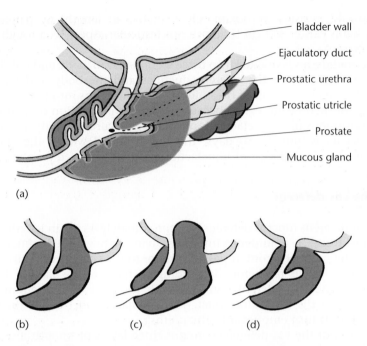

Bladder wall

Ejaculatory duct

Prostatic urethra

Prostatic utricle

Prostate

Mucous gland

(a)

(b)   (c)   (d)

Figure 1.19 *The normal prostate gland (a) showing the effects of hyperplasia of (b) the lateral and middle lobes, (c) the middle lobes and (d) the lateral lobes*

The prostate consists of a network of secretory tubules, surrounded by a capsule of smooth muscle. Each tubule is enclosed by contractile smooth muscle fibres and the whole gland is supported by connective tissue. Prostatic fluid from the gland empties via the prostatic ducts into the urethra, the milky secretion constituting approximately 10–20% of the total volume of the ejaculate. This secretion is watery in nature, slightly acidic and contains a variety of enzymes (e.g. acid phosphatase) and many additional components (e.g. citrate, calcium, fibrinolysin). It also gives semen its characteristic odour. The prostatic fluid is thought to stimulate sperm motility, cause coagulation of the secretion from the seminal vesicles and help neutralize the natural acidity of the vagina (Blandy, 1992).

The verumontanum lies on the posterior wall of the prostatic urethra and as mentioned earlier is a 'landmark' in endoscopic surgery. The two ejaculatory ducts pass through the posterior aspect of the gland, and open into the urethra on either side of the verumontanum. Sperm from the vas deferens enters the urethra at this point.

The main area of glandular tissue is situated within the lateral and posterior portions of the prostate (outer zone), and the mucosal glands are situated close to the urethra in the middle of the gland (inner zone). There are no true defined 'lobes' within the prostate, but for clinical purposes specific areas within the gland are identified using this categorization. In association with its rich network of smooth muscle fibres, the prostate serves an important contractile function during ejaculation and orgasm. During ejaculation the bladder neck and prostate undergo muscular contraction (therefore preventing retrograde ejaculation), and the external sphincter mechanism relaxes; these actions result in the passage of semen into the penile urethra.

The prostate is dependent upon adequate amounts of circulating testicular hormones being present for its secretory function, and both secretion and growth of the gland are intimately linked to changes in the plasma concentrations of these hormones.

Bulbourethral or Cowper's glands

The bulbourethral glands are approximately the size of a pea and lie between the prostate and the penis, and their ducts open into the urethra. The glands produce a mucus-rich secretion, which serves as a urethral lubricant, prior to ejaculation. The secretion is thought to neutralize traces of acidic urine present in the urethra.

The penis

The penis (Figure 1.20) along with the scrotum and its contents make up the external genitalia in the male. The penis consists of three spongy sacs, two above and dorsal to the penile urethra (the corpora cavernosa) and one in the lower part of the penis, surrounding the urethra (corpus spongiosum). The three corpora act as distensible storage reservoirs for blood, and are surrounded by a tough, rigid connective tissue layer known as Buck's fascia. The two reservoirs of the corpora cavernosa are able to intercommunicate and blood travels between them. The 'storage' property of the corpora allows them to fill and distend with blood which results in an increase in rigidity, resulting in a state of erection (Figure 1.21).

The enlarged head of the penis is referred to as the glans penis; it is an extension of the corpus spongiosum and the urethra opens at its end. The glans penis is covered by a retractable hood of skin (prepuce or foreskin), which is removed during the procedure of circumcision. The corpus spongiosum is expanded posteriorly to form the bulb of the penis. The bulb is covered by the bulbospongiosus muscle which has many fibres associated with the corpus spongiosum, and aids the propulsion of semen along the urethra.

The penis is a highly vascular organ and each corpus cavernosum receives its blood supply from a large artery that runs through its length. The corpus spongiosum receives blood supply from two arterial sources and the overall penile blood supply is further augmented by a network of smaller arteries. The penis also possesses several veins that facilitate drainage. The physiology of erection and ejaculation is discussed in Chapter 12.

Semen

Semen consists of a mixture of spermatozoa (male gametes) and secretions from the prostate and the other male accessory organs. Semen is also rich in the enzyme hyaluronidase, which breaks down mucopolysaccharides, thus helping the sperm pass through the cervical mucus. The bulk of the seminal fluid originates from the seminal vesicles and has a combined pH of about

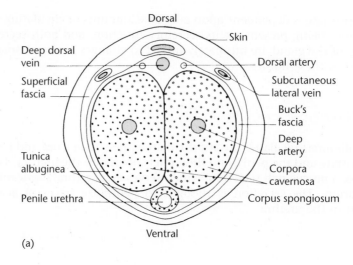

(a)

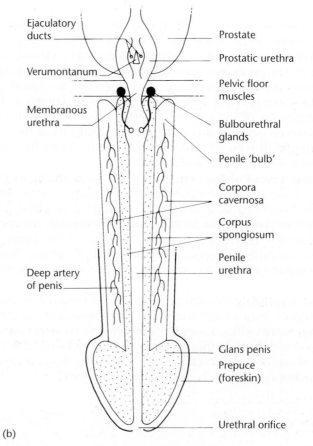

(b)

Figure 1.20   *The penis: (a) transverse section, (b) longitudinal section*

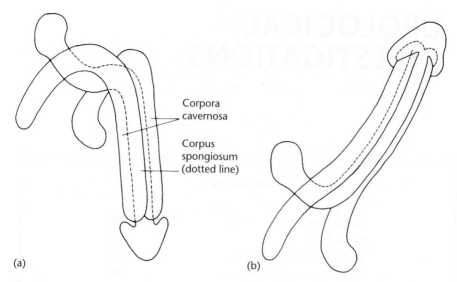

Figure 1.21 *Penile structure and associated changes on erection: (a) flaccid, non-erect penis; (b) penile erection*

7.2–7.4. This helps to neutralize the vaginal acidic pH, as the sperm become rapidly immobilized by an acid environment.

Spermatogenesis is discussed in Chapter 13.

REFERENCES

BERNE M R and Levy M N (1990) *Principles of Physiology*. St Louis: Wolfe.
BLANDY J P (1992) *Lecture Notes on Urology*, 4th edn. Oxford: Blackwell Scientific.
BULLOCK N, Sibley G and Whitaker R (1991) *Essential Urology*. Edinburgh: Churchill Livingstone.
GUYTON A C (1991) *Textbook of Medical Physiology*, 8th edn. Philadelphia: WB Saunders.
MARIEB E N (1995) *Human Anatomy and Physiology*, 3rd edn. Redwood City, California: Benjamin/ Cummings.
McLAREN S M (1996) Renal Function. In: Hinchliff S M, Montague S E and Watson R (eds) *Physiology for Nursing Practice*, 2nd edn. London: Baillière Tindall.

FURTHER READING

BLANDY J P (1992) *Lecture Notes on Urology*, 4th edn. Oxford: Blackwell Scientific.
HINCHLIFF S M, Montague S E and Watson R (1996) *Physiology for Nursing Practice*, 2nd edn. London: Baillière Tindall.
KARLOWICZ K ed. (1995) *Urologic Nursing, Principles and Practice*. Philadelphia: WB Saunders.
MARIEB E N (1995) *Human Anatomy and Physiology*, 3rd edn. Redwood City, California: Benjamin/ Cummings.
SMITH D R (1984) *General Urology*, 11th edn. Lang Medical.
THOMPSON F D and Woodhouse C R J (1987) *Disorders of the Kidney and Urinary Tract*. London: Edward Arnold.
ULDALL R (1988) *Renal Nursing*, 3rd edn. Oxford: Blackwell Scientific.

2 UROLOGICAL INVESTIGATIONS

Contents

Technological developments have created a variety of new investigative methods that can yield information regarding the urinary tract and its function, as well as a whole group of tests that have been of benefit for many years. These new aids to diagnosis, however, cannot replace the need for a thorough patient assessment, the most vital tool in which is the ability to listen to the patient's problems. Investigations should only be carried out when they are appropriate.

The purpose of this chapter is to outline the common investigations that play an essential role in attempting to discover why a patient presents with a particular urological problem.

TESTING THE URINE

Examination of the urine is a simple, non-intrusive test, which can yield a great deal of information regarding renal and urinary function. For hundreds of years, doctors have tested urine by taste, smell and vision. Urinalysis, using chemically impregnated squares (e.g. Multistix), in combination with macroscopic examination (looking at the colour, smelling the odour, for instance), makes a comprehensive urinary examination possible these days without having to resort to ingestion!

There is also much to be read from the simple recording of an accurate 'frequency–volume' fluid balance chart.

Urine samples should be tested while still fresh and free from contaminants (e.g. airborne dust). Urine is an excellent culture medium and at room temperature many bacteria will grow rapidly and thus make the sample invalid.

Urinalysis

The following five factors are particularly useful:

Urinary pH

Normal urinary pH should fall in the range 4–8, and this wide range underlines the role of the kidney in acid–base regulation (i.e. an acid or alkaline urine can be produced, according to bodily requirement). However, prolonged alkalinity of urine may be an indication of urinary tract infection. Certain organisms (bacteria) contain the enzyme *urease*, and are able to 'split' the urea molecules within urine, so releasing ammonium which causes the increased, alkaline pH. Such infection is commonly caused by *Proteus mirabilis*, or other gram-negative bacilli.

Protein

The kidney normally excretes up to 200 mg of protein per day but this small amount remains undetected by routine urinalysis. However, significantly larger amounts than this will provide a positive urinary Multistix test. Proteinuria may be an indication of urinary infection, or more seriously, of a kidney that is 'leaking' protein as a result of an underlying disease process (e.g. glomerulonephritis). Further investigation is likely to be required. However, proteinuria can be misleading in women, as the positive result may occur owing to vaginal cells shed into the urine sample.

Blood

The urinary Multistix test for blood is extremely sensitive, and may well prove positive in healthy individuals owing to the detection of very small numbers of red blood cells. This test has been responsible for a significant increase in the referral of patients to a urologist by general practitioners, or as result of pre-employment or insurance health screening. In the vast majority of cases, no underlying disease process is found. Nonetheless, blood in the urine (*haematuria*) can be highly significant and may point to an underlying urinary tract infection (with inflamed mucosal lining, which then loses red blood cells and leucocytes), stones within the kidney or urinary tract, a bleeding disorder or a more sinister condition such as urological cancer.

It is commonplace to find haematuria following instrumentation of the urinary tract or in patients who have indwelling urethral or suprapubic catheters. Haematuria in women may be the result of menstrual blood contaminating the urine sample.

Leucocytes

The newer urinalysis reagent strips allow the detection of leucocyte esterase (an enzyme within white blood cells) in urine. A positive leucocyte assay is an extremely reliable indicator of a urinary tract infection (Stevens, 1989). However, this may not imply a *significant* infection – rather, that a urinary pathogen is present; the patient may be otherwise asymptomatic and thus require no further treatment.

Nitrites

Many organisms, especially gram-negative bacilli, are able to reduce nitrate to nitrite, as a result of a specific metabolic pathway within their cells. Thus a positive nitrite assay, using Multistix, is again indicative of a urinary infection, but may not indicate significance. In combination with a positive leucocyte assay, a positive nitrite result is highly indicative of infection within the urine (Lowe, 1985; Stevens, 1989; Hiscoke *et al.*, 1990). Conversely, a negative nitrite and leucocyte result are approximately 97% reliable in excluding the presence of urinary infection. It therefore provides an effective emergency diagnostic screen, or for patients on admission to hospital prior to instrumentation of the urinary tract.

Urinary microscopy

Microscopy of urine is an underused and inexpensive test, which involves simple urinary examination under a bright field or by use of phase contrast microscopy (to enhance the background and therefore make visualization of bacteria easier). Centrifugation (an attempt to concentrate bacterial cells) is also used, but is both tedious to perform and inconvenient.

Bacteria can be seen in stained preparations of 90% of specimens containing more than 10^5 organisms (or colony-forming units) per ml. An additional Gram stain also allows the morphology and staining reaction to be determined and therefore provides a useful guide to antimicrobial therapy. Jenkins (cited in Stevens, 1989) carried out a review of urinary examination using this method, and concluded that stained, centrifuged urine provides the most sensitive screening test, and that unstained, non-centrifuged urine, which is more commonly used, is much less reliable.

Microscopic examination for pyuria (leucocytes in the urine) also provides an effective method for distinguishing between established urinary infection and simple contamination of the specimen. The presence of more than 10 leucocytes per ml of urine correlates well with established urinary tract infection.

Examination of the 'sediment', following centrifugation, may show evidence of *casts* or *crystals*. The term 'casts' refers to the 'squeezed-out' contents of the collecting tubules of individual nephrons, and may be either *clear* or *granular* in nature. Clear or hyaline casts are made of protein, whereas granular casts are formed either from red blood cells or leucocytes, or from a combination of the two. Casts are commonly found in urine as a result of infection (e.g. pyelonephritis), in renal diseases such as glomerulonephritis, or following either nephrotoxic or ischaemic lesions, which cause damage to the glomerular basement, and thus allow 'leakage' of large cells such as leucocytes.

Crystals are commonly found in the urine of patients with renal stones, and are characteristic of the type of material causing the stone. For example, calcium oxalate crystals are octahedral, cystine crystals are hexagonal and calcium ammonium phosphate ('*triple*' or '*infection*') crystals are square.

In cases of infection with organisms such as *Schistosoma*, ova may be seen on microscopy, especially in an early morning specimen of urine.

Early morning urine

Early morning urine (EMU) collection and examination is a further useful microscopic technique, especially when tuberculosis or cancer of the urinary tract is suspected. The principle is that the first urine voided in the morning is likely to be the most concentrated (owing to increased antidiuretic hormone secretion at night, and decreased fluid intake) and there is a greater chance of finding malignant cells, organisms or bacteria. Further, the urinary volume is generally smaller, and has been collected over a long period (7–10 hours). The tubercle bacillus will not grow on ordinary culture media, but an EMU can be centrifuged and the sediment then stained using a Ziehl–Neelsen stain, which penetrates the lipid outer layer of the bacteria (this layer prevents the uptake of more commonly used bacterial stains).

If cancer is suspected, the EMU should be voided into a sterile receptacle and then transferred into a bottle containing 10% formalin, which 'fixes' any malignant cells, preventing their breakdown. The urine is then centrifuged and stained with a Papanicolaou ('Pap') stain, allowing malignant cells, if present, to be identified.

Urinary culture

As urine is an effective culture medium for microbes, urine specimens must be obtained without contamination (e.g. bacteria from the prepuce or vulva, airborne dust particulates); it should be left at room temperature for as little time as possible (preferably refrigerated) if the laboratory is unable to plate and examine it immediately.

The laboratory can establish the number of individual colonies from a given specimen which can then give a figure for the number of colony-forming units (CFU) per ml of urine (thus a CFU can be either a single cell, or a group of identical cells). It is normally taken that more than 10^5 CFU per ml constitutes a significant urinary tract infection, which will then require intervention. However, studies by Stevens (1989) have shown that this figure is not completely reliable, though it has remained unchallenged for many years. The figure of 10^5 CFU ml^{-1} arose from work originally carried out by Kass (1957), who attempted to establish a diagnosis of a urinary tract infection (UTI) by examining the number of bacteria found within early morning samples of 'clean catch' specimens. Kass considered no other evidence of UTI at all, and thus many hold the figure of 10^5 as sacrosanct, even though a significant symptomatic UTI may be associated with lower numbers of bacteria. For example, Roberts (1986) found that 18% of patients with a UTI in conjunction with bacteraemia had counts of less than 10^5 CFU ml^{-1}, and similar results were reported by Strand *et al.* (1985). Further, these patients had serious life-threatening urinary infections, yet the 10^5 figure would classify such infections as insignificant. Catheterized patients may also have lower numbers of organisms per ml yet still have a symptomatic and often dangerous urinary infection (Kellogg *et al.*, 1987).

Overall the 10^5 figure is extremely useful and is used widely, but it does need to be seen within the context of the Kass study. It is probably more valid to categorize a urinary infection as significant if it is causing adverse symptoms for the patient.

Specimens for culture

Urinary specimens for culture are obtained in the following ways:

♦ *Midstream specimen of urine (MSU).* The patient is asked to clean the prepuce or vulva with a topical agent (according to local policy), and then asked to collect the middle part of the void in a sterile container; this is to reduce the number of contaminants in the specimen. However, many patients fail to understand what is required and the specimen is invalid. A number of researchers (Morris *et al.*, 1979; Immergut *et al.*, 1981; Brown *et al.*, 1991) have cast doubt upon the efficacy of cleansing prior to urine collection.

♦ *Catheter sample of urine.* A sterile needle and syringe can be used to puncture the sample port in the catheter drainage bag and 3–5 ml of urine are removed; this is transferred to a sterile container for transit to the laboratory. A chlorhexidine impregnated swab is used to clean the sample port before and after puncture according to local policies.

♦ *Suprapubic aspiration.* This is a quick and easy method to obtain a specimen of urine for culture, but must only be performed by a skilled practitioner. The anterior abdominal wall and then the bladder are punctured by a needle and syringe and the specimen is aspirated. This method is more commonly used in paediatric practice since it is more difficult to obtain sterile urine samples from babies and small children despite advances in the design of collecting bags.

The reliability of the results obtained from all the specimens described depends upon the technique of the collector, the sterility of the collecting vessel, and the length of time and storage temperature before the specimen is examined.

24-Hour urine collection

This is a simple yet important investigation, because it allows an assessment to be made of the 24-hour urinary excretion of a variety of key metabolites (e.g. sodium, potassium, calcium, phosphates, protein, creatinine, urinary catecholamines). The patient is asked to void (or the catheter drainage bag is emptied) and this first specimen is discarded; the time is noted and all urine voided over the subsequent 24 hours is collected. The collecting vessel may vary (either plastic or glass) and it may require the addition of a preservative according to the specifics of the assay being undertaken.

Urinary clearance estimation

The concept of renal clearance provides a reliable estimation of overall renal function. The value obtained is an expression of the theoretical volume of plasma that the kidneys are capable of clearing ('cleansing') of a specific substance in 1 minute. The substance is present within blood, and filtered by the nephron as it passes through the renal vasculature. The degree of intact renal function will be reflected in how much of the substance is filtered: i.e. how many ml of plasma per minute are effectively *cleared* of the chosen urinary metabolite. A 24-hour urine collection is required plus a specimen of venous blood taken during that period. The urinary metabolite normally used for the estimation of renal clearance is creatinine, a breakdown product of muscle metabolism (hence this test is sometimes referred to as 'creatinine clearance'). For clearance to be accurate, the substance passing through the kidneys must do so unchanged, i.e. none must be absorbed into blood, via the tubules, nor any excreted from the tubules into tubular fluid.

Creatinine, however, is not totally unchanged by the tubule. Some is excreted by the distal tubule, but this amount is insufficient to compromise the validity of the test. Conversely, glucose cannot be used for calculating urinary clearance, because in healthy individuals it is totally absorbed by the proximal tubule. Urea is also not particularly effective, as its daily urinary excretion varies according to liver function, protein intake and nutritional status. It is more effective if the urea excretion is estimated over a prolonged period and compared with changes in the glomerular filtration rate (GFR).

One of the most accurate substances for calculating renal clearance is the polyhydric alcohol inulin, which is freely filtered without any absorption or excretion. Thus a very close estimation of the GFR is possible, but the disadvantage of inulin is its high cost and it is therefore not widely used. The normal clearance figure for creatinine or inulin is dependent on age, as renal function progressively deteriorates with advancing years, owing to the loss of nephrons and disruption to renal blood flow. For a young, fit individual, a normal clearance figure would be approximately 125 ml per minute. Thus around 10% of the effective plasma flow per minute, through the kidney, is actually 'cleared' of unwanted metabolites, such as creatinine. By the age of 70 years, the normal clearance figure has fallen to approximately 60–70 ml min^{-1}. Clearance is calculated using the following formula:

$$Clearance = \frac{u \times v}{P}$$

where u is the urinary concentration of the designated metabolite per 24 hours, v is volume of the urine passed per 24 hours, and P is the plasma concentration of the designated metabolite. Renal clearance is therefore an inexpensive and very useful investigation, which causes minimal patient inconvenience.

BLOOD ASSAY

Blood assay is a crucial part of the investigative process. Table 2.1 illustrates some of the more important plasma constituents relevant to the urological patient which can be estimated from venous blood samples.

RADIOLOGICAL INVESTIGATIONS

Investigations that utilize imaging via X-ray, using either plain film or radio-opaque contrast dyes, form a large component of diagnostic assessment of the urinary tract. There are also now a number of more advanced methods, which are described later in this chapter. It must be noted that all radiological procedures are a hazard to pregnant women, and thus women of childbearing age must be questioned about the time of their last menstrual period prior to undergoing any X-ray procedure.

PLASMA CONSTITUENT	DIAGNOSTIC SIGNIFICANCE
Haemoglobin	Reduced in anaemia, severe haematuria, urological cancer, glomerulonephritis
White blood cells	Raised in UTI, pyelonephritis, glomerulonephritis, tuberculosis, cancer
Creatinine	Raised in renal impairment
Potassium	Relates directly to renal function
Sodium	Relates directly to renal function, raised levels also indicate dehydration
Calcium	High levels correlate to stone formation (owing to enzyme deficiency or high dietary intake)
Phosphate	Raised in renal impairment
Plasma proteins (e.g. albumin, globulin)	Severely reduced in renal disease (e.g. glomerulonephritis) or in malnutrition
Prostatic specific antigen	Significantly raised in prostate cancer – more reliable screen than acid phosphatase
Tumour markers (e.g. human chorionic gonadotrophin, α-fetoprotein)	Allow determination of metastatic tumour spread, and provide a reliable indicator of response to treatment

Table 2.1 Possible diagnostic significance of plasma constituents

Plain abdominal film

The normal plain film has limited use as it does not include the bladder. A 'kidney ureter bladder' film is of much greater value.

Kidney, ureter, bladder film

A kidney, ureter, bladder (KUB) film is an X-ray of the kidneys, ureters and bony pelvis, taken from both anterior and posterior aspects, without the use of contrast media. The patient is normally in the standing position, although if the patient is only able to lie supine, then a single anterior X-ray view is taken.

Indications

A KUB film is used to screen for renal calculi in symptomatic patients where a stone is suspected. However, not all stones are radiolucent. This film is also used prior to intravenous urogram (IVU), or prior to endoscopic stone removal, as a final check on the presence and location of the stone.

Information

A KUB film can readily demonstrate both of the renal outlines (shadows), thus providing an estimation of the number, size and position of the kidneys. It is also possible to observe the psoas muscle shadows, bony pelvis and spinal column, and therefore discover evidence of bony decalcification or damage caused by metastatic spread from bladder or prostatic carcinoma.

Patient preparation

Patient preparation is minimal, as the procedure is quick and painless. However, an explanation of the procedure is clearly necessary, particularly as a KUB film may form only part of a complex series of investigations.

Intravenous urogram

An intravenous urogram (IVU) is one of the mainstay urological investigations, and is commonly performed on an outpatient basis. It is wrongly referred to as an intravenous pyelogram (IVP), as it visualizes far more than just the renal pelvis, and also may then be confused with the completely separate pyelogram investigation.

The effectiveness of an IVU, within urological investigation, lies in the fact that it is able to image the entire urinary tract, including the urethra (although it is seldom used to do this, as a urethrogram provides a superior quality image). An IVU comprises a series of X-ray films, which use a renally excreted contrast medium to enhance the morphology of the urinary tract, when the contrast medium passes through the kidney and drains into the bladder. Thus detailed information can be obtained regarding the kidneys (number, size, position), the ureters (number, possible obstruction or duplex systems, carcinoma or retroperitoneal fibrosis) and the bladder (size, capacity, space-occupying lesions).

The process of urinary transport from kidney to bladder is evaluated using a series of sequential films, at set intervals of time following the intravenous injection of the contrast medium. The contrast medium chosen is usually based on the compound benzoic acid, and contains iodine atoms bonded to the ring structure of the benzoic acid molecule. Thus, the contrast contains virtually no 'free' iodine. The dosages administered vary, depending on individual patients: a patient with poor renal function will require far more contrast as the rate of excretion is much slower. Dosages are categorized as low, medium or high. A suitable adult dose is approximately 1 ml kg^{-1} body weight of the commercially available preparations. In the case of children, an intravenous contrast medium of lower strength is used, as this exerts less influence upon both blood volume and red blood cells. The dose is given over 2–3 minutes, so that there is no sudden shift of fluid between body compartments.

Indicators

An IVU is performed on a wide variety of patients, particularly where an underlying structural abnormality is thought to be present within the urinary tract. An IVU is also a valuable investigation in cases of renal, ureteric or bladder calculi, recurrent urinary tract infection or pyelonephritis, haematuria, suspected space-occupying lesions in the bladder or kidney, carcinoma within the urinary tract, urinary obstruction (e.g. prostatic hyperplasia) or in cases of congenital abnormality (e.g. horseshoe kidney, duplex kidney or ureter, or vesicoureteric reflux).

Precautions

An IVU is clearly contraindicated in patients who are allergic to iodine or those who are asthmatic. It should also be performed with care in patients who have renal impairment, and in those who have multiple myeloma or diabetes mellitus, since excessive dehydration could result in further renal damage and subsequent renal failure.

Patient preparation

◆   Screening for allergy to iodine-based preparations.
◆   Nil by mouth (NBM) for 4 hours prior to the procedure – to reduce nausea and enhance picture quality. If dehydration is contraindicated, the patient can be hydrated via a peripheral intravenous infusion and still 'starved' to avoid nausea during the procedure.
◆   Bowel preparation – this depends on the patient's age and tolerance, and also is not a priority in an emergency. However, since X-ray images must pass through the colon to

visualize the kidneys, the bowel should be as empty as possible. The commonly used purgative agents include castor oil, bisacodyl and senna, but this varies between centres.

◆ Information – IVU is performed with the patient lying down and the contrast is given via a single injection, as a bolus. There is an initial 'flushing' feeling of warmth which proceeds up the arm into the whole body, and a feeling of nausea which lasts only 20–40 seconds; patients may also experience an unpleasant metallic taste in the mouth. The patient will be in the radiology department for some time while the series of X-rays is taken and may feel quite anxious.

Complications

The major complication of IVU relates to hypersensitivity reactions. These can be rapid and life-threatening (including glossopharyngeal and tracheal oedema, bronchospasm, widespread vasodilation and cardiac arrest). Ninety per cent of severe reactions occur withn 5–15 minutes of injection (Doyle et al, 1989), and over 20% of patients experience some reaction to the contrast, though the majority of symptoms are minor (e.g. urticaria, nausea). It is vital that resuscitation equipment (and those trained to use it) is available in the radiology department.

Film sequence

An IVU consists of the following films.

Pre-contrast KUB

The precontrast KUB acts as a control film, and will illustrate any opacities such as stones or other areas of tissue calcification.

Immediate film

An immediate film (nephrogram) is taken as an anterior-posterior view of the kidneys. The film is taken 15–20 seconds after the injection of the intravenous contrast medium, the time delay reflecting the 'arm to kidney' transit time. The film aims to show the nephrogram, which consists of the renal parenchyma enhanced by contrast medium within the proximal tubules of the nephrons. The nephrogram film is dependent upon water absorption from the contrast.

The nephrogram displays the number, size and shape of the kidneys and allows assessment of renal scarring. If excretion from either kidney is delayed, owing to tubular obstruction (e.g. stones), or if renal circulation is reduced, a much more dense nephrogram will be seen and may last for several hours. If there are confusing overlying shadows on the film, caused by gas in the bowel, or if cancer or calculi are suspected, tomograms may be taken to enhance the view. Thus a series of films focus on a single plane of the kidney, effectively giving views of 'slices' through the kidney.

Five-minute film

The 5-minute film is taken as an anterior-posterior view of the renal areas. It allows the estimation of symmetrical contrast excretion, and also enables further contrast medium to be given if there is poor initial opacification of the kidneys.

Often a compression band is applied midway around the patient's abdomen (like a wide belt) over the point at which the ureters cross the pelvic brim (Doyle *et al.*, 1989). The aim of this is to temporarily occlude the drainage of the contrast medium down the ureters and result in an effective distension of the renal pelvis and calyces, giving an enhanced image. Compression is not used in cases of:

- ◆ recent abdominal surgery
- ◆ renal trauma
- ◆ suspected abdominal mass (potential for haemorrhage)
- ◆ a 5-minute film already displaying calyceal distension

Fifteen to twenty minute film

The 15–20 minute film is an anterior-posterior view of the renal areas. This film further displays the renal calyces and pelvis, showing further enhancement of the image as more contrast has, by this stage, been filtered.

Compression is released if adequate films have been obtained, and the contrast is allowed to proceed down the ureters into the bladder.

Release film

The release film (30 minutes) is taken supine, as an anterior-posterior view of the abdomen. In patients where abdominal compression is not used, this view is taken 15–20 minutes after injection. Prone abdominal films can be taken to enhance the visualization of the ureters.

This film allows visualization of the whole urinary tract including the ureters and bladder. It will display evidence of ureteric obstruction or trauma, or space-occupying lesions in the bladder. The 30-minute film is also useful in patients with urinary stomas to visualize the residual volume in the stoma 'loop', as well as the size of its lumen (a 'loopogram' or 'stomagram' is a more effective procedure, however).

Postmicturition film

The postmicturition film is taken supine and aimed at the bladder approximately 5 cm above the level of the symphysis pubis. The patient is asked to empty the bladder and as soon as possible after this an X-ray is taken, which allows assessment of the volume of contrast left in the bladder and thus is an accurate measure of the 'residual volume'. Bladder disorders such as diverticulum, carcinoma or calculi are seen much more clearly on this film.

A further film may be taken of the urethra during voiding (a 'voiding urethrogram'), although this is not common practice, as much greater opacification is achieved when contrast is instilled via the retrograde approach.

Delayed IVU films may be required in cases of obstructive uropathy, where excretion is very slow, or where renal function is poor. The film may be taken 6–12 hours later.

It is vital that fluids are taken normally after an IVU to redress the dehydration prior to the procedure.

Antegrade urography

Antegrade urography may be used when IVU has failed to provide the information desired.

The pelvis of the kidneys are located using ultrasound, and a fine-bore needle is then inserted through the skin, progressing down into the renal pelvis. A flexible, polythene cannula is then passed down the needle lumen and into the pelvis, and the needle is removed. Contrast can be injected directly into the renal pelvis and a number of X-rays can be taken, with the patient lying on his or her side, supine or prone.

If a previous IVU has revealed what appears to be an obstructed ureter, the cause of which is uncertain (it could be possibly swollen or oedematous, or there is retroperitoneal fibrosis inhibiting peristalsis), then the indwelling cannula can be used to perform Whitaker's test. Whitaker's test relies on the principle that in an unobstructed ureter (or tube), fluid will flow out of the tube at the same rate as it flows into it. Therefore, the patient is catheterized urethrally, and the nephrostomy cannula connected to an infusion pump which allows a constant flow of fluid into the renal pelvis. At the same time, the rate of fluid collection from the urinary catheter is measured. If the two rates of flow are equal, this will indicate that no secondary cause of obstruction is present, but if the rates are not equal then there is some obstruction.

The polythene cannula can be left in place or replaced with a wider-bore tube, which is sutured in place, an occlusive dressing is applied and the tube connected to a drainage bag. This arrangement draining urine directly from the renal pelvis is known as a 'nephrostomy' and provides a simple and effective method of decompressing an obstructed kidney. This will prevent further damage and loss of function of the nephrons, and thus preserve renal function.

If cancer is suspected, antegrade cannulation of the pelvis should be carried out with care as it is possible to cause the spread of tumour cells (particularly if there is bleeding). However, fluid samples can be taken directly from the renal pelvis and sent for cytological examination.

Information

Antegrade urography gives information about renal size, the integrity of the calyces, renal pelvis, pelviureteric junction and ureter. It can demonstrate the presence of tumours (or obstructive lesions) in any one of these locations and can be used to relieve outflow obstruction, via nephrostomy.

Patient preparation

◆ Nil by mouth for 3–4 hours prior to procedure – if dehydration is contraindicated then intravenous fluids may be given.

◆ Screening for allergy to iodine-based preparations.

◆ Full pre-procedure information: the patient is asked to lie on the opposite side to the kidney under investigation, and the skin site is shaved (if appropriate) and cleansed according to local policy. After visualizing the kidney by ultrasound, a mark is made on the skin, an incision is made and the cannula advanced into the renal pelvis.

◆ If the patient is nervous a pre-procedure sedative may be given, and analgesia will be required afterwards, particularly if the nephrostomy tube is left in situ.

◆ An accurate fluid balance chart will be needed after the nephrostomy tube insertion to monitor the diuresis, and thus calculate replacement therapy.

Renal arteriogram/angiography

A renal arteriogram is a highly invasive investigation, involving direct cannulation of the renal artery and a high-speed series of X-rays which allow detailed examination of the arterial supply of both kidneys.

Angiography is performed under local anaesthesia, often with some sedation. In the radiography department, following administration of the local anaesthetic and local skin preparation, a radio-opaque, flexible catheter is inserted into the femoral artery. The catheter is threaded into the abdominal aorta and from there to the renal artery. The catheter once in position is connected to a 50 ml syringe, located in a driver capable of emptying the syringe over 2–5 seconds.

The syringe driver is activated and simultaneously a series of X-rays is taken at automatic pre-set intervals, as the contrast is infused (the technique uses a rapid serial film changer and is thus known as 'serial radiography'). The first films are taken over the initial 2–4 seconds following injection, and allow visualization of the renal arteries (e.g. the interlobar and arcuate arteries). Normally, two films are taken per second for the first 2 seconds, one film per second for the next 5 seconds; during the 5–10 second period and the 15–20 second period a second series of films is taken: these provide visualization of the renal substance. The venous phase follows, but is more limited in the amount of information that can be obtained.

Digital subtraction angiography is a refinement of the above technique, and uses a computer to subtract images of surrounding tissues, and thus enhance the quality of the films.

Information

Renal angiography may show evidence of renal artery stenosis (in hypertensive patients), tumour, the nature of space-occupying lesions within the renal substance (which may have their own 'corrupted' blood supply that is different from the normal architecture of the kidney). Angiography is also undertaken prior to live related donor transplantation, as it is crucial to know how many branches there are from the renal arteries before attempting donor nephrectomy. Angiography may also be undertaken following renal trauma if laceration is suspected.

Patient preparation

- ◆ Screening for allergy to iodine-based preparations.
- ◆ Nil by mouth for 4 hours prior to procedure.
- ◆ Full pre-procedure information: including the groin shave in the radiology department, the 'flushing' feeling as the contrast media is injected (see IVU procedure), through to limitations after the procedure owing to the arterial puncture of a large high-pressure vessel.

The risk of haemorrhage is high and the patient is kept on bed rest for 8–12 hours after the procedure, with close monitoring of blood pressure, pulse, puncture site, pedal pulses and nail-bed flush. It is normal for some bruising to occur at the puncture site and occasionally a haematoma may form which should resolve spontaneously.

Renal venogram

Taking a renal venogram is very similar to angiography in method, except that cannulation is carried out via the right femoral vein, and the catheter is then advanced via the inferior vena cava to the left or right renal vein as necessary. The image may be further enhanced by injecting adrenaline into the renal artery approximately 10 seconds after contrast is injected into the vein; this will delay excretion of the contrast via the venous circulation owing to the vasoconstriction within the kidney.

Venography is performed in cases of renal vascular hypertension, and blood may also be sampled and assayed for plasma renin concentration. Venography may also be used in cases of renal vein thrombosis, or renal tumour.

Postprocedural care differs only from arteriography in that pedal pulses need not be checked; however, the colour and warmth of the lower limb must be monitored.

Retrograde pyeloureterography

A retrograde pyelogram is a series of radiographs, taken either as distinct films, or more commonly by using an image intensifier, with films taken of specific views. It provides detailed anatomical information about the ureter, the pelviureteric junction, renal pelvis and calyces. The investigation is performed while the patient is anaesthetized (general or spinal) in the lithotomy position.

Using a cystoscope the surgeon identifies the ureteric orifice and proceeds in one of two ways:

1. The classic approach is to insert a graduated ureteric catheter up the length of the ureter to the renal pelvis. Contrast is then gently injected or infused under gravity into the upper tract and X-rays taken.
2. The more modern approach is to use a bulb-ended catheter (e.g. a Prash bulb) which temporarily seals the end of the ureter prior to injection of contrast. This is particularly useful when ureteric catheterization is not possible, and is less traumatic to the ureter; pelvicalyceal filling may be incomplete, as filling occurs from the base of the ureter. The radiologist presses the bulb against the ureteric orifice and 2–3 ml of contrast is slowly injected. As contrast runs into the ureter, image intensification may show the renal pelvis to be filled with contrast, or the presence of calculi or tumour.

Indications

Retrograde pyelography can be used in patients who are allergic to iodine-bound contrast media, and in those who have non-functioning kidneys which are unable to concentrate and excrete contrast making IVU ineffective. Specific patient preparation is based around preparing for anaesthesia and the postoperative recovery. A full explanation of the procedure is nonetheless essential.

Contraindications and complications

Retrograde imaging must only be performed in patients who have a negative urinary screen prior to instrumentation, as any significant urinary tract infection could be inoculated into the blood stream. Other complications include mucosal damage to the ureter and possible ureteric perforation or perforation of the renal pelvis by the catheter.

Occasionally, contrast media may be absorbed and cause an allergic reaction, but the risk is far less than with excretion urography. Sterile pyelitis, caused by contrast stasis, and overdistension of the pelvis can also occur. Pyelonephritis as a result of instrumentation is also possible. Thus following the procedure the patient should be observed for loin pain, dysuria, fevers and rigors especially during the first 24–48 hours. Should infection occur the treatment should be aggressive, including urinary culture, intravenous antibiotics, additional fluids and analgesia as appropriate.

Contrast extravasation is also possible, but is temporary as the water-based contrast is absorbed from the surrounding tissue space.

Cystogram

A cystogram is a complex investigation which involves radiographic examination of the bladder using contrast media. It is normally performed as a single investigation (rather than as part of an IVU) when a problem such as vesicoureteric reflux is suspected. Usually a video film is taken via image intensification, so that reflux may be observed as it occurs.

Cystograms, flowmetry and their significance are discussed further in Chapter 3.

Ascending urethrogram

A urethrogram is a useful and commonly employed investigation which allows visualization of the length of the urethra. There are two methods; in each of these the patient lies supine on the X-ray table and three views (lateral, supine and oblique) are taken with the left leg abducted and the left knee flexed, and then again with the right knee flexed and right leg abducted.

1. A viscous contrast medium is gently injected into the urethral meatus, via a syringe and a penile clamp applied behind the glans. This effects greater urethral distension and thus enhances the images of the anatomy when X-rays are taken.
2. A water-based contrast solution is inserted into the urethra via a Foley catheter, positioned just outside the meatus. The catheter balloon can be inflated with 1–2 ml of water after insertion into the navicular fossa; X-rays are then taken. Film quality is not as good as urethral distension is limited.

Viscous contrast cannot be used with a catheter because the pressure created in the urethra would dislodge the catheter.

Chapman and Nakielny (1986) suggested that ascending urethrography should be followed by micturating cystourethrography or excreting micturating cystourethrography, to demonstrate the proximal urethra. Occasionally, it is only possible to see a urethral fistula or periurethral abscess on a 'voiding' examination, and reflux of contrast into dilated prostatic ducts is also better seen during micturition.

Information

The ascending urethrogram will demonstrate:

◆   urethral stricture
◆   false passage or urethral tear following traumatic catheterization
◆   congenital abnormalities (e.g. urethral valves)
◆   periurethral abscess or prostatic abscess
◆   urethral fistulae

The urethrogram is contraindicated in patients with a urinary tract infection or following recent instrumentation owing to the risk of bacteraemia.

Patient preparation

No specific preparation is required prior to urethrography, but adequate information must be given as this investigation may be uncomfortable and is potentially embarrassing.

Downagram

A 'downagram' is a variation upon the ascending urethrogram, but is used following urethral surgery (e.g. urethroplasty) to assess urethral patency and healing 10–14 days after surgery. A water-based contrast medium is used in case there is any leakage from an anastomosis.

Such patients usually have both urethral and suprapubic catheters in place; contrast is injected into the suprapubic catheter and allowed to drain out of the fenestrated urethral catheter. Therefore contrast drains around the catheter as well as through it and the urethral outline can be visualized; extravasation of contrast indicates that the surgery has not yet made the urethra 'watertight' and the catheters should be left in situ for longer to allow further healing.

An 'up-and-downagram' is a combination of classic urethrogram and downagram.

Patient preparation

There is no specific preparation other than a full, clear explanation of the procedure.

Lymphangiogram

Lymphangiography is now used much less frequently owing to the availability of computer-assisted tomography, nuclear magnetic resonance scanning and ultrasonography. Results are often of poor quality and are difficult to assess reliably and accurately.

Indications

Lymphangiography is a lengthy investigation used to search for abnormalities in the lymphatics caused by metastatic deposits or lymphoma (i.e. blockages) or filling defects within otherwise normal-looking nodes. It was commonly used to assess the spread of testicular cancer but improvements in less invasive technology have made it almost obsolete. It is not a good method of assessing the spread of prostatic or bladder cancer either and carries with it a number of risks.

Lymphangiography is contraindicated if:

♦ The patient has pre-existing respiratory disease – the contrast will end up in the lungs and may cause small pulmonary emboli which appear as fine 'pinpoint' opacities on a chest X-ray 24 hours after the procedure; these are normally asymptomatic but if a large volume of contrast reaches the pulmonary circulation, more significant emboli may occur. Systemic oil emboli are also possible and may cause cerebral emboli, since the contrast is slowly absorbed.

◆ Radiotherapy to the lung within 3 weeks of lymphangiography can disrupt the normal pulmonary architecture and allow contrast into the circulation.

◆ The patient has active thrombophlebitis, localized sepsis or iodine sensitivity.

◆ The patient is undergoing cytotoxic therapy – the lymph glands may be already damaged and thus allow more contrast into the circulation.

Procedure

The two medial web spaces of both feet are injected with a mixture of 2 ml of 1% lignocaine and 2 ml of 2.5% patent blue dye; the feet are then exercised for 30–60 minutes until the lymphatics are visible on the dorsum of each foot.

Under local anaesthesia, a small incision is made over a lymphatic vessel, which is then cannulated and the needle secured with silk ties or a suitable tape. The vessel is aspirated to check that a vein has not been cannulated. This procedure is repeated for the other leg. An 'oily' contrast (10–20 ml volume) is then injected under pressure via a syringe driver. Films are taken in sequence:

◆ ankle – 10 minutes
◆ knees – 15 minutes
◆ thighs, pelvis and femora – 30 minutes
◆ supine abdomen – 40 minutes
◆ a further supine film is taken every 15 minutes until the contrast reaches the level of the third lumbar vertebra (L3)
◆ 2 hours after the injection a chest X-ray is taken, supine abdominal film, and anterior/posterior films of pelvis and upper femur; these are repeated after 24 hours

The contrast should fill up the lymphatic vessels of the leg, the nodes in the groin and the iliac and para-aortic nodes.

Patient preparation

◆ Full, clear and concise information – the co-operation of the patient is obviously required.
◆ If oedema is present the limbs should be elevated for the preceding 24 hours to aid cannulation.
◆ Children may require general anaesthesia.
◆ It is probably advisable that the patient empty the bladder prior to the procedure.

After the procedure the skin and the urine may be blue. An overnight hospital stay is advised for monitoring (observation for allergic reactions, infection, lymphangitis or pulmonary problems); no general anaesthesia, radiotherapy or cytotoxic drugs is advised for at least one week.

NON-INVASIVE INVESTIGATIONS

Computer-assisted tomography

Computer-assisted tomographic (CT) scanning has been used for over 15 years. It provides a high-resolution tomographic image, which provides films of 'slices' taken transversely at different levels through areas of the body (e.g. thorax, abdomen, head).

A CT scan provides an estimate of the densities of various tissues, which it calculates in Hounsfield units (named after the inventor). Normal parenchymal tissues have a value of 80–100 units, bone + 1,000 units, air − 1,000 units, fat − 100 units, and water is 0 unit.

Indications

For urological use, CT scanning is employed to give computer-generated images of the abdomen (to examine the kidneys, ureters, bladder and renal blood vessels); of the thorax (to examine the lungs, para-aortic nodes for evidence of metastatic tumour spread); and CT scanning is also being used to search for enlarged lymph nodes which may be indicative of metastatic disease.

Nuclear magnetic resonance imaging

Nuclear magnetic resonance (NMR) imaging has many similarities in its methodology to CT scanning, but the image obtained is produced in a completely different way. Because the number of protons (positively charged particles, present in the nucleus of atoms) differs within living tissue of different types, each tissue creates a minute, unique magnetic field. If exposed to a magnetic field of greater magnitude, the protons align themselves along the direction (lines of force) of the stronger field at the lowest energy state possible (the 'ground' state). If the tissues under study are then exposed to a brief pulse of radio waves, a brief rise is seen in the energy state of the proton particles (owing to the processes of interference and resonance). When the radio waves are removed, this increase in energy from the ground state is lost, and the protons return to the ground by releasing the energy in the form of electromagnetic radiation. It is this energy signal the NMR scanner detects, and computer enhancement and processing produces images which can be studied.

Views can be generated from sagittal, coronal and transaxial planes; NMR scanning is not effective for detecting calculi or tissue calcification.

Indications

As for CT scanning.

Contraindications

Nuclear magnetic resonance scanning is contraindicated in patients with pacemakers (it may cause interference) and in patients with other metallic implants (staples may move during the procedure) as they should not be exposed to strong magnetic forces. Claustrophobic patients may also find both NMR and CT scanning disturbing as they are required to lie still in an enclosed tube-like structure.

Patient preparation

◆ Careful information and teaching – some patients may require sedation (e.g. elderly confused or claustrophobic patients and children).
◆ All metal objects must be removed (e.g. earrings, watches, rings, underwired bra) prior to the procedure.

Ultrasonography of the urinary tract

Ultrasound is entirely non-invasive, and a measure of its safety is indicated by the way it is used to monitor fetal growth and position during antenatal care. Ultrasonography uses a probe which is placed upon the patient's skin above the area to be imaged. The probe emits high-frequency sound waves (5–20 kHz) which enter the body and are reflected back from the organ being studied. The degree of reflection is dependent on the density of the tissue acting as reflector. Thus a dense structure like bone would reflect more than a fluid-filled cyst. The sound waves returning to the probe are detected, and fed to a computer which analyses the difference between the sent and returning signal to produce an image on a screen.

The equipment can also be used to take still photographs or moving film. Since no radiation dose is involved, ultrasound has many advantages over X-rays: multiple images can be produced, from several angles; repeat studies are not dangerous and can be carried out away from the X-ray department; and bowel preparation is not required.

Indications

Ultrasound is used in numerous ways in urology; a few applications are listed below:

◆ to image the renal pelvis, calyces and renal outline, and to measure bladder capacity and postmicturition residual volume
◆ to show upper tract dilatation and hydronephrosis

- ◆ to distinguish cystic structures from solid tumour
- ◆ to locate urinary calculi
- ◆ to locate collections of fluid (e.g. subphrenic abscess)
- ◆ to assist in insertion of nephrostomy
- ◆ transrectal ultrasound can assess prostatic growth

Patient preparation

1. Explanation that ultrasound is quick, painless and simple.
2. A conducting jelly is placed on the skin to improve transmission and enhance the quality of the image.

RADIONUCLEOTIDE IMAGING OF THE KIDNEY (RENAL SCANNING)

Isotopic nuclear imaging of the kidney and urinary tract uses a radioactive tracer molecule (e.g. technetium 99m) which is either bound to a substance freely filtered by the kidney (e.g. diethylene briamine penta-acetic acid, DTPA) or which is bound to a substance that binds directly to the tubular cells (i.e. is taken up and not filtered). Thus, the first approach yields information regarding function of the kidney, whereas the second provides more information concerning the structure of the kidney. The radionucleotide (e.g. ^{99m}Tc-EDTA) is injected intravenously, and its activity (or handling by the kidney) is then detected and measured by a computer-enhanced detection system, such as a gamma camera (sensitive to gamma radiation), which allows comparison between the kidneys to be made simultaneously.

A renal scan can thus provide useful information regarding both structure and function of the kidneys, as well as providing a quantitative comparison of renal function. Such functional information is given the generic term of 'renogram'.

The approaches that may be used are shown in Table 2.2. The normal

NAME	USE
DTPA scan (renogram)	Differential renal function
	Suspected obstruction
	Assessment of single kidney function
DMSA scan	Differential function and detection of structural damage (e.g. cortical scarring)
Sodium ortho-iodohippurate (Hippuran) scan (renogram)	As for DTPA scan

Note: DMSA, dimercaptosuccinic acid; DTPA, diethylenetriamine penta-acetic acid.

Table 2.2 Methods of renal scanning

renogram, using a tracer substance, produces a graphical result, which can be divided into three phases. These are:

1. *Vascular phase.* This represents the uptake function of the kidney and relates directly to renal blood flow (0–2 minutes).
2. *Filtration phase.* This reflects the transport of the isotope from the nephron to the renal pelvis, and will be clearly prolonged if there is renal damage (e.g. acute tubular dysfunction from acute renal failure) or poor renal perfusion, when the renal blood flow is reduced (2–6 minutes).
3. *Excretion phase.* This phase reflects the passage of the isotope from the renal pelvis down the ureter, and will clearly be lengthened by any pelviureteric junction or ureteric obstruction (6–15 minutes). (Thus, the excretion phase will lengthen in hydronephrosis, caused by a ureteric stone, or in cases of a large, 'baggy' renal pelvis, or in cases of a tumour at the ureterovesical junction.)

Because some of the isotope is taken up by the soft tissues, it is normal to place an additional detector over an adjacent part of the loin or over the arm, which measures the background uptake, and automatically subtracts this figure from the value obtained over the kidney.

Technetium-99m diethylenetriamine penta-acetic acid scan

The radioactive compound ^{99m}Tc-DTPA is mainly excreted via glomerular filtration and can therefore be used to image kidneys, ureters and bladder. Its primary use is to assess any upper tract obstruction, although glomerular filtration rate and differential renal function may also be estimated.

Following an intravenous bolus injection, an initial film (similar to the nephrogram of an IVU) may be taken at 30 seconds, to provide an estimation of renal cortical blood flow. Subsequent pictures are then taken at 1, 5, 10, 15 and 20 minutes.

Scanning with DTPA provides more functional information than structural detail. Further, if pelviureteric junction (PUJ) or ureteric obstruction is suspected, radionucleotide washout can be imaged from each kidney, following the administration of an intravenous diuretic such as frusemide. If obstruction is present, a slower rate of removal or no removal of isotope will be seen. If a large, baggy, unobstructed pelvis is present, which is thought to be collecting urine and/or causing urinary tract infection, the use of intravenous diuretic will result in an increased excretion rate, and the baggy pelvis will be seen to empty.

Technetium-99m dimercaptosuccinic acid scan

The mercurial compound ^{99m}Tc-DMSA is taken up and 'held' by the nephrons, where it binds to the basement membrane of proximal tubular cells. It therefore allows evaluation of renal cortical structure. Following intravenous injection, it is usual to take a series of images using a gamma camera, approximately 45–60 minutes later, and these will readily display any evidence of renal cysts, scarring or space-occupying lesions.

Iodine-131 orthoiodohippurate scan

The compound ^{131}I-OIH is excreted by both glomerular filtration and tubular excretion. It can yield the same information as DTPA, but emits far more gamma radiation (Brundage, 1992). Its use is therefore limited, but it may be of value where renal function is poor and relatively little isotope is being filtered.

Isotopic measurement of GFR

Radioactive tracer (isotope) studies can also be used to measure glomerular filtration rate, by accurately detecting and quantifying the clearance from blood of a designated tracer molecule. After the dose is administered intravenously, serial measurements of vascular radioactivity are taken (over a 60 minute period) either by serial sampling or by the use of a counter placed over the forearm, which is less invasive. Isotopic GFR measurement is especially useful in patients where a conventional 24-hour urine collection is hard to obtain, and has the advantage of being extremely accurate.

Bone scan

A useful application of radioisotope imaging is in screening for cancer of the prostate and bladder, which may present with possible bony metastases. The specific investigation is called a bone scan, and normally uses Tc-99m methylene diphosphonate (^{99m}Tc-MDP).

The isotope is taken up by vascular areas of bone, and will readily detect bony metastases because the vascularity of such areas is increased, owing to the higher metabolic rate. Metastatic deposits can therefore be observed before they are visible on conventional radiographs, by the use of isotopic imaging. Further, because of the low dosage of radiation, this investigation can be performed repeatedly over a prolonged period, to assess response to treatment.

A problem with this technique, however, is that inflammation due to recent bony injury, arthritic conditions or other degenerative changes will also increase vascularity within those bony areas affected, and thus will also display increased uptake of isotope. There is, therefore, a potential for false-positive results to be obtained, although, in the hands of a competent radiologist this is unlikely, as such areas can be easily distinguished; further, these conditions tend to occur within defined areas of the bony skeleton. Because spread of prostatic cancer is primarily to the bony pelvis, femurs and lower spine, a bone scan provides an effective method for assessing tumour growth and patient response to treatment (Maisey *et al.*, 1991). No specific patient preparation is required.

Contraindications

Isotopic imaging is contraindicated during pregnancy, because of the emission of gamma radiation.

Patient teaching and nursing care

Radioactive tracer substances are administered via intravenous injection, and therefore care of the site after the procedure is important, as irritation can result.

There is no other specific preparation, and no requirement for bowel preparation as gamma radiation will readily pass through the bowel, including any faecal material or gas. Also, the radiation dosage is significantly less than for an IVU, which is a great advantage of isotopic study, and the half-life of the tracer is only hours in length.

The patient's urine, following the procedure, should be disposed of in accordance with hospital policy. Because of the nature of the investigation, patients require careful explanation and information, particularly as the method will be more effective in a co-operative patient. Patients also need reassurance that the dose of radiation administered is very small.

DIRECT VISUALIZATION METHODS

Direct visualization of parts of the urinary tract relies upon endoscopy, using a precision optical telescope containing an intrinsic light source (e.g. nephroscope, ureteroscope, cystoscope). Nephroscopy allows visualization of the renal pelvis and calyces via an antegrade approach, whereas ureteroscopy and cystoscopy both employ a urethral approach, ureteroscopy then proceeding further to cannulation of the ureteric orifice in question.

For nephroscopy, a percutaneous tract is first made under radiographic control, with the patient under anaesthesia. The track is made using an image intensifier and the use of contrast and either a rigid metal sheath inserted into the track followed by a rigid endoscope (rigid endoscopy) or a smaller-bore, flexible endoscope (flexible endoscopy). Either method allows biopsy specimens to be taken, and often is combined with endoscopic stone removal. Nephroscopy, although its principal use is for percutaneous nephrolithotomy, can also be of value in cases of recurrent urinary tract infection or congential abnormality, where direct visualization of the renal substance is therefore possible.

All endoscopic methods are contraindicated in patients with established urinary tract infection, as they could easily result in an inoculation of the causative organism into the blood stream. Urine must therefore be suitably screened, prior to investigation.

Nursing care

Patients require work-up for either general or spinal anaesthesia, and must have non-infected urine. Any urinary infection must be treated, although with stone disease it may be impossible to eradicate all bacteria completely.

Following the procedure, patients require routine postoperative care, plus observation for haematuria (this is expected, but should not be heavy or prolonged) and infection. Because of the possibility of mucosal damage and the spread of bacteria into the circulation, any evidence of fever or systemic infection must be aggressively treated.

Patients require adequate preoperative information, reassurance and preparation for the anaesthetic of choice. The nephroscopic track will close in 48–72 hours, unless a nephrostomy tube is left in position following the procedure.

Ureteroscopy is becoming more common, as it forms part of laser-assisted endoscopy for ureteric stones (lasertripsy). Here, a laser fibre (or extrahydraulic lithotripsy probe) is passed up the ureter, under direct visualization, using a narrow-bore fibreoptic telescope. The stone is visualized, and then broken up using either laser or sound waves.

Following the procedure, the ureteroscope allows examination of the whole length of the ureter, and therefore any obstruction or areas of oedema (which may be hard to distinguish from obstructive lesions on radiographs) can readily be seen. Ureteroscopy is thus very versatile, and allows video film or photographs to be taken.

Patient preparation is the same as for cystoscopy, and is performed under general or epidural anaesthesia, with the patient in the lithotomy position. Patients require information and reassurance, especially as they may have back pain on the side visualized after the procedure. Ureteroscopy is invasive and the urine must again be infection-free.

After the procedure, the patient should be observed for evidence of infection, haematuria or excessive pain. Ureteroscopy is an increasingly common procedure, owing to its use in the treatment of stones.

Cystoscopy

In many ways, cystoscopy is one of the best known of invasive urological investigations, allowing direct observation of both the urethra (especially in the male, where the urethra is a far more complex structure than in the female) and the interior of the bladder.

The cystoscope used can be either a rigid, metallic telescope or a flexible, polymer-based telescope, both using an intrinsic or fibreoptic light source. Cystoscopy is generally performed in theatre, under general anaesthesia, with the patient in the lithotomy position; glycine irrigation fluid is used to maintain a clear visual field for the operator. However, many patients who have frequent cystoscopic examinations (e.g. for follow-up after treatment of bladder cancer) are now being successfully treated as outpatients, under local anaesthesia in a suitable clinic environment. This eliminates the need for hospital admission. Outpatient cystoscopy is performed with a flexible cystoscope, with the patient sitting in a specialized chair, after the use of a suitable intraurethral anaesthetic agent.

For either method, the urine must have no infection.

Indications

Cystoscopy is one of the 'mainstay' urological investigations and, in cases of unexplained haematuria, allows visualization of the bladder, ureteric orifices, trigone, sphincters and urethra.

Cystoscopy is also performed to investigate bladder dysfunction, obstruction (e.g. strictures or bladder neck obstruction) and for both the diagnosis and staging of bladder cancer, where it allows mucosal biopsy to be taken for histology as well as the depth of spread (and thus 'staging') assessed. Cystoscopy takes approximately 5–15 minutes.

Contraindications

There are few contraindications, as even frail patients or those with cardiac or respiratory compromise can be cystoscoped with suitable precautions (e.g. by the use of flexible cystoscopy under local anaesthesia).

Patient preparation and teaching

Patients require preparation for general or epidural anaesthesia, and reassurance and information is important, especially if they have never experienced cystoscopy before. Often patients have some urethral discomfort postoperatively, and should be observed for significant haematuria and reestablishment of voiding.

The urine must be screened preoperatively, and any postoperative infection treated aggressively.

REFERENCES

BROWN J, Meikle J and Webb C (1991) Collecting mid-stream specimens of urine: the research base. *Nursing Times* **87** (13): 49–52.

BRUNDAGE D (1992) *Renal Disorders*. St Louis: Mosby.

CHAPMAN S and Nakielny R (1986) *A Guide to Radiological Procedures*, 2nd edn. London: Baillière Tindall.

DOYLE T, Hare W S C, Thomson K and Tress B (1989) *Procedures in Diagnostic Radiology*. Edinburgh: Churchill Livingstone.

HISCOKE C, Yoxall H, Greig D and Lightfoot N F (1990) Validation of a method for the rapid diagnosis of urinary tract infection suitable for use in general practice. *British Journal of General Practice* **40**: 403–405.

IMMERGUT M A, Gilbert E G and Fresilli F J (1981) The myth of the clean catch urine specimen. *Urology* **17**: 339–340.

KASS E H (1957) Bacteriuria and the diagnosis of infections of the urinary tract. *Archives of Internal Medicine* **100**: 709–714. Cited in Stevens M (1989) Screening urines for bacteriuria. *Journal of Medical Laboratory Sciences* **46**: 194–206.

KELLOGG J A, Manzella J P, Shaffer S N and Schwartz B B (1987) Clinical relevance of culture *versus* screens for the detection of microbial pathogens in urine specimens. *American Journal of Medicine* **83**: 739–745.

LOWE P A (1985) Chemical screening and prediction of bacteriuria – a new approach. *Journal of Medical Laboratory Sciences* **42**: 28–33.

MAISEY M N, Britton K E and Gilday D L (1991) *Clinical Nuclear Medicine*, 2nd edn. London: Chapman & Hall.

MORRIS R W, Watts M R and Reeves D S (1979) Perineal cleansing before midstream urine: a necessary ritual? *Lancet* **ii**: 158–159.

ROBERTS F J (1986) Quantitative urine culture in patients with urinary tract infection and bacteremia. *American Journal of Clinical Pathology* **85**: 616–618.

STEVENS M (1989) Screening urines for bacteriuria. *Journal of Medical Laboratory Sciences* **46**: 194–206.
STRAND C L, Bryant J K and Sutton K H (1985) Septicaemia secondary to urinary tract infection with colony counts less than 10^5 CFU ml. *American Journal of Clinical Pathology* **83**: 619–621.

URODYNAMICS

Contents

Urodynamics is the study of the neuromuscular function and dysfunction of the lower urinary tract. It is more simply described as the study of pressure and flow relationships in the lower urinary tract (Norton 1986).

Not everyone with urinary symptoms, such as frequency or incontinence, requires a full urodynamic evaluation of all phases of their bladder filling and voiding cycles. Often the cause of the problem can be diagnosed following a full history and medical examination (Chance, 1994). Less invasive tests, such as urinalysis (Laker, 1994), frequency and volume voided charts (Duffin, 1992) and a pad test (Abbott, 1992), which measures the volume of urine lost over a stated period, can also be used to aid diagnosis. If these tests do not identify a cause or if conservative treatment is unsuccessful, then the patient may need to undergo additional urodynamic tests. Urodynamic tests will also be required for patients with mixed symptoms such as frequency and stress incontinence, underlying neurological diseases and those considered for some urological surgery.

Urodynamic studies can be divided into three groups:

1. Urinary flow studies (uroflowmetry).
2. Pressure studies of both bladder and urethra (cystometry).
3. Video studies (video cystometrogram).

UROFLOWMETRY

Uroflowmetry measures the rate and volume at which urine is expelled from the urethral meatus in millilitres per second (ml s^{-1}). It is the simplest form of clinical urodynamic test and is useful as a preliminary investigation (Stephenson *et al.*, 1984). It can also be combined with pre- and post-micturition ultrasonography for a cystodynamogram (Chapple and Christmas, 1990). In addition it forms an integral part of the voiding phase of the cystometrogram.

Different types of equipment can be used to measure flow rates: dipstick, weight transducer and a rotating disc. However, all involve the person either sitting on a commode seat or voiding directly into the funnel of the machine.

Dipstick method

The dipstick is usually made of Perspex with a metal plate on either side. As the level of urine in the jug rises, the electrical capacitance changes. This information is then fed into the computer which produces a tracing.

In order to obtain accurate results, the nurse needs to ensure the correct jug and dipstick combination is used. The bottom of the dipstick should be immersed in water prior to use (unless the metal plates touch the bottom of the jug) in order to ensure that all the urine voided is recorded. The rest of the dipstick should be dry and fitted in the jug vertically.

Weight transducer method

The collecting jug sits on a weight transducer. As the jug fills with urine, the weight increases and from this the flow rate can be calculated. Unlike the dipstick method, the type of jug can vary as the machine is zet to zero *after* the jug is placed on the transducer.

Rotating disc method

A disc at the bottom of a funnel spins continuously as urine is voided onto it. As this happens the motor demands more power in order to keep the disc rotating at a constant speed. The change in power required is then used to calculate the flow rate. Again, the collecting device is not important and the machine can therefore be directly plumbed into the sewerage system.

The equipment should be prepared before carrying out the investigation, ideally in a room set aside purely for measuring flow rates, with the equipment plumbed in and a lockable door to maintain privacy.

Patient preparation

The investigation must be explained to the patients before they attend the clinic so that they arrive with a full bladder. The patient should be asked to void when comfortably full. Ideally the flow rate tests should be performed in a flow rate clinic where the patient produces a series of three consecutive measurements over several hours, and is able to leave the clinic between tests. A series of recordings gives a far more reliable picture than a single recording. However, if only a single recording is made it is essential to ask the patient if the flow and volume were normal. If not, this should be noted on the recording and the study should be repeated (Stephenson 1994). Inhibition can greatly increase hesitancy and slow the flow, hence the importance of maintaining privacy at all times.

Following the final flow rate test the residual urine may be determined. This is especially useful if the flow rate has been poor owing to either obstruction or poor detrusor function. The residual urine can be estimated either by bladder ultrasonography or by passing a urethral catheter. Some typical flow rate profiles are shown in Figure 3.1.

CYSTOMETRY

For many years cystometry has been the main method of investigating bladder function. Simply put, when performing a cystometrogram (CMG) we are looking at the bladder pressure both when filling the bladder and while voiding. A straightforward non-video CMG is performed if it is felt that seeing the outline and neck of the bladder is not necessary to make an accurate diagnosis. It therefore follows that a video CMG is performed if it is necessary to see bladder outline and neck, for example if bladder diverticula are suspected.

Non-video CMG

Prior to the investigation a history of the patient's voiding problem is taken to ensure an accurate current picture of the problem, as the situation may have changed since the initial referral.

Investigation

The patient should arrive for the CMG with a full bladder, and as soon as the procedure has been explained, the patient will be asked to void into the flow rate machine. This action indicates the patient's bladder capacity and uninhibited flow rate. After this the patient is urethrally catheterized with a Jacques catheter to allow filling and with an intravesical pressure catheter. The patient has both catheters inserted at the same time using a sterile technique. Any residual urine is noted, except where there is a known neuropathic bladder (having been completely emptied it may give an abnormal reading).

The suprapubic route can also be used, although this is rarely done unless there is a suprapubic catheter already in situ. Children, however, will often have suprapubic lines (filling and pressure) inserted under general anaesthesia, usually at the same time as cystoscopy.

The pressure line is filled with water and connected to a pressure transducer, which is wired to a recorder. The filling catheter is connected to normal saline (at room temperature) via an irrigation or intravenous giving set.

The bladder pressure line records the intravesical pressure, i.e. the detrusor pressure together with the abdominal pressure caused by the position of the bladder in the body. In order to exclude a pressure rise due to an extravesical component, e.g. intra-abdominal pressure rise due to straining or coughing, a rectal line is inserted. This records the intra-abdominal (rectal) pressure

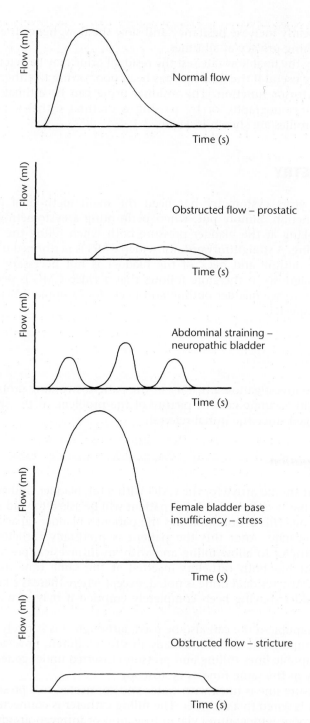

Figure 3.1 *Typical flow rate profiles*

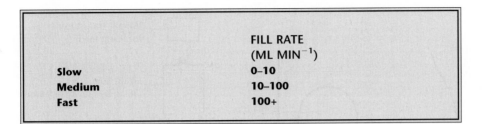

	FILL RATE (ML MIN^{-1})
Slow	0–10
Medium	10–100
Fast	100+

Table 3.1 *Accepted fill rates*

separately, which is then electronically subtracted from the intravesical pressure, giving the intrinsic intravesical pressure or detrusor pressure.

Both the bladder pressure line and the rectal line are flushed with water to allow recordings to be taken. Once the tubes are in and flushed, the patient is asked to cough: this will raise the abdominal pressure and therefore the total bladder pressure. However, the subtracted pressure (the detrusor pressure) should show no rise. The filling of the bladder can then commence.

A 'physiological' fill rate of 1 ml per minute is impractical and would make routine cystometry impossible. A medium fill rate is therefore generally used (Table 3.1). In patients with a suspected neuropathic bladder, the filling is reduced to 10–20 ml min^{-1} as filling too quickly may give an abnormal reading. The liquid may be pumped into the bladder at a predetermined speed or else the bladder can be filled by gravity. The fluid bag or bottle will hang on a weight transducer so that the volume of fluid entering the bladder can be measured. The patient is asked to inform the examiner when the 'first sensation' or first desire to void is experienced, and the volume at this stage is noted. However, the filling continues. When the patient has reached full capacity, the filling catheter is removed, leaving both the bladder and rectal pressure lines in place. The patient will then be asked to cough to check for subtraction and signs of leakage.

The examiner may try other methods to induce leakage such as asking the patient to jog on the spot, or turning on a water tap. Once the examiner is satisfied that all is being recorded the patient is asked to void into the flow rate funnel. Halfway through voiding the patient may be asked to stop. After the stop test, the patient continues to void until completion. The pressure lines are then removed and the patient is given the opportunity to freshen up and change prior to seeing the doctor. At this point the doctor may be able to prescribe medication or explain possible surgery if required. The nurse continence adviser will also be able to give advice.

Figure 3.2 illustrates a typical cystometrogram investigation.

Video CMG

The video procedure is essentially the same as the basic CMG except that a radio-opaque contrast is used as the filling medium. Fluoroscopy is then done intermittently throughout the procedure and shown on a TV monitor together with the pressure and flow recordings. This information is then stored on videotape. The additional video information means that the bladder and urethra can be observed during filling and voiding.

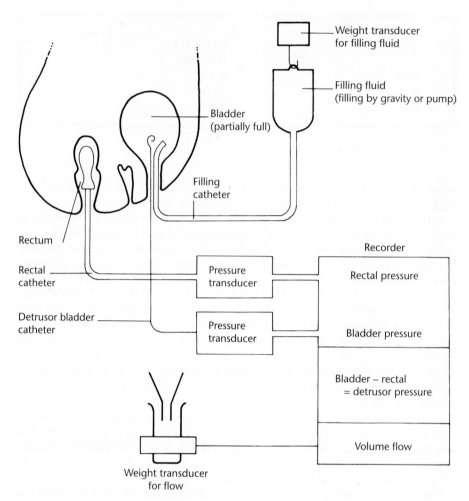

Figure 3.2 *Cystometrogram investigation*

If outflow obstruction is suspected (although a straight CMG would indicate this) a video would indicate where the obstruction was (i.e. prostate, bladder neck or urethral stricture). A video would also show evidence of bladder trabeculation diverticula or ureteric reflux, and this significantly enhances the diagnostic capability of the procedure. Some common CMG profiles are illustrated in Figures 3.3–3.7.

Typical cystometric values

Normal CMG

A normal CMG result is shown in Figure 3.3.

◆   *Filling*:
        first sensation about 150 ml

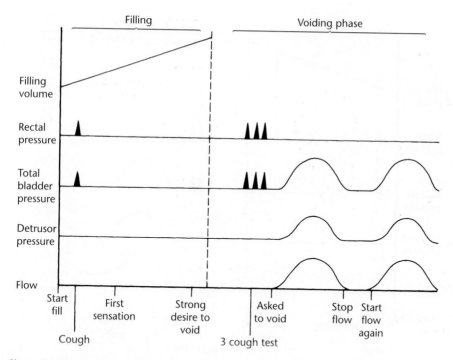

Figure 3.3 *Normal cystometrogram*

    strong desire about 400 ml
    no rise in detrusor pressure; no urgency or leakage
   ◆   *Voiding*:
    no leakage on pre-test cough
    voiding pressure 40–60 cmH$_2$O for male, less for female
    able to stop and start
    maximum flow rate 27 ml s^{-1}
    volume voided 400 ml; no residual urine

Stress incontinence

Figure 3.4 illustrates a CMG showing stress incontinence.

   ◆   *Filling*:
    first sensation about 150 ml
    strong desire about 400 ml
    no rise in detrusor pressure
    no urgency or leakage
   ◆   *Voiding*:
    leaks on three-cough test
    voiding pressure 30 cmH$_2$O
    unable to stop test
    maximum flow 35 ml s^{-1}
    volume voided 400 ml, therefore no residual urine

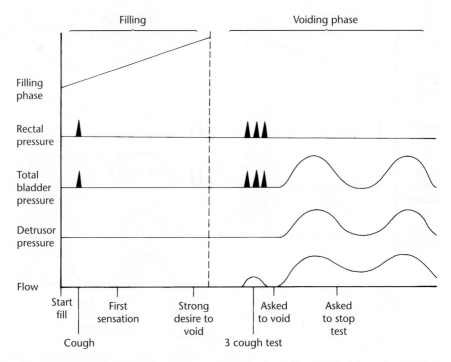

Figure 3.4   Cystometrogram showing stress incontinence

Atonic bladder

A typical atonic bladder CMG is shown in Figure 3.5.

◆   *Filling*:
no first sensation
no desire (strong)
no rise in detrusor pressure
no urgency or leakage
filling stopped at 800 ml
◆   *Voiding*:
no leakage on coughing
no detrusor pressure when asked to void, although total pressure exceeds 100 cmH$_2$O
voids with abdominal straining
voided volume 150 ml, residual 650 ml at least (residual not drained at start)

Bladder instability with detrusor overactivity

A CMG showing bladder instability is illustrated in Figure 3.6.

◆   *Filling*:
first sensation early
strong desire early

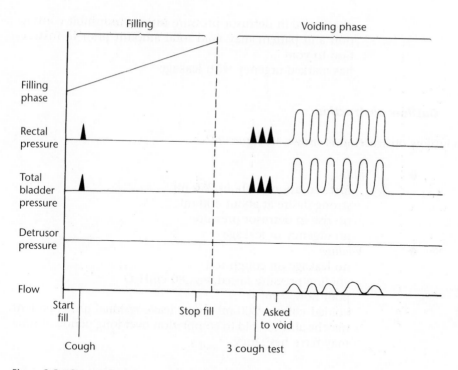

Figure 3.5 *Cystometrogram showing bladder atonia*

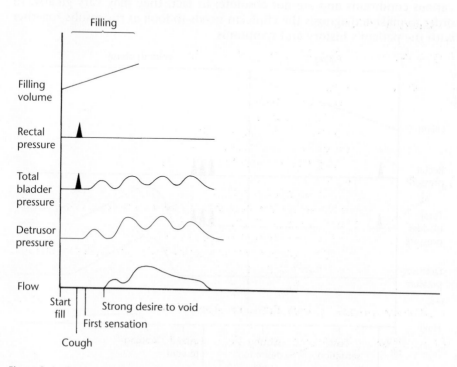

Figure 3.6 *Cystometrogram showing bladder instability*

phasic rise in detrusor pressure unable to inhibit contraction and patient may void total amount prior to instruction to void

has marked urgency with leakage

Outflow obstruction

Outflow obstruction is shown in Figure 3.7.

◆ *Filling*:
   first sensation at about 250 ml
   strong desire at about 400 ml
   no rise in detrusor pressure
   no urgency or leakage
◆ *Voiding*:
   no leakage on cough test
   voiding pressure raised, e.g. 80 cmH$_2$O
   poor flow, 7 ml s^{-1}
   voided volume 200 ml – may leave residual urine; patient may be able to void to completion over long period of time
   may have hesitancy

It is important to note that the figures quoted above are typical examples for various conditions and are not absolute; in fact, they may vary greatly. In order to make a diagnosis the clinician needs to look at the results together with the patient's history and symptoms.

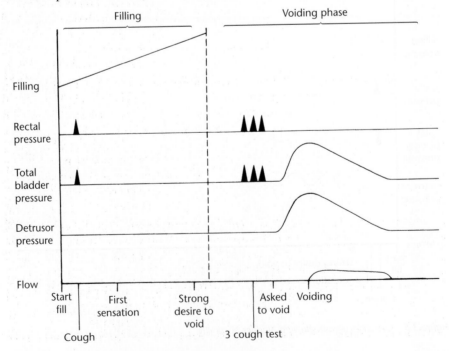

Figure 3.7 Cystometrogram showing bladder outflow obstruction

Nursing care

The examiner needs the behaviour of the bladder to be consistent with non-test conditions. However, the presence of equipment and the personnel necessary to undertake urodynamic studies can be very inhibiting for the patient and may affect the investigations. The nurse has an important role in helping to relieve the potential anxiety and inhibitions of the patient. Some anxiety can be relieved by explaining the test. The nurse will also explain the benefits of the test, i.e. that the results will help the doctor make a diagnosis and enable the appropriate treatment to be given.

The nurse will also act as the patient's advocate and ensure that only essential personnel are present during the investigations to ensure that the patient's privacy and dignity are maintained. The nurse should be prepared to answer any questions the patient may have regarding advice on continence aids and appliances and other measures that may be required after the test, such as pelvic floor exercises.

The urodynamic tests will provide the clinician with valuable information which may be useful in aiding diagnosis and planning the first line of treatment (Table 3.2).

URODYNAMIC FINDINGS	CONSERVATIVE MANAGEMENT	SURGICAL MANAGEMENT
Stress incontinence	Pelvic floor exercises Vaginal cones Electrotherapy	Bladder neck suspension (various types) Bioplastic injection Artificial sphincter
	Oestrogen replacement	Bladder neck closure and catheter or catheterizable stoma
Outflow obstruction	Prostatic drug therapy e.g. indoramin Urethral dilation Self-catheterization	Remove obstruction: prostatectomy urinary stent urethrotomy bladder neck incision Catheter insertion Catheterizable stoma (continent urinary diversion)
Atonic bladder	Self-catheterization Electrical nerve stimulation Indwelling catheter	Catheterizable stoma (continent urinary diversion)
Bladder instability	Bladder retraining Anticholinergic drugs	Cystoplasty with or without self-catheterization

Table 3.2 Management of urinary problems

FURTHER URODYNAMIC STUDIES

Ambulatory urodynamics

Ambulatory urodynamic measurement enables the detrusor pressure to be monitored while the patient is mobile. Both the bladder and rectal pressure catheters are inserted as with a CMG. However, the bladder is filled physiologically. Continuous pressure recordings are monitored over several hours into a portable unit. The patient records any significant symptoms, such as urgency, with the use of an 'event button'. The markings on the trace can then be correlated with the pressure recordings. This investigation appears to be particularly useful in diagnosing instability where a CMG study has not demonstrated any abnormalities.

Electromyography

Electromyography (EMG) monitors the electrical activity within a muscle – in this case the sphincter – and is useful when a neurological abnormality is suspected (Abbott, 1992). The electrical activity is monitored by passing a very fine needle into the sphincter via the perineum.

Urethral pressure profile

The urethral pressure profile (UPP) is the measurement of the intraurethral pressure from bladder neck to external meatus. The procedure involves passing a urethral pressure catheter into the bladder urethrally (rather than suprapubically). The catheter is then mechanically withdrawn at a constant rate and the pressure along the urethra recorded. The test will normally be repeated three times for an average recording.

REFERENCES

ABBOTT D (1992) Objective assessment ensures improved diagnosis. Principles and techniques of urodynamics. *Professional Nurse* **7** (11): 738–742.
CHANCE R (1994) A problem we need not take for granted. *Professional Nurse* **9** (7): 498–504.
CHAPPLE C and Christmas T (1990) *Urodynamics Made Easy*. Edinburgh: Churchill Livingstone.
DUFFIN H (1992) Assessment of urinary incontinence. In: Roe B (ed.) *Clinical Nursing Practice: The Promotion and Management of Continence*. London: Prentice-Hall.
LAKER C (1994) Urological investigations. In: Laker C (ed.) *Urological Nursing*, p. 37. London: Scutari.
NORTON C (1986) *Nursing for Continence*, p. 45. Beaconsfield: Beaconsfield Publishing.
STEPHENSON T P (1994) The interpretation of urodynamics. In Mundy A, Stephenson T P and Wein A J (eds), *Urodynamics: Principles, Practice and Application*, 2nd edn. Edinburgh: Churchill Livingstone.

CONSERVATIVE MANAGEMENT OF UROLOGICAL PROBLEMS

Contents

Urology is viewed as a surgical specialty; however, many conditions are successfully treated or managed using non-surgical treatments such as drug therapy.

Conservative treatment of such conditions as stress incontinence has long been recognized, with Kegal (1948) introducing formalized education of the pelvic floor using muscle exercise programmes. The expanding role of the clinical nurse specialist in continence care in the UK, along with Department of Health recommendations in 1977 that continence advisors should be appointed, has meant that much conservative management has been undertaken by nurses.

In this chapter conservative management is seen to extend beyond that relating to urinary continence and into other areas such as the treatment of urinary tract infections. Some of the therapies mentioned have long histories, whereas others are new developments.

URINARY TRACT INFECTION

Recurrent urinary tract infections (UTI) are common both in the hospitalized patient and in the community. Studies in the USA indicate that 3% of women experience one or more episodes of UTI a year (Ronald and Pattullo, 1991). Symptoms associated with bacterial infection are dysuria, frequency and urgency.

Certain individuals appear to be more susceptible to UTI, with the incidence in women greater than in men. With a few exceptions most urinary tract infections arise from ascending bacteria; infection via the blood stream occurs rarely. In the majority of the population, urinary tract infection is prevented largely by the washout mechanism. If bacteria enter the urethra or bladder, subsequent efficient voiding ensures that they are expelled with the urine. Rarely urinary tract infection may be due to fungi such as *Candida* or chlamydia. Factors associated with UTI can be divided into those associated with the host and the microbial features, and those associated with behaviour.

Microbial factors

Susceptibility to infection is dependent upon the interaction between the immune system and bacterial virulence. *Escherichia coli* cells have the ability to adhere to uroepithelial cells at special host receptor sites. It would appear that many women suffering from recurrent UTIs have an abnormally high number of these receptor cells (Leiner, 1995).

Behavioural factors

The strongest behavioural link with the development of UTI is sexual intercourse (Leiner, 1995). This appears to be the case in both acute UTI and recurrent infection. Some studies have indicated a link with the use of spermicidal agents and diaphragms. No other behaviour is consistently associated with UTI.

Prevention

Little empirical evidence exists to suggest that any change in behaviour will limit the number of urinary tract infections; however, the following advice may be helpful.

Urinary stasis allows colonization of bacteria: by increasing fluid intake and voiding more frequently the patient will prevent stasis and help to prevent colonization.

Cranberry juice has long been used by North Americans to prevent and treat urinary tract infections. It has been found to inhibit the adherence of bacteria to mucosal cells (Beachy, 1981). It is recommended that those susceptible to urinary tract infection drink 200–400 ml a day.

Propolis, a flavonoid derived from bees, has been shown to have antibacterial (Vilanueva *et al.*, 1970) and antifungal properties (Metzner *et al.*, 1975, 1977). Propolis is available commercially in healthfood stores; it has no known side-effects and may prove to be useful in preventing recurrent infections.

Women using spermicides and diaphragms may like to switch to alternative methods of contraception in order to prevent cystitis.

Several studies have suggested that susceptible women should void within 10–15 minutes following sexual intercourse in order to expel any bacteria (Adatto *et al.*, 1979; Foxman and Frerichs, 1985; Foxman, 1990). There is no evidence to suggest that changing other behaviours, such as wearing tight underclothes or synthetic underclothes, or using bath additives, has any impact on the number of urinary tract infections experienced (Leiner, 1995).

Treatment

Not all urinary tract infections require antibiotic therapy; however, each patient must be assessed and treatment options discussed with a microbiologist if there is any doubt. Before initiating any antibiotic therapy the following guidelines should be followed:

- ◆ Send a midstream urine sample for culture and sensitivity.
- ◆ If there is severe dysuria, then administer an agent to alkalinize the urine, e.g. potassium citrate, or one teaspoon bicarbonate of soda dissolved in a glass of water (omit if the patient is suffering from hypertension or heart failure).
- ◆ Advise the patient to drink cranberry juice.
- ◆ Administer mild painkillers, e.g. aspirin, paracetamol. Provide local pain relief such as a heat pad.
- ◆ Increase fluid input to 3–4 litres a day, if there is no cardiac or renal impairment.

Traditionally women who have recurrent UTIs undergo a variety of investigations to determine if they have any structural abnormality of the urinary tract. There is little evidence to suggest that this is beneficial. Nickel *et al.* (1991) stated that investigation is indicated where there is gross haematuria, microscopic haematuria in the absence of infection, symptoms of obstruction, renal tract stones or infection with *Proteus mirabilis*.

Although for most women UTIs are not dangerous, infection can cause much distress. If the conservative therapy outlined above is not effective, then prophylactic antibiotics may be indicated.

INTERSTITIAL CYSTITIS

Interstitial cystitis was first described by Skene in 1878. Also known as Hunner's ulcer, it remains a debilitating condition of unknown aetiology despite much research. The sufferers are predominantly women. The main symptoms are urinary frequency, urgency, suprapubic pain (often relieved by voiding) and nocturia. Biopsy of the bladder is essential for confirmation of the diagnosis (Raz and Leach, 1983).

Reaching the diagnosis

For many sufferers a diagnosis is not easily reached; this delay in diagnosis can result in the patient feeling isolated and losing confidence in the medical team. The following investigations are helpful in making a correct diagnosis.

PREVENTING AND TREATING CYSTITIS: ADVICE FOR SUFFERERS

There are several different causes of cystitis. Often the cause is a bacterial infection; other reasons you might suffer from cystitis-like symptoms include thrush or an irritable bladder. The advice below is in addition to any treatment your general practitioner or specialist may be giving you.

- ◆ Drink at least 2500 ml (4 pints) of fluid every day. This may need to be increased in hot weather. This will help to flush out any germs that are in your bladder, before they can cause an infection.
- ◆ Drink 200–400 ml of cranberry juice a day. If you find this bitter, try mixing it with another fruit juice.
- ◆ Do not allow your bladder to get overfull. Pass urine whenever you feel the need, aiming to empty your bladder every 4 hours. Holding on will encourage the growth of germs.
- ◆ Try to ensure that you empty your bladder completely when you visit the toilet. It may help to try to pass urine again after finishing passing urine.
- ◆ If you suffer from cystitis following intercourse, try to empty your bladder within 10–15 minutes afterwards.

If you have an acute attack of cystitis, the following advice may be helpful.

Recognizing the signs of an attack

In an attack you may notice the following:

- ◆ A desire to pass urine more often than usual, although the amount passed may be small
- ◆ An urgent desire to get to the toilet for fear of losing control
- ◆ A burning pain in the urethra when passing urine
- ◆ Pain in the lower abdomen or the back
- ◆ Fever, a feeling of being generally unwell
- ◆ Cloudy urine or blood in the urine.

Treatment

◆ Immediately start drinking extra fluid, a glass as often as possible, e.g. every half an hour. Try to include some cranberry juice.

◆ Take a teaspoon of bicarbonate of soda in a glass of water. *If you have high blood pressure or heart problems, do not do this without first consulting your doctor.*

◆ Take some of the tablets you usually have for a headache, e.g. aspirin or paracetamol.

◆ Try to keep warm; you may find that using a hot-water bottle is helpful.

◆ Take a specimen of urine to your doctor, and arrange to be seen as soon as possible.

Urinary culture

The urine of those with interstitial cystitis is generally not infected; however, any underlying urinary tract infection should be treated.

Urinalysis

Fewer than 10% of sufferers have haematuria (Frye, 1994). Symptoms of frequency and urgency may be suggestive of carcinoma in situ, and urine should be analysed to exclude this.

Videocystometrogram, cystometrogram

Urodynamic studies are useful to exclude detrusor instability. The cystometrogram in sufferers of interstitial cystitis will display an urgency not associated with a rise in detrusor pressure during filling and a small bladder capacity.

Cystoscopy and biopsy

The diagnosis of interstitial cystitis is dependent upon a positive biopsy result, revealing a higher than normal number of mast cells (indicative of an inflammatory response) and detrusor mastocytosis. Cystoscopy will also reveal a reduced bladder capacity; if hydrodistension is performed (which can relieve symptoms in 20–50% of people) a hallmark lesion of petechial haemorrhages will be seen (Messing, 1987).

Living with interstitial cystitis

Conservative measures are employed when managing interstitial cystitis; however, major surgery (for example augmentation or substitution cystoplasty and formation of ileal conduit) can be indicated in those who do not respond. A team approach to management should be employed, involving the urologist, the chronic pain specialist and the continence advisor or urology nurse.

Treatment

Cystoscopy and dilation

Hydrodistension of the urinary bladder can give some symptomatic relief, although the mechanism for this is not clear.

Drug therapy

Both oral drug treatment and intravesical agents can be useful in the control of symptoms. Anticholinergic therapy can be helpful for some sufferers who find that it has some analgesic effect and helps to reduce frequency. Tricyclic antidepressants can have beneficial effects, helping to block pain receptors as well as reducing urinary frequency. Urinary analgesics may also be used.

Intravesical agents have been used in the management of interstitial cystitis. Anticholinergic agents can be given intravesically on a named patient basis, thus reducing the side-effects, and anti-inflammatory agents can be delivered directly in this manner. Sant (1987) reported a 50–70% effectiveness of dimethyl sulphoxide (DMSO) when used intravesically. New developments in drug treatment are being investigated.

Bladder retraining

Bladder re-education using planned voiding schedules with increasing intervals between voids can be useful to achieve a reduction in urinary frequency and urgency. The individual with interstitial cystitis may well need concurrent drug therapy with anticholinergics.

Diet

It has been found that many sufferers benefit from reducing their intake of foods that are metabolized via the citric acid cycle, e.g. alcohol, citric fruit and carbonated drinks. Other foods implicated are those that use the dopamine cycle, e.g. yoghurt and cheese (Richmond, 1994). Drinks high in caffeine such as coffee and tea can also be an irritant and increase urinary frequency and urgency. Cranberry juice may be helpful.

Other methods

Mild to moderate symptoms may be helped by such strategies as wearing loose clothing, using a heat pad and avoiding constipation.

POSTMICTURITION DRIBBLE

Postmicturition dribble is an embarrassing condition for its male sufferers who may be of any age. It is characterized by the loss of urine after the main stream, typically when the man is replacing his penis in his clothing or walking away from the toilet. Normally at the end of voiding the bulbospongiosus muscle contracts, causing urine to be 'milked' back into the bladder. The function of the bulbospongiosus can be impaired by trauma, surgery or as a result of muscle weakness, resulting in the pooling of urine in the bulbar urethra.

The man can be taught how to evacuate this urine manually at the end of his stream in the following manner (Figure 4.1):

◆　　　At the end of the stream, wait a few seconds to allow for bladder emptying.
◆　　　Apply pressure using the fingers behind the scrotum, then

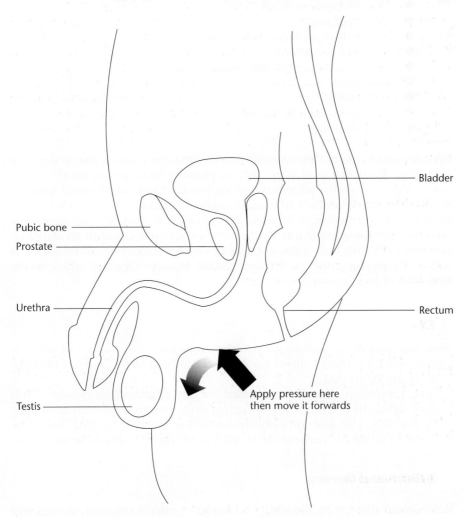

Figure 4.1　*Postmicturition dribble: method of manual evacuation*

♦ maintaining this pressure draw the fingers slowly forward in the midline. This forces the urine into the penile urethra, where it can be removed by shaking or squeezing the urethra. This can be repeated before leaving the toilet.

URGENCY AND FREQUENCY

Urgency and frequency are urinary symptoms often suggestive of some underlying disorder, and an individual complaining of these symptoms should undergo investigations to eliminate any sinister cause. Causes of urinary frequency are listed below:

- Urinary tract infection
- Detrusor instability
- Drugs, e.g. diuretic therapy
- Diabetes mellitus
- Pregnancy
- Constipation, pelvic mass
- Inflammation
- Calculi, e.g. bladder stone
- High fluid intake
- Habit
- Neurological disease
- Tumours

Urgency and frequency may result from an unstable bladder, that is detrusor instability diagnosed urodynamically by pressure increases within the detrusor on filling, when the patient is making no effort to void. Detrusor instability may develop secondary to bladder outflow obstruction; when there is no evidence of obstruction, it is defined as idiopathic. Urgency and frequency may also develop without any rise in detrusor pressure, but with an early first sensation of filling and reduced capacity due to bladder discomfort, this is called 'sensory urgency' or 'hypersensitive' bladder. Urgency when severe may lead to urge incontinence.

Treatment

First, any underlying pathology must be excluded. Urine should be sent for culture and for cytology. Blood glucose levels should be measured. Constipation should be treated.

Next, the patient should be assessed for any contributing factors. A full history should be taken, including current drug therapy, especially treatment with diuretics. The level of mobility, including access to toilets, should be assessed. Fluid intake, particularly of caffeine-rich drinks, should be measured.

Behavioural therapy

Behavioural therapy in the form of bladder re-education aims to help sufferers of urinary frequency and urgency to relearn control over their bladder.

Bladder re-education is effective for those with both detrusor instability and sensory urgency. Various techniques exist for retraining the bladder. The author uses the following regimen based on the work of Frewen (1978).

1. A baseline assessment of voiding and incontinence episodes is made using a simple frequency chart (urinary volumes are not requested) by the patient in the week prior to the appointment.
2. At the consultation the patient is asked to void with a full bladder into a flowmeter, the volume of urine passed is recorded and the maximum flow rate compared to a flow nomogram (to exclude outflow obstruction).
3. The frequency chart is discussed with the patient, with attention paid to the background of any increase or decrease in frequency.
4. A simple explanation of bladder filling and emptying is made, using diagrams.
5. The rationale of bladder retraining is explained.
6. The patient is asked to void at set times only, determined by their own frequency chart. The patient must not pass urine any earlier even if it means becoming wet.
7. When the patient is dry and comfortable with this regimen, the interval between voids can be increased. This is repeated until an acceptable amount of time between voids has been achieved.
8. A normal fluid intake should be maintained (approximately 1.5 litres a day). A trial without caffeinated drinks is encouraged.
9. The patient is taught distraction techniques to use when experiencing urgency.
10. Positive feedback is given at all stages of the programme.
11. The patient is told not to follow the regimen overnight, in order to maximize sleep.
12. The patient is regularly reviewed, with new targets for the time between voids being set.

Bladder retraining programmes have proved to be very effective in the management of these patients. Frewen (1982) reported a 86.6% cure rate, with an additional 11.1% seeing an improvement in their symptoms. Other studies have been less impressive: Pengelly and Booth (1980) reported only a 44% cure rate, with an additional 28% improvement.

Anticholinergic therapy can act as an adjunct to the programme. If the frequency is not too severe, or the voiding pattern is very irregular, bladder retraining can be undertaken by the patient delaying voiding by increasing intervals, i.e. holding on for 10 minutes initially.

Electrical stimulation

Electrical stimulation was originally developed for the treatment of stress incontinence; early studies indicated that it also had a beneficial effect on urge incontinence (Alexander and Rowan, 1968). It is thought that stimulation helps to inhibit the afferent pudendal nerve (Sundin and Carlsson, 1972). This can be used therapeutically in the individual with an unstable bladder to help reactivate 'lost' functional patterns (Plevnik et al., 1989).

Electrical stimulation is administered using a vaginal or anal electrode, and has been found to be effective as a home treatment. Home therapy consists of a daily application of anal or vaginal stimulation (10 Hz) lasting 20 minutes, for 3–4 weeks. This therapy is contraindicated in those with pacemakers and in pregnancy. It has been found to be as effective as bladder retraining with a 50% cure rate and an additional 33% seeing significant improvement in symptoms (Eriksen *et al.*, 1989). The initial outlay for the necessary equipment may be prohibitive for some.

Drug therapy

Many different drugs have been tried in the treatment of frequency and urgency, particularly when detrusor instability is present. No drug has proved to be universally acceptable. Drug therapy has a short duration of action and withdrawal of treatment will mean a return of symptoms. Drugs that are useful in the control of these symptoms are those that either inhibit detrusor contraction or increase bladder outlet resistance, or decrease urine production. Cardozo (1989) suggested that the following groups of drugs may be useful.

- ◆ Drugs that inhibit detrusor contraction:
  anticholinergic agents
  musculotropic relaxants
  tricyclic antidepressants
  calcium channel blockers
  beta-adrenergic agonists
  alpha-adrenergic antagonists
  prostaglandin inhibitors
- ◆ Drugs that increase outlet resistance:
  alpha-adrenergic stimulators
  beta-adrenergic blockers
- ◆ Drugs that decrease urine production:
  antidiuretic hormone analogues

STRESS INCONTINENCE IN FEMALES

The term 'stress incontinence' can be used either as a medical diagnosis – incontinence caused by incompetence of the urethral sphincter – or as a symptom, when it is used to describe the experience of leaking urine upon physical exertion.

The urethral sphincter and pelvic floor muscles normally work together in keeping urethral pressure higher than bladder pressure during bladder filling, thus maintaining continence. If either muscle group is functioning with less than complete efficiency, the urethral pressure will be lowered. Under ordinary circumstances the pressure will still remain higher than that of the bladder. However, if the bladder pressure rises owing to an extravesical stimulus such as coughing or sneezing, the urethral pressure may not be sufficient to withstand this and leakage of urine may occur.

The conservative (non-surgical) methods of treating stress incontinence are based on increasing the urethral pressure either by strengthening the pelvic floor muscles or by mechanical aids causing occlusion.

Pelvic floor exercises

Kegel (1948) was one of the earliest doctors to advocate the teaching of pelvic floor exercises as a cure for females with incontinence. Since then numerous papers have been written on pelvic floor exercises by nurses, physiotherapists and urologists; much recent work has been written by a physiotherapist, Josephine Laycock (1991). The following programme is based on her work.

Assessment

The assessment is explained to the patient and consent for examination obtained. The patient lies on the couch in the supine position with knees bent and dropped apart. The examiner's gloved and lubricated index finger is then inserted into the vagina. The middle finger can then be introduced if it can be accommodated. If the introitus allows it the fingers can be opened in a scissor-like manner with fingers on top of one another. The patient is then asked to squeeze the fingers together. The modified Oxford grading system as described by Laycock (1991) is then used to record strength of contraction (Table 4.1).

The length of time in seconds that the contraction is held is also recorded. The patient then has a short rest of 4 seconds (Laycock, 1991) before repeating the squeeze. The patient continues repeating the squeeze with a rest between each one. When the examiner feels the contraction has weakened in strength or duration, the number of exercise repeats for that patient can be determined.

The examiner will then have completed the assessment of the slow-twitch muscle fibres (see Chapter 1). The fast-twitch fibres are then assessed by the examiner keeping the fingers in the vagina and asking the patient to relax and contract quickly – for 1 second's duration. The number of contractions performed before the strength of the contraction lessens will be recorded. The assessor can then record the following information:

- strength of contraction
- length of contraction

0	Nil
1	Flicker
2	Weak
3	Moderate
4	Good
5	Strong

Table 4.1   *The Oxford grading system for assessing the strength of the pelvic floor*

◆ number of contractions
◆ number of 1-second fast-twitch contractions

This will then form the basis of the teaching programme.

In addition to digital examination, vaginal cones can also be used as an assessment tool. A typical assessment might reveal the following results:

strength of contraction – 3 (moderate)
length of contraction – 4 seconds
number of contractions – 5
number of fast-twitch contractions – 6.

Exercise plan

The exercise routine should be repeated eight times a day (Laycock, 1991). The exercise consists of contracting the pelvic floor and holding for 4 seconds. Relax for 4 seconds, and repeat four more times.

In view of the amount of information the patient has to absorb at this stage it is advisable to delay instructions on fast-twitch exercises until a follow-up session.

Progress should be evaluated at the same point in the menstrual cycle as the initial assessment is made as pelvic floor muscles are under hormonal influence (Bhalia *et al.*, 1989, cited by Laycock, 1991). After the second assessment the exercise regimen can be replanned. The client continues on the exercise plan until the symptoms subside or until no further progress is being made. She will then go onto a maintenance programme so that improvements are maintained. If symptoms remain, other conservative treatments should be explored before surgery is considered.

Vaginal weights

The use of vaginal weights was first proposed by Plevnik (1985). These are tampon-like weighted cones that are inserted into the vagina. The pull of gravity gives the user the feeling that they will fall out, causing her to contract the pelvic floor in an effort to keep the weight in place.

The weights can also be used as an objective tool for assessment.

Cone assessment

The lightest cone is lubricated with a little K-Y jelly and then inserted into the vagina. The user retains this weight for a minute while gently walking around. If she manages to retain it, it is then removed by pulling on the string. The next weight is then inserted. This process continues until she finds the weight that cannot be retained for a minute. This weight will then be used to perform the exercises. The heaviest weight that can be retained for a minute will be recorded as a measure of the strength of the pelvic floor.

Exercise programme using weights

The patient inserts the starting weight twice a day and tries to keep it in place for up to 15 minutes. Once she is able to hold on to it for 15 minutes she will

INFORMATION SHEET
UNDERSTANDING PELVIC FLOOR
EXERCISES: INFORMATION FOR WOMEN

This information is designed to help you:

- Understand why you need to exercise your pelvic floor
- Learn how to do pelvic floor exercises

What and where is the pelvic floor?

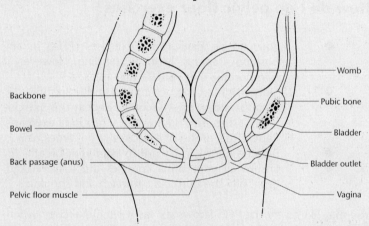

Backbone

Bowel

Back passage (anus)

Pelvic floor muscle

Womb

Pubic bone

Bladder

Bladder outlet

Vagina

The pelvic floor is a sling of muscles rather like a hammock which goes from the pubic bone at the front to the tail bone (coccyx) at the back. Its function is to support the pelvic organs and it also prevents leakage of urine or faeces from the bladder or bowel by keeping the outlets closed.

Why exercise the pelvic floor?

The pelvic floor muscles need regular exercise (like other muscles of the body) to retain good muscle tone. If they are not exercised they may become slackened, stretched and weak and no longer work effectively. For example, you may leak urine when you cough, laugh, sneeze or even when you get out of a chair. This is known as stress incontinence. This may also happen following childbirth or in later years following the menopause. If carried out correctly and regularly, pelvic floor exercises will help to prevent leakage from bladder or bowel and may also have other benefits.

How to identify the pelvic floor

There are a variety of ways in which to identify your pelvic floor. This is important so that you know you are exercising the right muscles.

- ◆ Vaginal examination – this involves tightening around two fingers inserted into the vagina. The nurse may use a vaginal probe in addition to this.
- ◆ Try to stop the flow of urine midstream – the stop test.
- ◆ Imagine trying to avoid passing wind/flatus.
- ◆ Imagine trying to prevent a tampon from falling out of the vagina.

How do I do pelvic floor exercises?

- ◆ You can do pelvic floor exercises (PFEs) in any position – sitting, lying or standing. However, it is important that you are fully relaxed.
- ◆ Slowly tighten the pelvic floor and hold for _____ seconds. Relax for 4 seconds. Repeat this exercise _____ times. This is known as a group of exercises. Repeat this group of exercises _____ times daily.
- ◆ Breathe normally, try not to hold your breath.
- ◆ Ensure all your other muscles are fully relaxed, especially the buttocks, stomach and shoulders.

You may like to try the PFEs known as 'fast-twitch exercises' where you tighten and release the pelvic floor muscles as quickly as you can at the end of each set of slow PFEs. As a general guide, carry out five fast-twitch exercises 5–10 times a day.

If you are doing PFEs as part of a preventive programme this should be a lifetime habit. If this is an individually planned programme your nurse will advise you on a maintenance regimen after your course of exercises is complete.

The length of the course will vary from person to person depending upon your progress. It may be some time before you see any improvement – don't be disheartened, don't give up.

How will I know if the muscles are getting stronger?

- ◆ You may find it easier to stop the flow of urine midstream. Don't do this more than once a week.

◆ You may notice that you leak less urine when you cough, laugh, sneeze, etc. Do not hesitate to discuss your PFE regimen with your nurse who can be contacted at:

_____

Pelvic Floor Exercises Personal Programme
Name: _____
Date: _____

◆ Slowly tighten your pelvic floor and hold for _____ seconds. Relax for 4 seconds.
◆ Repeat this exercise _____ times.
◆ Repeat this group of exercises _____ times a day.
◆ Ensure that all your other muscles are fully relaxed, especially your thighs, buttocks, stomach and shoulders, and breathe normally.

Date of next appointment: _____

Acknowledgement: The combined Continence Advisory Services of Camden and Islington Community Health Services NHS Trust and University College London Hospitals NHS Trust.

move on to the next weight. Some women find they are able to hold heavier weights in the morning than in the evening, in which case they can exercise using the two different weights.

The manufacturers recommend that the weights should not be used when the patient is menstruating or pregnant, or if a vaginal infection is present. One manufacturer of vaginal cones has written guidelines for the sterilization of cones so that they may be used by different patients. They advocate steam sterilization, which can be done in hospital by sterile supply services.

This exercise programme may be accompanied by the teaching of pelvic floor exercises, even if they have previously been undertaken without success.

Electrostimulation

Faradism and interferential therapy have traditionally been undertaken by physiotherapists. However, there are now several electrostimulation devices available which are commonly used by continence advisers. They all work by passing an electrical current through the pelvic floor muscle.

The electrostimulator helps to restore and strengthen muscle tone and function in the pelvic floor (Rigby, 1996) by helping the muscles develop new fibres and increasing the number of capillaries which supply blood to them (Eriksen *et al.*, 1989). The frequency and duration of treatment will vary with the particular device chosen, ranging from 20 minutes a day for 4 weeks, to 4–6 hours a day for 16 weeks. The current can be generated from external patches or an internal probe.

Occlusion devices for women

The Contrelle sponge (see address list at end of chapter) uses the principles behind the tampon for its use. Made from polyvinyl foam (PVF), it is first softened in warm water and then inserted into the vagina in the same way as a tampon, where it is then able to support the bladder neck. It is not intended to absorb urine.

The Fem Assist personal urine control device (see address list) is an external device which helps prevent small amounts of urine leakage by supporting the tissue around the urethra. It is soft and flexible, and stays in place by vacuum with the aid of the sealing ointment supplied with the device. It is removed each time the woman voids.

The Reliance (see address list) is a small plug-like device which is inserted into the urethra. It is kept in place by inflating a tiny balloon just above the bladder neck and is removed each time the woman voids.

A ring pessary can be used if the incontinence is associated with a prolapse of the anterior wall of the vagina. The woman is measured and the correct size of pessary is fitted. The pessary is not suitable for women who are sexually active.

STRESS INCONTINENCE IN MALES

Men rarely present with genuine stress incontinence (GSI). They are not normally dependent on the pelvic floor to maintain continence. Therefore, if a man presents with symptoms of stress incontinence the assessor must establish that urine retention is not the cause. However, GSI can be found in men with open bladder necks such as in bladder exstrophy, and in a few men following surgical procedures such as transurethral resection of the prostate and radical prostatectomy.

Assessment of the male pelvic floor

Owing to anatomical differences between the sexes it is harder to assess the male pelvic floor, although it is possible by digital examination of the rectum which allows palpation of the puborectalis. Two fingers behind the scrotum and pressed into the perineum will detect a pelvic floor contraction (Laycock, 1991).

Many men find the stop test when passing urine the easiest way of identifying their pelvic floor. However, as in females, this should not be performed more than once daily. Once the pelvic floor has been identified patients can follow a similar exercise plan to the women.

INFORMATION SHEET
UNDERSTANDING PELVIC FLOOR
EXERCISES: INFORMATION FOR MEN

This information is designed to help you:

◆ Understand why you need to exercise your pelvic floor
◆ Learn how to do pelvic floor exercises

What and where is the pelvic floor?

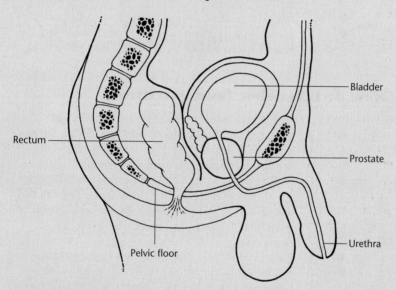

The pelvic floor is a sling of muscles rather like a hammock which goes from the pubic bone at the front to the tail bone (coccyx) at the back. Its function is to support the pelvic organs and it also prevents leakage of urine or faeces from the bladder or bowel by keeping the outlets closed. In most men the pelvic floor acts as a safety mechanism and continence is maintained chiefly by a sphincter muscle at the bladder neck.

Why exercise the pelvic floor?

The pelvic floor muscles need regular exercise (like other muscles of the body) to retain good muscle tone. If they are not exercised they may become slackened, stretched and weak and no longer work effectively. For example, you may leak urine when you cough, laugh, sneeze or even when you get out of a chair. This is known as stress incontinence. Following surgery the bladder neck sphincter may become weakened, making you more reliant on your pelvic floor. If carried out correctly and regularly, pelvic floor exercises will help to prevent leakage from bladder or bowel.

How to identify the pelvic floor

There are a variety of ways in which you can identify your pelvic floor. This is important so that you know you are exercising the right muscles.

- Try to stop the flow of urine midstream – the stop test.
- Imagine trying to avoid passing wind/flatus.
- Rectal examination – your nurse may ask to examine you while you contract your pelvic floor.

How do I do pelvic floor exercises?

- You can do pelvic floor exercises (PFEs) in any position – sitting, lying or standing. However, it is important that you are fully relaxed.
- Now, slowly tighten the pelvic floor and hold for _____ seconds. Relax for 4 seconds. Repeat this exercise _____ times. This is known as a group of exercises. Repeat this group of exercises _____ times daily.
- Breathe normally, try not to hold your breath.
- Ensure all your other muscles are fully relaxed, especially the buttocks, stomach and shoulders.

You may like to try the PFEs known as 'fast-twitch exercises' where you tighten and release the pelvic floor muscles as quickly as you can at the end of each set of slow PFEs. As a general guide, carry out five fast-twitch exercises 5–10 times a day.

If you are doing PFEs as part of a preventive programme this should be a lifetime habit. If this is an individually planned programme, your nurse will advise you on a maintenance regimen after your course of exercises is complete.

The length of the course will vary from person to person depending upon your progress. It may be some time before you see any improvement – don't be disheartened, don't give up.

How will I know if the muscles are getting stronger?

- ◆ You may find it easier to stop the flow of urine midstream. Don't do this more than once a week.
- ◆ You may notice that you leak less urine when you cough, laugh, sneeze, etc. Do not hesitate to discuss your PFE regimen with your nurse who can be contacted at:

_____

Pelvic Floor Exercises Personal Programme

Name: _____

Date: _____

- ◆ Slowly tighten your pelvic floor and hold for _____ seconds. Relax for 4 seconds.
- ◆ Repeat this exercise _____ times.
- ◆ Repeat this group of exercises _____ times a day.
- ◆ Ensure that all your other muscles are fully relaxed, especially your thighs, buttocks, stomach and shoulders, and breathe normally.

Date of next appointment: _____

Acknowledgement: The combined Continence Advisory Services of Camden and Islington Community Health Services NHS Trust and University College London Hospitals NHS Trust.

CONCLUSION

This chapter has described the more traditional conservative treatments for urological problems. The urology nurse should also be aware that homoeopathy, osteopathy, acupuncture, reflexology and aromatherapy may have a role to play in the treatment of urological conditions.

USEFUL ADDRESSES

Self-help and support groups

Interstitial Cystitis Support Group, c/o Sandra Bell, Council for Voluntary Service, 13 Hazelwood Rd, Northampton NN1 1LG

Incontact, 2 Doughty Street, London WC1N 2PH (telephone 0191 213 0050)

Suppliers of equipment

Aquaflex cones are available from:

Depuy Healthcare, Millshaw House, Manor Mill Lane, Leeds LS1 9YY

Femina cones are available from:

Colgate Medical Ltd, 1 Fairacres Estate, Dedworth Rd, Windsor, Berks SL4 4LE

Contrelle sponges are available from:

Coloplast Ltd, Peterborough Business Park, Peterborough, Cambs PE2 6BR (Customer Service Dept telephone 01733 392009)

Fem Assist personal urinary control device is available from:

Insight Medical UK Ltd, Asmec Centre, Eagle House, The Ring, Bracknell, Berks RG12 1HB (telephone 01344 382086)

Reliance is available from:

Astra Tech Ltd, Stroudwater Business Park, Brunel Way, Stonehouse, Glos GL10 3SW (telephone 01453 791763)

REFERENCES

ADATTO K, Doebeke K G, Galland L and Granowetter L (1979) Behavioral factors and urinary tract infection. *Journal of the American Medical Association* **241**: 2525–2526.

ALEXANDER S and Rowan D (1968) Electrical control of urinary incontinence by radio implant: a report of 14 patients. *British Journal of Surgery* **55**: 358.

BEACHY E H (1981) Bacterial adherence; adhesion receptor interactions mediating the attachment of bacteria to mucosal surfaces. *Journal of Infectious Diseases* **143**: 325–345.

CARDOZO L (1989) Drug treatment for detrusor instability. In: Freeman R and Malvern J (eds) *The Unstable Bladder.* London: Wright.

ERIKSEN B, Bergmann S and Eik-Nes S H (1989) Maximal electrostimulation of the pelvic floor in female idiopathic detrusor instability and urge incontinence. *Neurology and Urodynamics* **8**: 219–230.

FOXMAN B and Frerichs R R (1985) Epidemiology of urinary tract infection: 1. Diaphragm use and sexual intercourse. *American Journal of Public Health* **75**: 1308–1313.

FOXMAN B (1990) Recurring urinary tract infection: incidence and risk factors. *American Journal of Public Health* **80**: 331–333.

FREWEN W K (1978) An objective assessment of the unstable bladder of psychosomatic origin. *British Journal of Urology* **50**: 246–249.

FREWEN W K (1982) A reassessment of bladder training in detrusor dysfunction in the female. *British Journal of Urology* **54**: 372–373.

FRYE K (1994) Understanding interstitial cystitis. *Journal of Urological Nursing* **12**: 367–371.

KEGAL A H (1948) Progressive resistance exercise in the functional restoration of the perineal muscles. *American Journal of Obstetrics and Gynecology* **56**: 238–248.

LAYCOCK J (1991) Pelvic floor re-education for the promotion of continence, chapter 5. In: Roe B (Ed.) *Clinical Nursing Practice: The Promotion and Management of Continence.* London: Prentice-Hall.

LEINER S (1995) Recurrent urinary tract infections in otherwise healthy adult women. *Nurse Practitioner* **20**(2): 48–56.

MESSING E M (1987) The diagnosis of interstitial cystitis. *Urology* **23**: 4–7.

METZNER J, Bekemeier H, Schneidewind E and Schwaiberger R (1975) Bioautographische Erfassung der antimikrobeill wirksamen inhaltsstoffe von propolis. Cited in Graham J (1992) *The Hive and the Honey Bee*. Hamilton: Dadant.

METZNER J, Schneidewind E and Friedrich E (1977) Zur wirkung von propolis and Pinocembrin auf sprosspilze. Cited in Graham J (1992) *The Hive and the Honey Bee*. Hamilton: Dadant.

NICKEL J C, Wilson J, Morales A and Heaton J (1991) Value of urologic investigation in a targeted group of women with recurrent urinary tract infections. *Canadian Journal of Surgery* **34**: 591–594.

PENGELLY A and Booth C (1980) A prospective trial of bladder training as treatment for detrusor instability. *British Journal of Urology* **52**: 463–466.

PLEVNIK S (1985) New method of testing and strengthening of pelvic floor muscles. *Proceedings of the International Continence Society* (London): 267–268.

PLEVNIK S, Vodusek D and Janez J (1989) Electrical stimulation treatment for detrusor instability. In: Freeman R and Malvern J (eds) *The Unstable Bladder*. London: Wright.

RAZ S and Leach G (1983) Interstitial cystitis. In: Raz S *Female Urology*. Philadelphia: W B Saunders.

RICHMOND J (1994) The tyranny of interstitial cystitis. *Nursing Times* **90**(43): 72.

RIGBY D (1996) Promoting continence with electrostimulation. *Professional Nurse* **11**(7): 431–434.

RONALD A R and Pattullo L S (1991) The natural history of urinary infection in adults. *Medical Clinics of North America* **75**: 299–312.

SANT G R (1987) Intravesical 50% dimethyl sulfoxide (RIMSO-50) in the treatment of interstitial cystitis. *Urology* **29**: 17.

VILANUEVA V R, Barbier M, Gonnet M and Lavie P (1970) Les flavonoides de la propolis. Isolement d'une nouvelle substance bacteriostatique; la pinocembrine (dihydroxy 5, 7-flavone). Cited in Graham J (1992) *The Hive and the Honey Bee*. Hamilton: Dadant.

WEBSTER D and Brennan T (1994) Use and effectiveness of physical self-care. Strategies for interstitial cystitis. *Nurse Practitioner* **19**(10): 55–61.

URINARY DRAINAGE SYSTEMS

Contents

It has been estimated that 12.6% of patients admitted to hospital in the UK will be catheterized (Crow *et al.*, 1986). More recently, Colley (1994) reported that 7.9% of inpatients over a 1-week period had a catheter in situ, of which 96.8% were urethral catheters and 3.2% were suprapubic catheters. Roe (1989a) found that 4% of community patients known to the District Nursing Services in one district used a long-term catheter. Thus catheterization is still a common procedure despite the trend towards a reduction in use of urethral catheters, thought to be due to the implications of their use (Roe, 1992a), and an apparent increase in popularity of alternative forms of bladder drainage such as suprapubic catheterization and intermittent catheterization.

The management of urinary drainage systems has traditionally been the domain of nursing staff who are responsible for the majority of catheterization procedures and subsequent management of the urinary drainage system (UDS) (Crow *et al.*, 1988). Despite this, studies have found that nurses' knowledge of the establishment and management of urinary drainage systems is poor and rarely underpinned by relevant research, (Roe and Brocklehurst, 1987; Crow *et al.*, 1988; Crummey, 1989; Barnett, 1991; Henry, 1992). McCullough (1989), in a small study of 12 male patients being discharged with long-term catheters, found that their preparation for discharge was poor and that information given was inconsistent. It is interesting to note that Crummey (1989) found that the majority of the nurses questioned in her study expressed dissatisfaction with their knowledge levels. Few had received even a little instruction during their training, and none had received any since qualifiying. These findings were supported by Henry (1992) who also found, among a small sample of doctors interviewed, a reliance on nursing staff for provision of the correct urinary catheter.

There is now an increasing body of research surrounding this area of nursing practice and the above findings emphasize the need for nurses to utilize this. Thus, the aim of this chapter is to provide nurses with the knowledge required to establish and manage a urinary drainage system safely, and to present the research available to support this practice.

A urinary drainage system can be defined as comprising a catheter, to ensure complete bladder emptying, to which is attached a collecting bag or catheter valve. The need for such a system may be temporary or permanent, and the catheter is inserted into the bladder via the urethra or a suprapubic cystotomy. If permanent, the catheter is referred to as 'indwelling'. Intermittent catheterization does not require a drainage bag since the catheter is removed directly after drainage has ceased.

Indications for catheterization are as follows:

- ◆ To ensure complete bladder emptying prior to surgery or an investigative procedure
- ◆ For the relief of acute and chronic urinary retention
- ◆ For postoperative drainage when intermittent catheterization is inappropriate or stenting of the urethra is required
- ◆ To measure accurately urine output in the critically ill patient
- ◆ To manage intractable urinary incontinence when other methods of urine collection are inappropriate

PREPARATION FOR THE ESTABLISHMENT OF A URINARY DRAINAGE SYSTEM

The prospect of catheterization is almost always alarming for the patient and it is important that the procedure is handled sensitively. Roe and Brocklehurst (1987) reported on an investigation into patients' understanding and acceptance of their catheters, taking a sample of 36 male and female patients living in the community within one health district. Patients stated that it took a median of up to 1 year to get used to having a catheter, accepting it and coping with its management. The authors concluded that a long-term catheter should be considered as a prosthesis about which both users and carers require education. Thus the significance of catheterization in the lives of patients, particularly where use is long-term, cannot be overemphasized, and patients should be counselled about this prior to insertion.

In hospital, most catheters are inserted on a temporary basis as indicated by the median duration of catheterization of 4 days reported by Crow *et al.* (1986). They found the most common reason for catheterization in both sexes to be facilitation of drainage to aid surgical repair. The patient should be prepared for and reassured by the temporary nature of the catheterization. A patient who has a catheter inserted while unconscious should be told about the catheter as soon as possible.

In a community setting, Roe and Brocklehurst (1987) found the most common reasons for catheterization to be management of urinary incontinence and retention, and the median duration of catheterization to be 4 years. Thus it is even more important that these patients are helped to cope with and accept this form of management.

Except in an emergency, the decision to catheterize should be a joint one between medical and nursing practitioners in discussion with the patient. With all its attendant complications, catheterization is best avoided if at all possible and should never be considered for the convenience of the nurse. However, in the community it may be the only acceptable way for a person to retain an independent lifestyle, and it can thus be a very positive form of management.

Thought should be given early in the planning stage as to whether the patient will be able to manage the equipment and procedures required, and whether the necessary care and support will be available. An example of an area in which difficulty may arise is that of male catheterization which traditionally has been the domain of male nurses and doctors. Although it is now widely accepted practice for female nurses to undertake male catheterization, until this skill becomes as much a part of nurse training as female catheterization there will remain instances where a catheter change means a visit to hospital. Alternatively, the patient, a friend or relative may be taught the catheterization procedure.

Only once the correct equipment is available should catheterization proceed. The use of inappropriate equipment is poor practice and, particularly in the case of the catheter itself, could be harmful and cause unnecessary discomfort to the patient. It is pertinent to note at this point that equipment should only be used according to instructions issued by the manufacturer and that the operator, in this case the nurse, is liable if products are used inappropriately.

The selection of individual products is discussed in detail below. However, at all times the patient's lifestyle, social circumstances and personal preferences should be taken into account. Restricted choice of products in hospitals is usually due to the limited range that the stores department is able to hold. If there are no suitable stock items available, others can often be obtained by special order. It is important to remember that an extensive range of products for urinary drainage systems is available in the community on prescription, and it is preferable that patients are set up initially with systems with which they are likely to continue, especially if hospital discharge is imminent.

The technique of catheterization is an aseptic procedure and the local policies for aseptic technique and hand-washing should be followed. Catheterization policies vary slightly between areas but should follow the same principles.

CATHETER SELECTION

Design

A catheter is a thin, hollow tube which may be passed intermittently into the bladder or held permanently in situ, originally by suturing it to the skin. In the 1930s, Dr Foley invented the first retention catheter with two channels, one for drainage and the second as a means by which to inflate a balloon which is positioned around the proximal end of the catheter immediately below the drainage eyes (Figure 5.1a). The balloon is inflated immediately after the catheter has been inserted into the bladder, allowing retention in the bladder, and can be deflated to facilitate removal.

Three-way catheters are available with a third channel to facilitate continuous bladder irrigation after urological surgery. Nelaton and Scott catheters are made from polyvinyl chloride (PVC) without a retention balloon and are for intermittent use only (Figure 5.1b,c).

An innovation in catheter design is the Conformacath (Figure 5.1d), described by Brocklehurst *et al.* (1988). This is a development of the Foley catheter which incorporates a collapsible urethral portion. This aims to conform to and reduce distortion of the urethra, which is a twisting, spiralling slit. It has been designed to increase comfort and reduce urethral trauma and

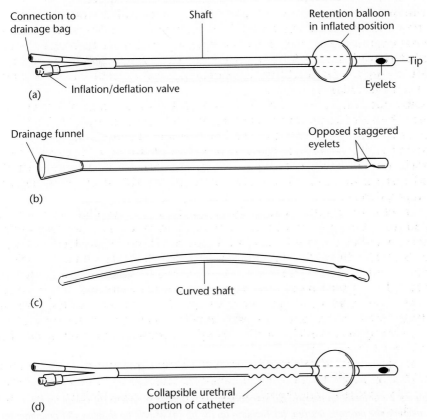

Figure 5.1   *Urinary catheters: (a) Foley catheter; (b) Nelaton catheter; (c) Scott catheter; (d) Conformacath*

related complications for female patients. The authors found, in a controlled crossover trial, that the conformable catheters remained in situ for longer periods than the Foley catheters, which they concluded was due to reduced levels of encrustation in the intraurethral portion of the Conformacath (this catheter is available only in female length and size 14 Charrière). This type of catheter has been recommended for use in all situations requiring continual bladder drainage except in the presence of strictures (Brocklehurst *et al.*, 1988), although Pomfret (1992) found it suitable for selected patients only.

Catheter tip design

The standard tip is rounded, with two staggered drainage eyes. However, there are a number of variations available (Figure 5.2). These are designed for specific uses normally within urology departments.

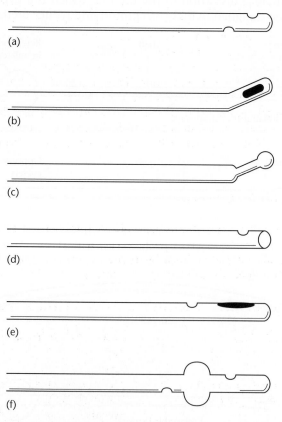

(a)

(b)

(c)

(d)

(e)

(f)

Figure 5.2 *Catheter tip designs: (a) standard tip with staggered eyelets; (b) Coudé tip for negotiating the prostatic urethra; (c) Tiemann tip (as b); (d) whistle tip to allow clot drainage; (e) Couvelaire tip to allow clot drainage with the option of continual irrigation; (f) Roberts tip for drainage of residual urine*

Material

Catheters are available in a variety of base materials and surface coatings which determine the length of time for which they are recommended to be left in situ (Table 5.1). Thus the length of time the catheter is required to remain in situ will, to a large extent, determine which type of catheter is used.

The earliest catheters were fashioned from dried reeds and palm leaves (Roe, 1992b). The first Foley catheters were made from red rubber which caused severe urethral irritation, ultimately leading to stricture formation. This was superseded by latex, which caused fewer problems but was still toxic and led to the procedure of 'coating' catheters. Manufacturers in the UK are now bound to ensure that their catheters meet the specifications laid out in British Standard 1695.

Catheters for short-term use

Plastic or PVC catheters, because of the inert nature of the material and the low rate of absorption of water, have been found to exhibit low toxicity (Blacklock, 1986) and to retain the widest internal diameter (Ryan-Woolley, 1987). However, plastic catheters do remain rigid even at body temperature which, although making this the material of choice for postoperative drainage of clots and debris, has been found to cause bladder spasm, pain and leakage of urine (Blannin and Hobden, 1980).

Latex provides a more flexible material but chemicals within latex can leach out causing cytotoxic reactions (Nacey *et al.*, 1985; Ruutu *et al.*, 1985) leading to acute and chronic inflammation (Wilksch *et al.*, 1983). Encrustation with mineral deposits (Blannin and Hobden, 1980) and absorption of up to 40% of its weight in water resulting in increased external diameter and reduced lumen (Ryan-Woolley, 1987) supports the use of latex in the short-term only.

Catheters for long-term use

Coated catheters were introduced in an effort to improve the surface smoothness of the catheter and provide insulation for the urethra against the latex (Blacklock, 1986). Catheters have been coated with polytetrafluoroethylene (PTFE), recommended for use for up to 4 weeks only, silicone-elastomer and

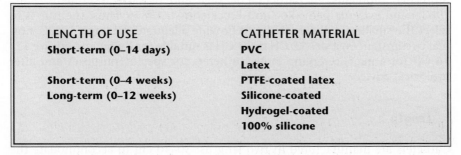

LENGTH OF USE	CATHETER MATERIAL
Short-term (0–14 days)	**PVC**
	Latex
Short-term (0–4 weeks)	**PTFE-coated latex**
Long-term (0–12 weeks)	**Silicone-coated**
	Hydrogel-coated
	100% silicone

Table 5.1 *Catheter materials for short-term and long-term use*

hydrogel. Cox (1990) found silicone-elastomer to have a smoother surface than PTFE-coated or latex catheters and thus may encourage less encrustation. Hydrogel-coated catheters, the most recent innovation in coatings, have been found to produce minimal inflammatory changes to the urethral mucosa (Nacey and Delahunt, 1991), to have a longer life in situ and be preferred by patients over a silicone-elastomer catheter (Bull *et al.*, 1991). Hydrogel also has hydrophilic properties and thus hydrates when in contact with the urethra, making insertion easier (Cox, 1990).

Catheters manufactured from 100% silicone (previously also known as 'all-silicone') produce minimal changes in the urethra owing to the inert nature of the material (Edwards *et al.*, 1983). However, Cox *et al.* (1988) found little difference in encrustation when comparing 100% silicone and hydrogel-coated catheters, although Kunin *et al.* (1987) found 100% silicone catheters to result in less encrustation in patients who commonly experienced blockage. The 100% silicone catheters are expensive but, as they are uncoated, do have a relatively large lumen compared with their Charrière size (Kennedy, 1984a). The extra expense may prove beneficial where blockage with debris is a problem. Catheters of different materials and manufactured by different companies are produced in a range of colours. Therefore, it is important that catheters are not identified solely by their colour.

Catheter size

Width

Catheters are measured in the Charrière scale (CH) or French gauge (FG), one unit of which equals 0.3 mm. Thus a size 12 CH catheter actually measures 4 mm in external diameter. Sizes range from 8 CH, for paediatric use, to 30 CH. Nelaton catheters are also available in size 6 CH. Although the diameter of the lumen, i.e. the inner dimension, varies between coated and uncoated catheters, it does not increase significantly with Charrière size between coated catheters. Therefore, inserting a larger Charrière catheter does not necessarily ensure a wide drainage channel. Indeed, Edwards *et al.* (1983), comparing flow rates through a range of catheter types in different sizes, concluded that the smaller sizes were capable of transporting the volumes produced by the average human being over a 24-hour period.

The urethral mucosa contains elastic tissue which will close around the catheter. Larger catheters have been found to be associated with more catheter-related problems, in particular leakage and blocking (Kennedy *et al.*, 1983a) and extreme pain (Roe and Brocklehurst, 1987). Thus, the rule is to select the smallest catheter that will provide adequate drainage. Under normal circumstances, a size 12 CH or 14 CH is suitable for a woman and size 12–16 CH for a man, reserving larger catheters for specific purposes and after urological advice.

Length

Catheters are manufactured in two lengths: 30–40 cm to accommodate the male urethra, and 23–26 cm for female use only. The shorter catheter provides an alternative for females, reducing the external length of catheter which could be tugged or pulled. However, the longer catheter often remains preferable for women, particularly where obesity exists, because it allows easier access to the junction between the catheter and the drainage bag. Despite the choice in catheter length, Crow *et al.* (1988) found that out of 165 females in five district general hospitals, female length catheters were used by only 5 patients. This is not surprising since many nurses remain unaware of this choice (Crummey, 1989).

Balloon size

Retention balloons come in three sizes: 3–5 ml for paediatric use; 10 ml for standard use; and 30 ml for use after some urological procedures. The larger balloon size is used to provide traction haemostasis on the bleeding prostatic bed after transurethral resection of the prostate. For adults, a 10 ml balloon should always be used as standard practice. The use of larger balloon sizes is mistakenly believed by many nurses to be a solution to bypassing of urine around the catheter (Crummey, 1989), whereas they have actually been implicated in catheter-related complications including leakage of urine (Roe and Brocklehurst, 1987) and bladder spasm (Blannin and Hobden, 1980).

The retention balloon should only be inflated once the catheter is in the bladder. Sterile water should be used for this as diffusion of some of the contents of the balloon into the bladder is likely. Several catheter materials have been found to lose water from the inflated balloon in the bladder, with 100% silicone catheters losing as much as 50% of their volume within 3 weeks (Barnes and Malone-Lee, 1986).

The valve at the distal end of the inflation channel connects to a water-filled syringe to enable inflation and deflation of the balloon. Some coated catheters are now available with prefilled balloons. These should always be used when available since they ensure that the correct amount of sterile water is inserted, reduce the amount of equipment required for the procedure and mean that there are no 'sharps' to deal with afterwards.

Packaging and markings

Each catheter is double-wrapped and sterile. Information written on both the outer packet and the catheter includes the size of the catheter, a code number and the names of both manufacturer and product. The outer packet also has printed on it the sterilization and expiry dates. Out-of-date catheters should be discarded. The person performing the catheterization is responsible for ensuring that the equipment used is in a satisfactory state. The code number is important and should be recorded in the patient's notes so that faulty items can easily be traced by the manufacturers.

Cost

The price of catheters ranges from the fairly inexpensive Nelaton catheter to the more costly catheter with special features. The cost of the catheter should not be the primary factor in the selection process. However, all else being equal, the nurse should be aware of the different costs and select accordingly. Where more frequent catheter changes are required it is recommended that a cheaper catheter designed for short-term use is used rather than the repeated disposal of the more expensive long-term catheters (Blannin and Hobden, 1980). Individual health districts will make their own contractual arrangements with specific companies which will reduce the cost per item.

Storage

Catheters should be stored flat in the boxes in which they are dispatched and should not be tied in bundles with elastic bands which might damage the wrapping and or the catheters, compromising sterility. Catheters should not be exposed to direct heat or sunlight and should be kept in a dry, cool environment.

Catheter supports

Many of the problems discussed later in this chapter are related to urethral trauma and can be minimized if the urinary drainage system is well supported. Although there is little research available to inform on supporting the catheter itself against the leg, Burkitt and Randall (1987) stated that urethral pressure necrosis can occur if the catheter is not fixed distally. Pomfret (1991) investigated the practice of attaching the catheter to the leg in nine hospital wards and among continence advisors in one health region. He found inconsistency in both areas with regard to the frequency of this practice as well as the methods used, although the practice was more common in the community units. Despite the availability of specially designed supports, he found the practice of using adhesive tape to be common. He also reported concerns of catheter manufacturers that not only could catheter fixation impede drainage but that, in the case of silicone or silicone-elastomer catheters, it is unlikely that adhesive tape would stick to the catheter, since such materials are used as 'release systems' for medical adhesive tapes.

There are now a number of catheter supports available either on prescription or by special order. These aim to provide a firm, secure support for the catheter without impeding drainage or restricting movement while ensuring that the catheter cannot be tugged. It would therefore seem sensible to use such an appliance if a catheter support is felt to be necessary and it seems this is largely dependent on the preference and comfort of the patient. In any event, there should be ample room for movement, different reclining positions and penile erection without the catheter becoming taut.

DRAINAGE BAG SELECTION

Indwelling catheters are normally used in conjunction with an attached urine collection bag to allow periodic emptying, although catheter valves now provide an alternative. Previously, catheters drained into open glass

Winchester bottles on the floor (Roberts *et al.*, 1965). Modern drainage bags are made from moulded plastic and are designed to be worn either attached to the leg or supported on a stand. There are design elements common to all drainage bags: each bag has an inlet tube, the proximal end of which is connected to the catheter, a collecting chamber and drainage tap (Figure 5.3).

If the drainage bag is to be connected directly to an indwelling catheter it should be sterile, since the use of 'closed' drainage systems using a sterile bag has been associated with reduced levels of bacteriuria (Gillespie *et al.*, 1967). Although drainage bags have been sterilized for reuse in the laboratory (Hashisaki *et al.*, 1984), it is unlikely that this is practical for everyday management by patients. Non-sterile and sterile free-standing bags are available for connection to a body-worn bag in a 'link' system, and non-sterile body-worn bags are available for use with urinary drainage sheaths.

Body-worn or leg bags should be used whenever possible and have been found to be recommended by nurses for ambulant patients (Roe, 1989a). They allow maximum freedom of movement and can be concealed beneath clothing. This is an essential feature for patients in the community, but is important during any period of rehabilitation.

Most drainage bags are available on prescription in the community, but availability in hospitals is subject to local purchasing agreements. However, as for catheters, the patient's needs must determine provision and it may be necessary to look further than this for the most appropriate appliance. Since there are many different types of bag available (Ryan-Woolley, 1987; Association of Continence Advisors, 1988) and no single bag will suit all users (Roe *et al.*, 1988; DoH, 1993) it is recommended that the individual needs of patients should be taken into account when selecting a system (Kohler-Ockmore, 1992) and that patients should be given an opportunity to try different systems to determine which best suits their needs (Roe *et al.*, 1988).

Length of inlet tube

Inlet tubes range in length from about 4 cm to 45 cm, so that the bag can be attached to the thigh, knee or calf and thus be concealed under various garments while still remaining accessible for emptying. The length of the inlet tube can be adjusted on some body-worn bags to suit individual needs by adding pieces of extension tubing, or by cutting the existing tubing and reapplying the connecting piece.

Capacity

Most leg bags come in capacities ranging from 350 ml to 800 ml, although bags are now available that can hold up to 1,300 ml. Which size is most suitable depends on how frequently the bag is to be emptied, and in practice the 500 ml bag is most popular. When selecting the volume of bag, opportunity for bag emptying should be taken into account as well as the visibility and weight of the full bag.

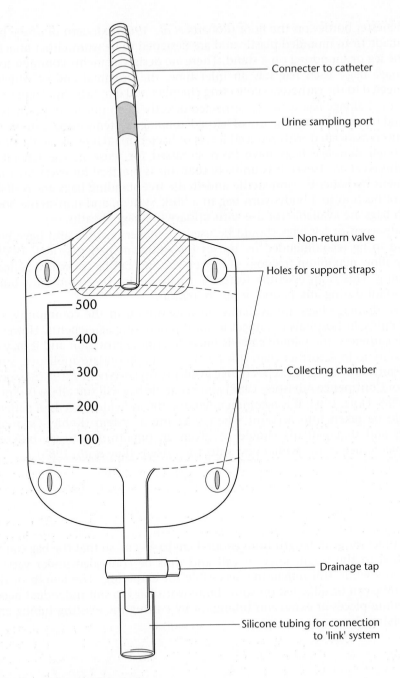

Connecter to catheter

Urine sampling port

Non-return valve

Holes for support straps

Collecting chamber

500

400

300

200

100

Drainage tap

Silicone tubing for connection to 'link' system

Figure 5.3 *Body-worn drainage bag*

Outlet tap

Tap design is a feature of urinary drainage bags which has been implicated in cross-infection, particularly with regard to ease of emptying and contamination of the operator's hands (Glenister, 1987). There are various tap designs available (Figure 5.4) and it has been found that taps that can be used with

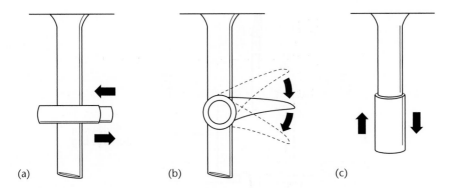

Figure 5.4 *Outlet tap designs: (a) barrel tap; (b) lever tap; (c) push–pull tap*

one hand without the fingers becoming wet with urine are preferred (Roe *et al.*, 1988). It is particularly important that the patient can manage the tap where manual dexterity is compromised and this should be taken into account during selection.

Collecting chamber design

Originally all leg bags were designed with a single chamber which, as the bag begins to fill, can result in 'sloshing' of urine and can cause an unsightly ballooning of the bottom of the bag. A design modification intended to reduce this effect by compartmentalizing the urine was the introduction of bonded vertical lines. However, a study of patient preference between four designs of leg bag, two of which incorporated a 'segmental' design, did not identify this as a particularly positive feature since some patients complained specifically of the bulge when the bag was full with one of the segmented bags, and that the compartments could be seen beneath clothing with the other (DoH, 1993).

A new shape of leg bag has now been designed for wheelchair users in which the inlet tube enters the collecting chamber at an angle, providing a curved shape intended to conform to the knee.

Link system connector

Most leg bags now have a facility for connection to a free-standing drainage bag when a larger capacity is required without having to break the closed drainage system (see below and Figure 5.5). This connection is usually a piece of silicone tubing which is attached to and extends beyond the drainage tap. Patients have been reported to have experienced difficulty in managing the connection as well as disconnection of the night bag (Roe *et al.*, 1988), and it is recommended that the additional tubing is bonded onto the leg bag to encourage the use of a 'link' system and reduce the risk of accidental disconnection.

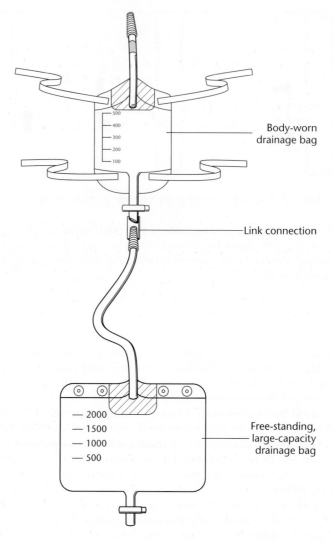

Figure 5.5 *Link system for connecting a larger-capacity bag*

Sampling port

Most drainage bags have a facility for the aspiration of urine for analysis. This is usually an area of inlet tube covered by a sleeve of resealable rubber through which a needle can be injected. However, there is a risk of needle-stick injury if the needle is pushed out through the back of the tubing. This resulted in the development of a rigid plastic backing to the aspiration area. Another concern is the integrity of the resealable portion since bacteria must not be able to gain access to the urinary tract via this route (Ryan-Woolley, 1987).

A sampling port has now been developed that accepts a Luer-Lok syringe, thus dispensing with the requirement for a needle for this procedure and significantly reducing the risk of injury. However, it is unclear how efficient this system is at preventing access by bacteria.

Backing material

Drainage bags are made from soft plastic and this can be uncomfortable, causing perspiration when worn next to the skin (DoH, 1993). Some bags have a woven coverstock on their posterior surface although this has been reported as becoming damp and stained, hard to dry and peeling off (Roe et al., 1988; DoH, 1993). One manufacturer has produced a separate coverstock backing held in place by the leg-bag straps, which can be easily removed prior to bathing or showering.

Support systems

It is extremely important that a body-worn bag is properly secured so that it cannot suddenly drop, thereby pulling the catheter and potentially trauma-tizing the urethra. The traditional method for this uses straps which are slotted through either end of the bag and fixed around the leg. However, there are a number of alternative methods available (Ryan-Woolley, 1987; Association of Continence Advisors, 1988) and a system should be sought which the patient and carers can manage and in which they have confidence (Figure 5.6).

Packaging and markings

Most bags and outer packaging carry details of the manufacturer, product name, prescription details, sterilization and expiry date. Most bags also have the capacity in millilitres marked on the front of the bag. Glenister (1985 unpublished thesis) reported the unnecessary emptying of urinary drainage bags to record even small amounts of urine and, having identified bag emptying as a potential source of contamination, recommends that accurate volume markings would enable nurses to reduce the frequency of this practice. Efforts have been made recently by manufacturers to tone down the colouring of the markings on the bags to make them less visible through light clothing.

FREE-STANDING BAGS

Free-standing drainage bags are constructed in a similar way to body-worn bags but are much bulkier, with capacities ranging from 2 litres to 4 litres, and thus are used for overnight drainage or the bedbound patient. Modified free-standing bags are available with an inner measuring chamber which allows accurate measurement of urine in the critically ill patient. In hospital, because of the risk of nosocomial infection, night drainage bags should not be reused in link systems (Roe, 1993) and cheaper, non-drainable bags should be used instead. In the community, it is common practice for patients to reuse free-standing or night drainage bags and so there is a requirement for a drainage tap. Slade and Gillespie (1985) recommended that these be rinsed through with soapy water and then dried thoroughly. Free-standing drainage

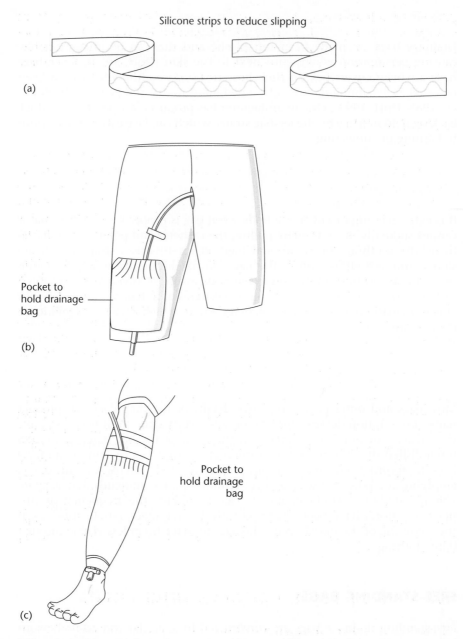

Figure 5.6 *Drainage bag support systems: (a) pair of elasticated straps; (b) catheter pants; (c) calf support garment*

bags only have to be sterile if they are to be attached directly to a catheter, not if they are used in a link system.

Free-standing bags require a stand for support, to reduce the risk of dislodging the link system. These stands range from cardboard or plastic, available free to patients from the manufacturers, to plastic-covered metal stands which are generally more substantial. However, Roe *et al.* (1988) found several different stands and support systems for free-standing drainage bags to be suboptimal. An appropriate stand should always be used, preferably that recommended by the manufacturer for their particular bag, and the failure to use such stands has been implicated in leakage of urine from around the catheter during periods in bed (Kennedy, 1984b).

CATHETER VALVES

While the variety of drainage bags now available helps to ensure maximum freedom and independence, they are nevertheless an encumbrance. Catheter valves, as an alternative to drainage bags, allow more discreet drainage and maximum freedom and movement. They may also assist in the maintenance of a degree of bladder tone since the bladder is able to fill and empty in a manner akin to the normal micturition pattern, although there is no published research available to date about their use.

There are now several commercially available valves and recently two have become available on prescription. They are designed either for single or repeated use, although none of those available for reuse is supplied with cleaning instructions suitable for community use. Standard spigots have been used to plug catheters but these are unsuitable because the closed drainage system has to be repeatedly broken to allow bladder drainage. Catheter valves can be opened without having to break the closed drainage system and are designed for use with one or both hands.

The successful use of a valve depends upon the manual dexterity of the patient who must also be able to recognize the need to empty the bladder either through sensation or on a timed schedule to ensure that the bladder does not overdistend. If bladder distension is allowed to occur the patient may be at risk from urinary tract infection and dilatation of the upper urinary tract (Lapides *et al.*, 1972). As for urinary drainage bags, it would seem to constitute good practice that a sterile catheter valve be connected each time the junction between catheter and valve is broken. Not all catheter valves have a secure facility for connection to a drainage bag (either body-worn or free-standing) which may restrict their use, since periods of free drainage may be required, for example, overnight or during a period of reduced dexterity.

MANAGEMENT OF THE URINARY DRAINAGE SYSTEM

Management is based on reduction of the risks of the complications that are well documented as occurring in association with indwelling catheterization (Roe, 1993; Getliffe, 1995) and resulting in frequent referrals to hospital (Kohler-Ockmore, 1992). Some of the complications of catheterization are inevitable, but with careful management the effects of these can be minimized.

Urinary tract infection

Urinary tract infections (UTI) accounted for 30% of all nosocomial infections reported during a UK prevalence study (Meers *et al.*, 1981). Indwelling catheterization has been found to be a significant cause of UTI increasing morbidity and mortality (Kunin *et al.*, 1992) and causing extended hospitalization and increased patient care costs (Givens and Wenzel, 1980; Platt et al, 1989).

Urine leaving the bladder should remain sterile until it passes through the non-return valve of the drainage bag. However, it may become contaminated with bacteria which adhere to the surfaces of the catheter and drainage bag inlet tube once in contact with urine. The result is the formation of a biofilm which has been defined by Mulhall (1991) as a collection of micro-organisms and their extracellular products bound to a solid surface. The biofilm appears to afford protection against antibiotics and antiseptic agents, including chlorhexidine (Stickler *et al.*, 1987) commonly used in the form of a bladder washout. Indeed, the use of such agents has been implicated in the development of resistant organisms (Dudley and Barriere, 1981). Biofilms have been found on the surfaces of several different catheter materials (Mulhall 1991). Thus it would seem sensible that the only way to remove the biofilm is to recatheterize the patient.

The incidence of urinary tract infection has been shown to be directly proportional to the number of days that a catheter is left in situ (Crow *et al.*, 1986), and the most common infecting organisms are *Escherichia coli*, *Streptococcus faecalis*, *Proteus mirabilis* and *Staphylococcus epidermidis*. Infection with urease-producing bacteria can lead to encrustation and subsequent catheter blockage, and related problems such as bypassing of urine around the catheter and catheter-associated pain. Thus all efforts should be made to delay the onset of UTI and reduce its impact when it occurs.

Bacteria are thought to be able to enter the bladder at the time of catheterization, via the periurethral space or the catheter lumen (Falkiner, 1993), having gained access either during a break in the closed drainage system or from the drainage bag itself.

Principles of management for reducing bacterial access

Closed drainage

Prior to the use of closed drainage systems, almost 100% of catheterized patients developed urinary tract infections within 96 hours (Kass, 1957). Closed drainage has been shown to reduce this rate of infection substantially (Gillespie *et al.*, 1967) and is now widely accepted as good practice.

If the catheter and the drainage bag are disconnected the closed drainage system will be broken, allowing bacteria access to the system, and thus this should only occur if absolutely necessary either to change the drainage bag or to perform a bladder washout. Frequent changing of drainage bags has been found to increase the risk of bacterial infection, resulting in more catheter-related problems (Kennedy *et al.*, 1983). It is recommended that drainage bags, attached directly to a catheter, should not be changed more often than weekly since no advantage was found in more frequent changes (Reid *et al.*, 1982). Exceptions to this are after bladder washout, or if the drainage bag leaks or smells.

The link system

Before the importance of closed drainage was realized, the connection between the catheter and the body-worn bag would be broken regularly to allow connection of a larger capacity, free-standing night bag. Although this method is still in use in some areas (Crow *et al.*, 1986), the use of a link system whereby the night drainage bag is connected to the outlet tap of the body-worn bag, which is then left in the open position, is now recommended practice (Roe *et al.*, 1988). It is important that the large-capacity bag is supported on a stand by the bed to reduce disconnection and leakage (Kennedy, 1984b), but there must be slack in the tubing if the patient turns. If the bag is tied to the bed this cannot occur and may thus traumatize the urethra (Lowthian, 1989).

Bag emptying

It is important to note that empptyting of the drainage bag also constitutes a break in the closed system. The importance of contamination of nurses' hands as a cross-infection hazard has been highlighted by Glenister (1987). She found nurses' hands to be contaminated after bag emptying with organisms from the urine and other sources, possibly the outer aspects of the bags. Bradley *et al.* (1986) also found that bacteria can gain entry to the drainage bag after contamination of the tap and concluded that escalating air bubbles, urinary stasis or accidental pressure applied to the bag would increase the risk of the bacteria ascending to the bladder. Effective hand-washing is important before and after bag emptying, and the use of drainage taps which allow emptying without contamination from urine is recommended. Disposable gloves may be worn and changed in between patients, although this should not be a substitute for hand-washing. Crow *et al.* (1986) having identified the reuse of containers for the collection of urine from drainage bags without cleansing in between, recommended the use of a disposable urinal, one for each patient to reduce the risk of cross-infection. At the very least, reusable containers should be cleaned between uses.

Gravity drainage

The free flow of urine through the drainage system is important to prevent areas of stagnant urine collecting in the tubing proximal to the non-return valve. This provides a suitable medium for bacterial multiplication and can also result in unexpected disconnection of the system. The positioning of night drainage bags too high for the bed has resulted in drainage failure (Kennedy, 1984b; Roe *et al.*, 1988). The drainage bags should always be positioned below the level of the bladder and the catheter, and inlet tubing should be secured in a downward position.

Meatal cleansing

Meatal cleansing refers to cleaning around the urethral meatus, where the catheter enters the body (Roe, 1993). Increased urethral secretions, due to irritation of the urothelium by the catheter, collect at the meatus and may form crusts which, when removed, expose areas of damaged tissue susceptible to bacterial colonization which may then ascend to the bladder. The practice of using antiseptic agents for meatal cleansing has been shown not to reduce bacterial infection (Burke *et al.*, 1981; Gibbs, 1986) and, although it has been reported by patients as giving greater comfort (Gibbs, 1986), has been found to predispose to the emergence of multiresistant bacterial strains (Dance *et al.*, 1987). Despite these findings, observation of meatal cleansing procedures has shown that there is still confusion and inconsistency in practice (Crow *et al.*, 1986). It is recommended that secretions are removed using soap and water and clean washcloths (Roe, 1993). The frequency of this procedure is dependent upon the amount of secretions produced and, therefore, will vary between individuals, although once or twice a day should normally be sufficient.

Treatment of UTI during periods of catheterization

Eradication of bacteria from the bladder during periods of indwelling catheterization is extremely difficult owing to the presence of biofilms. Where urine is in direct contact with the catheter a biofilm will form. Organisms seem particularly resistant to antimicrobial agents in this state (Mulhall, 1991) and thus short courses of antibiotics have not been found particularly useful against catheter-associated urinary tract infections. However, despite having large numbers of bacteria in the urine, the patient may remain asymptomatic and not require treatment. It is only when symptoms occur that active treatment should be considered after removal of the catheter. If the reason for catheterization is urinary retention a period of intermittent catheterization will allow drainage to continue and antibiotics to take effect in the absence of an indwelling catheter.

The type of antibiotic used will depend upon the organism implicated. However, this may not be determined for up to 48 hours and so a broad-spectrum antibiotic may be prescribed initially.

Urine specimens

A catheter specimen of urine should be collected using a needle and syringe from the aspiration port of the drainage bag situated along the inlet tubing. A leg bag is now available with a sampling port which has a connecting point designed to accept a Luer syringe tip and thus a needle is not required. Hands should be washed before and after collection to reduce the risk of contamination and cross-infection. Urine should never be collected from the drainage bag as it should be fresh and uncontaminated. The specimen should be clearly labelled and sent immediately to the microbiology laboratory for analysis. If this is not possible, a specimen may be kept in a refrigerator designated for specimens overnight. The laboratory will culture the organisms and examine them under the light microscope, and the antibiotics to which the organisms are sensitive will be determined.

Blockage of the urinary drainage system

There are a number of ways in which the UDS can become blocked and these can be hard to correct. The result is a build-up of urine proximal to the blockage which may lead to detrusor spasm and leakage of urine. High-pressure bladder distension may compromise vascularity and leave the bladder vulnerable to infection (Lapides et al., 1972). In the event that urine does not leak around the catheter, the risk is of high-pressure dilation of ureters and renal pelves resulting in pyelonephritis and hydronephrosis (Lowthian, 1989). If urine is prevented from entering the drainage bag, the result may be disconnection from the catheter.

A blockage in the drainage bag may be due to a design fault, in which case the manufacturers should be informed and the bag changed. If there does not appear to be a problem with the drainage bag and the blockage is intermittent, it is possible that the inlet tubing is becoming kinked and this should be observed for during a range of movements. The patency of the inlet tubing can easily be disrupted if metal clamps or toothed forceps are applied. If it is necessary to disrupt the flow of urine then either non-toothed forceps should be used or gauze should be wrapped around the jaws of the forceps first. Clamping of the catheter itself should be avoided as compression of the inflation channel may lead to difficulty with balloon deflation later.

Blockage of the lumen of the catheter is common. Clues as to the nature of the blockage may be found in the urine if it contains debris or clots which can block the catheter lumen and the inlet tubing. This type of obstruction can often be shifted by repeatedly squeezing and releasing ('milking') the tubing distal to the blockage. However, this technique should not be used on a regular basis as it may cause damage to the urothelium.

Catheter encrustation

Encrustation has been found to occur on all catheter surfaces to a greater or lesser extent and is the most common cause for occlusion of the catheter lumen (Getliffe, 1995) affecting up to 50% of long-term catheter users. The principal components of encrustations are struvite (magnesium ammonium phosphate) and calcium phosphate (Bruce et al., 1974; Cox et al., 1988). Deposits are able to precipitate in urine which has become alkaline as a result of infection with micro-organisms which produce urease and release ammonia from urinary urea (Getliffe, 1993).

The amount of encrustation has been found to be related not only to the presence of urease-producing organisms but also to individual factors such as urinary composition (Hedelin et al., 1991). More recently, Getliffe (1994) has identified further characteristics associated with blockage due to encrustation. She found that 'blockers' were more likely to be female, catheterized for incontinence and significantly less mobile than 'non-blockers', but could not be characterized by medical condition, medication or dietary habits.

However, 'blockers' were found to have a high urinary pH and ammonia concentrations.

Bladder washouts

Intermittent use of bladder washouts is a common form of management for dealing with and preventing catheter blockage. Despite this, nurses have been found to have a poor level of knowledge with regard to type of fluid for specific use and the frequency of administration (Roe, 1989b; Bailey, 1991). Chlorhexidine has been reported as the most widely used solution, despite findings that it is ineffective in dissolving encrustations (Flack, 1993) and as an antiseptic against many infecting organisms.

In recent years, the use of prepacked, sterile washouts in a range of solutions has gained popularity. The advantages of these are that fewer items of equipment are required, they are available on prescription and they allow the bladder washout to be more easily performed using an aseptic technique. The use of prepacked solutions has been reported as preferable by nurses, who found them quick to use, and by patients, who found them less traumatic than other methods. Once the connection with the catheter has been made, removal of the clamp and elevation of the bag allows gravity drainage of the irrigation fluid into the bladder. The bag is then lowered to allow the irrigation fluid to drain out. This method does not allow active flushing of the bladder and thus may be more use for prophylactic washouts.

The following solutions are suitable for bladder washouts:

- Saline 0.9% – recommended for mechanical flushing to remove tissue debris and small blood clots.
- Suby G solution – a citric acid solution (3.23%) aimed at preventing and dissolving crystallization in the catheter or bladder.
- Mandelic acid 1% – aimed at preventing the growth of urease-producing bacteria through acidification of the urine.
- Solution R – a citric acid solution (6%) aimed at dissolving persistent crystallization in the catheter or bladder.
- Chlorhexidine 0.02% – aimed at preventing or reducing the growth of bacteria in the bladder and particularly contamination with *E. coli* and *Klebsiella*.

Traditionally, bladder washout has been performed using isotonic saline (0.9%) and a 60 ml bladder syringe with a tip that fits the funnel end of a catheter. This method allows active flushing of the bladder using a push-pull action which, when repeated, disturbs the debris so it can drain. However, by withdrawing the plunger forcefully urothelium may be sucked into the eyes of the catheter, actually preventing drainage of the irrigation fluid as well as the debris. This practice can also cause discomfort, pain and trauma which may predispose to infection. Therefore, once the fluid has been instilled, the syringe should be removed and the catheter allowed to drain freely into a sterile kidney dish and input and output measured. The amount of debris obtained and subsequent urinary flow should also be noted.

To date, there has been no research to advise specifically on the frequency with which washouts should be used. However, Getliffe (1993) advised the regular use of 'mini-washouts' of 10–20 ml in patients whose catheters regularly block. Since the lumen of the catheter holds 4–5 ml, a small washout would bathe the inner surface of the catheter and the outer aspect of the catheter tip while minimizing the risk of large volumes of potentially irritant solution coming in contact with the urothelium. Dilute acid solutions have been shown to remove the surface layer of mucus in the bladder (Parsons *et al.*, 1970) and increased exfoliation of bladder mucosal cells has been observed to follow washouts (Elliott *et al.*, 1989).

Isotonic saline (0.9%) has been shown to have no effect in dissolving encrustations but may assist in dislodging debris through the mechanical effect of flushing (Flack, 1993). Suby G solution, mandelic acid and Solution R have been shown to be active in the dissolution of mineral deposits (Flack, 1993; Getliffe, 1993). Getliffe (1993) recommended the use of Suby G solution as it contains magnesium oxide which reduces tissue irritation. Chlorhexidine, although reported as the solution of choice by over 50% of nurses (Roe, 1989b), has been shown to be ineffective in reducing the urinary bacterial count (Davies *et al.*, 1987) although it may be active against some bacteria in the normal urethral flora (Stickler *et al.*, 1987), removal of which may allow colonization by resistant organisms. It should be noted that certain solutions may be contraindicated after some urological procedures, for example bladder augmentation, and it is recommended that medical advice is sought in such cases.

If used inappropriately, bladder washouts can be hazardous and expose the patient to increased risk of urinary tract infection. Therefore, the current lack of knowledge of nurses about the use of individual solutions and the technique of bladder washout (Roe, 1989b; Bailey, 1991) must be corrected. Although bladder washouts should only be performed when absolutely necessary as the procedure involves breaking the closed drainage system, the use of regular, prophylactic bladder washouts in patients whose catheters are prone to encrustation and regularly block is recommended as a means by which to extend catheter life (Roe, 1989b; Getliffe, 1993), although nurses should be fully cognisant of the manufacturer's recommendations when selecting the most suitable solution.

If bladder washout does not relieve the blockage it may be necessary to change the catheter. When the catheter has been removed, it should be inspected to ascertain the nature of the blockage. This may not be evident from external examination and it may be necessary to dissect the catheter.

If blockage is an ongoing problem, thought should be given to the type of catheter used and the lumen size. The hydrogel-coated and all-silicone catheters are recommended as providing a surface more resistant to encrustation, and the uncoated, all-silicone catheter will provide a slightly larger lumen relative to the Charrière size than a coated catheter. Whether or not a catheter blocks and after how long depends on the individual and the catheter. The frequency of recatheterization in the long term will thus be determined by the lifespan of a catheter. The determination of 'catheter life' can assist in planning a regimen of catheter changes of an appropriate frequency, thus minimizing the risk of catheter blockage and emergency changes. If a catheter continues to block, cystoscopy may be required to identify the nature of the blockage.

After urological operations that involve heavy blood loss, the bladder will require continuous irrigation. This is facilitated by the insertion of a three-way Foley catheter, usually made out of plastic for extra rigidity, and the bladder is continuously flushed with isotonic saline (0.9%).

Vitamin C and cranberry juice

The use of high doses of ascorbic acid to reduce debris formation in the bladder is not new, although it is unclear what actual role it plays. Ascorbic acid acidifies the urine, reducing the formation of mineral deposits, although a bacteriostatic effect remains unproved (Kunin, 1989).

Cranberry juice is now widely recommended for ingestion by catheterized patients and in the management of urinary tract infection, although its method of action remains unproven. Sabota (1984) found that it reduced bacterial adherence to the urothelium after periods of ingestion of only a few hours. Avorn *et al.* (1994) found that, amongst a group of elderly women, cranberry juice led to a reduction in the prevalence of bacteriuria and pyuria after a period of 4–8 weeks and concluded that the method of action is through a bacteriostatic effect. However, neither of the above studies supported the theory that cranberry juice works through a reduction in urinary pH.

Rogers (1991) studied a small group of physically disabled children whose bladders emptied through intermittent catheterization, clean intermittent self-catheterization and via urinary diversions. She found that the ingestion of two or three glasses of cranberry juice per day led to a reduction in odour attached to the urine and a reduction in mucus, and was well tolerated. However, she does warn against ingestion of more than a litre per day which can result in uric acid stone formation. Cranberry juice is now widely available in liquid form and as tablets from some healthfood stores.

Detrusor spasm

Spasmodic contraction of the detrusor muscle is a common response to the presence of a foreign body in the bladder and may also occur secondary to blockage of the catheter. Large catheters with large-capacity balloons can cause bladder contractions (Kennedy *et al.*, 1983; Kunin *et al.*, 1987). Often referred to as 'bladder spasm', these contractions can cause considerable discomfort to the patient, leading to bypassing of urine from the space between the urethra and the catheter, and occasionally are strong enough to cause expulsion of the catheter from the bladder. Catheterization of an already unstable bladder is likely to worsen the situation so, if time permits, treatment of the detrusor instability should commence prior to catheterization and may need to continue during the period of catheterization.

Management is based on removal of the cause of the spasm whenever possible and by ensuring that the catheter is not blocked. Oxybutynin hydrochloride and propantheline bromide are two drugs used to treat detrusor instability for their anticholinergic and antispasmodic effect on the detrusor muscle.

For some people, however, the spasm may be resistant to treatment, and removal of the catheter may have to be considered. Spasm occurring immediately after catheterization may be a temporary response and may settle down after 24–48 hours.

Catheter expulsion

The simplest reason for a catheter leaving the bladder unexpectedly is that the retention balloon has become deflated. It may not have had the correct amount of water inserted in the first place, hence the importance of recording the volume inserted. Also, it has been shown that the water is gradually lost from retention balloons at different rates according to the catheter material, but most rapidly from 100% silicone catheters (Studer *et al.*, 1983; Barnes and Malone-Lee, 1986).

Occasionally, a catheter will be expelled with the balloon fully inflated. This may be due to detrusor spasm which should be dealt with as above. If the catheter is not fully expelled but lodged in the urethra, the retention balloon should be deflated and the catheter removed. No attempt should be made to reinsert the original catheter without deflating the balloon as this would cause urethral trauma. A fresh catheter should be used for the recatheterization.

If the support system for the catheter and drainage bag is inadequate the catheter may accidentally be pulled out. A more secure system should then be set up prior to recatheterization. Occasionally the catheter will be removed deliberately by the patient. This is most likely to happen when the patient is confused, and recatheterization should not be attempted while the confusional state remains. The chronically confused patient may repeatedly remove the catheter, which is a traumatic event. Complaints of discomfort, therefore, should never be ignored, because, if severe enough, may drive even the most rational patients to remove the source of the pain if they do not feel they are being listened to.

Pain

Catheter-related pain is varied and may be felt in the suprapubic region or be referred to the tip of the penis or labia. Temporary discomfort may be experienced immediately after catheterization and should settle in 24–48 hours with mild analgesics.

Severe pain immediately after catheterization should arouse suspicion that the catheter is not properly sited in the bladder and that the retention balloon is inflated in the urethra. If not corrected immediately, this can lead to pressure necrosis of the surrounding urethral tissue. Therefore, the catheter should be inserted up to the bifurcation in men and a further 25 mm after urine has drained in women prior to balloon inflation.

The pain of detrusor spasm can range from a dull ache to severe pain. The spasm should be dealt with and the patient given analgesics. If this situation continues and cannot be controlled, it may be necessary to remove the catheter.

If the drainage bag is allowed to drag on the catheter, this in turn will pull on the bladder neck and the urethra, causing pain. Pain is always a warning that something is amiss and, particularly when it cannot be felt, as with some neurological lesions, it is vital that the nurse checks that the drainage bag and the catheter are well supported.

Phimosis and paraphimosis

For the purpose of catheterization or cleansing of the glans, the foreskin must be retracted. After these procedures, it should be replaced over the glans or else it may become oedematous and fixed in the retracted position, constricting the penis. This condition is known as paraphimosis. Phimosis is a condition where the foreskin cannot be retracted and the glans exposed, preventing adequate cleansing and, in extreme circumstances, visualization of the urethral meatus. Both of these can be remedied through manipulation but may require surgical correction by circumcision.

LONG-TERM COMPLICATIONS OF URETHRAL CATHETERIZATION

Urethral strictures are the most serious of the late complications. The most common cause is repeated instrumentation of the bladder, and the early complications of trauma, bleeding and inflammation may also result in stricture formation. Inflammation may also be caused by infection, chemical irritation or ischaemia (Burkitt and Randall, 1987).

Too large a catheter will block the paraurethral glands, resulting in paraurethral abscesses. These will either heal with scar tissue formation or burst outside the urethra, allowing urine to escape into the surrounding tissues and thus causing urinary fistulae. Too large a catheter can also cause blockage of and subsequent infection in the ejaculatory ducts, resulting in epididymitis. Similarly, blockage and subsequent infection of the prostatic ducts can result in prostatitis or prostatic abscesses (Blandy and Moors, 1989).

An unsupported catheter will traumatize the urothelium which will heal to form scar tissue. In severe cases, pressure can result in complete destruction of the urethra (Bearman, 1985). Mucosal damage termed 'polypoid cystitis' has been reported as caused by long-term catheterization (Ekelund *et al.*, 1983).

Perhaps a less obvious complication relates to the self-perception of the catheterized patient. Alteration of body image (Roe and Brocklehurst, 1987) and a feeling of dependence may result. It is very important that the nurse listens to the anxieties of the patient and takes into account lifestyle when planning a UDS. It may be appropriate to include the patient's partner in this discussion.

GENERAL CARE

Lack of mobility, particularly in patients in the community, has been found to be of major significance in catheter-related problems. Immobile patients may be on their own all day without access to fluids, and unable to change their position and improve the flow of urine (Kennedy *et al.*, 1983). Close proximity of the bowel to the bladder means that constipation can affect free drainage. Constipation can also worsen detrusor instability and result in bypassing of urine and catheter expulsion.

Maintaining adequate fluid intake can be difficult, particularly for elderly people, and should be realistic rather than prescriptive. Gradual increases relative to the patient's normal intake are more likely to achieve a positive outcome. An intake of 1,500–2,000 ml per day to replace fluid lost is considered adequate. It has been suggested that diuresis may assist in voiding micro-organisms from the bladder, although it may not reduce encrustation (Getliffe and Mulhall, 1991).

CATHETER REMOVAL

For most people, catheterization will be temporary and the timing of catheter removal will depend on the general condition of the patient or the healing time after a specific urological operation. The increased risk of urinary tract infection with time (Crow et al., 1986) means that the need for the catheter should be assessed on a daily basis during the initial period after catheterization.

If the catheter has been inserted with the intention that it be permanent, for example for the containment of incontinence, the decision to decatheterize may not be easy. Catheterization should be viewed as a last resort, to be used when all other attempts at management have failed. The longer-term consequences of indwelling catheterization require the need for a permanent catheter also to be regularly reviewed.

There are a number of alternatives to urethral catheterization including suprapubic and intermittent catheterization. If the initial bladder dysfunction was urinary retention, one of these alternatives will be required. However, if the bladder empties completely and incontinence was the initial reason for catheterization, management with an aid or appliance may be preferable (Association of Continence Advisors, 1988).

Catheters have traditionally been removed at 6 a.m., thereby allowing the whole day for normal voiding to resume. However, removal is often followed by a period of urinary frequency and urgency which can be stressful to the patient. Removal of catheters at midnight has shown a significant increase in the time to the first void after removal and consequently a greater initial volume, resulting in a faster return to a regular voiding pattern. This has the added advantage of allowing earlier discharge (Noble et al., 1990; Chillington, 1992).

Retention balloon deflation

Actual removal of the catheter is normally a straightforward procedure although occasionally problems will be experienced when trying to deflate the balloon. It should be remembered that there is likely to be less water in the retention balloon than was initially inserted (Studer et al., 1983; Barnes and Malone-Lee, 1986) and that the diameter of the catheter shaft is likely to have swollen through water absorption (Ryan-Woolley, 1987).

Once the syringe has been attached to the valve of the inflation channel, the pressure of the water draining from the balloon should push the plunger out. Thus it should be unnecessary to pull on the plunger, avoiding the risk of additional suction resulting in the inflation channel collapsing, and preventing further water from being withdrawn.

If water does not drain out, a different syringe should be tried, and if this fails aspiration of the sterile water from the balloon through insertion of a syringe and needle into the inflation arm proximal to the valve can be tried. The insertion of a further 1–2 ml of water and its subsequent withdrawal will indicate patency of the inflation channel. Encrustation around the catheter balloon can affect its ability to deflate. This may be helped by the use of a 'mini-washout' to dissolve deposits and, if similar problems have been experienced previously with a particular patient, can be a planned part of the decatheterization procedure. Deflation may be prevented by compression on the inflation channel by debris within the drainage channel, and 'milking' the catheter may dislodge this. Constipation may have the same effect and should be eliminated as a cause. Cutting the inflation arm of the catheter proximal to the valve is no longer recommended practice.

If the catheter remains in situ medical referral will be necessary, and there are a number of methods that can be used by urologists to burst the balloon. A fine, ureteric catheter stylet can be passed up the inflation channel and the balloon punctured from within. An alternative method of bursting the balloon is to introduce a needle transvesically (Moisey and Williams, 1980) or via a perineal approach using ultrasound. However, free fragment formation has been reported after such procedures, only identifiable by cystoscopy (Chrisp and Nacey, 1990).

One method that is no longer advocated is the insertion of ether up the inflation channel to dissolve the balloon. Ether is harmful to the urothelium and vaporization may expand the balloon to a point at which the balloon ruptures. Stones may then form around the fragments of balloon left in the bladder which also will require cystoscopy for removal.

Clamping the catheter

Periods of indwelling catheterization may result in reduced bladder capacity leading to urinary frequency and loss of detrusor muscle tone, resulting in poor bladder emptying after decatheterization. One method used to overcome this involves the clamping and intermittent release of the catheter for a period prior to removal. A review of the research on this practice suggests that it may result in the earlier resumption of normal voiding only after short periods of catheterization of up to 6 days (Roe, 1990). If there is any doubt about the patient's ability to empty the bladder after the catheter has been removed, the residual urine volume after voiding can be established using ultrasound.

The current trend is to remove the catheter immediately and to use intermittent catheterization to drain any significant residual amounts of urine. A hazard of this type of decatheterization programme is that the patient may be forgotten and left in urinary retention. Therefore, the patient should be made aware of the timing for voiding and measurement of residual volume, and the timing may need to be adjusted so that the amount of urine voided plus the residual volume does not exceed 400–500 ml. It should be remembered that intermittent catheterization in the hospital setting is an aseptic procedure and requires a sterile catheter.

Potential problems after removal

Urinary retention can be dealt with using intermittent catheterization. Occasionally retention continues, and the patient may need to be taught the technique of clean intermittent self-catheterization. This is preferable to a further episode of indwelling catheterization which does not provide an opportunity for the bladder tone to improve, although recatheterization will be more appropriate in some circumstances.

Slight bleeding may occur, particularly if the catheter tip has become calcified. The patient should be warned to expect some blood loss when next passing urine. If the bleeding persists or becomes heavy, cauterization of the bleeding vessels will be required.

Similarly, slight pain may be experienced during and after removal, particularly when the bladder starts to fill, and may be due to reduced detrusor compliance. The associated urinary frequency and urgency usually subsides as the bladder becomes used to holding increased volumes of urine. The patient can speed up this process by attempting to extend the time intervals between voids, a process known as bladder retraining. If the pain is due to trauma on removal, mild analgesics should be used until it subsides.

PREPARATION FOR DISCHARGE

As the numbers of patients cared for in the community grows and non-professional carers are expected to provide more care, it is increasingly important that all parties involved are provided with adequate instruction on various aspects of catheter care. However, it has been found that many patients are being discharged to the community with little idea about how to care for their catheters (Roe and Brocklehurst, 1987) and that this results in frequent telephone calls to the ward and may result in increased admissions (Kennedy, 1983a; Kohler-Ockmore, 1992).

Studies of what information is in fact given by nurses to patients and their carers have shown that it is neither comprehensive nor consistent with research literature (McCullough, 1989; Roe, 1989a). Further work has shown that patients do benefit from education programmes, and that these should be consistent and continued after discharge. To aid education, several manufacturers of urinary drainage equipment produce illustrated booklets written specifically for patients. These can be obtained, free of charge, by contacting the appropriate company.

Although much of this literature is also useful for staff, it has been recognized that they need information which is more technical and research-based (Wright, 1989). Thus it may be useful to have written guidelines for nurses and staff which act as an adjunct to practice policies and procedures.

The information patients require includes the following:

- ◆ Simple anatomy of the urinary tract
- ◆ The position of the catheter in the bladder in relation to function
- ◆ How to empty and change a body-worn bag
- ◆ How to set up a 'link' system and care for a free-standing bag
- ◆ How to recognize the onset of problems such as blockage and infection
- ◆ How to deal with specific problems
- ◆ Where and when to seek further advice (names and telephone numbers)

Some patients and their relatives or friends will also need to be taught how to recatheterize and perform bladder washouts. This process cannot be completed overnight and, if the person is an inpatient, discharge planning should reflect this. Liaison with the community nursing staff is vital, and it may well be more appropriate for them to teach some of the catheter-related skills in the patient's home environment. Only when patients are confident and support from the community nursing staff has been arranged should they be sent home.

Similarly, if a patient is to be admitted to hospital, the community nursing staff should inform the ward staff of the care given for that particular urinary drainage system. It is advisable that the patient bring in a catheter and spare leg bag or night bag to ensure that the correct equipment is available; this is especially important if the patient is going to the accident and emergency department for an emergency catheter change. Inpatients should be discharged with 2 weeks' supply of the correct equipment. Prescription details should be given so that further supplies can be obtained.

The date of recatheterization should be arranged and (if the patient is male) it should be established whether the community nurse is able to do this procedure, and the outpatient appointment adjusted as necessary.

SUPRAPUBIC CATHETERIZATION

Bladder drainage by suprapubic catheterization involves the insertion of a catheter into the bladder via an incision through the anterior abdominal wall (Hilton and Stanton, 1980). This artificial entrance into the bladder is known as a cystotomy. Suprapubic catheterization is preferable to urethral catheterization in all situations requiring long-term drainage or where the urethra cannot be catheterized, for example because of stricture or previous urethral closure.

As an alternative method of bladder drainage, suprapubic catheterization has some distinct advantages over urethral catheterization:

- ◆ The integrity of the urethra is retained
- ◆ Sexual intercourse can occur with less impediment
- ◆ The risk of UTI is reduced as the urethral defence mechanisms are not compromised (Norton, 1986)
- ◆ Access to the catheter entry site is easier for cleansing purposes
- ◆ It allows the resumption of normal voiding after surgery – the suprapubic catheter can be clamped to allow urethral voiding and released if voiding is incomplete

Suprapubic catheterization is gaining in popularity particularly as an alter-native where clean intermittent self-catheterization has failed or is inap-propriate (Barnes *et al.*, 1993). Griffiths (1985) reported the cheaper cost of materials and the fact that management of a suprapubic catheter is less time-consuming as reasons for such a preference, although she warned against the long-term use of suprapubic catheters because of potential cellular changes in the tract.

Hammarsten and Lindqvist (1992) found suprapubic catheters to be asso-ciated with lower rates of stricture formation in the anterior urethra and increased patient satisfaction. Barnes *et al.* (1993) also found that although catheter-related problems were common, patients preferred this method to urethral catheterization or intermittent catheterization because of the greater level of independence, particularly where carers would otherwise have been required.

There are a number of different types of suprapubic catheter available. Some are specifically designed for this purpose and require a suture to secure them in place. However, for long-term use, a Foley catheter is adequate. Sizes ranging from 18 CH to 22 CH with a 10 ml retention balloon have been recommended in 100% silicone or hydrogel-coated catheters (Winder, 1994), but smaller sizes can provide acceptable drainage.

Some of the potential problems associated with this type of drainage are:

- ◆ Urinary tract infection – although the onset may be delayed compared with urethral catheterization
- ◆ Vesical calculi, which are thought to be more common than with urethral catheterization (Winder, 1994),
- ◆ Discomfort, particularly from the tip of the catheter irritating the sensitive trigone area of the bladder
- ◆ Urethral leakage in females in association with catheter blockage or clamping (Barnes *et al.*, 1993)

Care of the suprapubic catheter

The nursing care is the same as for urethral catheters and exactly the same principles of management apply. Secretions which often occur around the catheter site can be removed during bathing with soap, water and a clean cloth. A dressing may be required if secretions soil clothing but this is not essential. Overgranulation of the tissue at the puncture site can be eradicated through the use of silver nitrate sticks.

Changing the catheter is a simple procedure which can be easily under-taken by nursing staff on the ward or in the patient's home, according to local policy. In some cases, the patient or carers may be taught to change the catheter. Care should be taken when inserting a suprapubic catheter that the catheter tip does not migrate into the urethra (Motiwala *et al.*, 1992). If this occurs, the catheter may be palpated in the male urethra, and visualized extruding from the urethral meatus in the female. In some instances, urethral closure may be performed after insertion of the suprapubic catheter if ure-thral leakage is a problem (Feneley, 1983).

Barnes *et al.* (1993) also recommended the use of anticholinergic drugs with a regimen of daily clamping and release of the catheter to maintain bladder capacity, thereby reducing the risk of ureteric reflux. Ineffective use of anticholinergic drugs to suppress bladder contractions was found to relate directly to increased urethral loss. After removal of the catheter, the channel should heal rapidly under a dressing.

SEXUALITY AND BODY IMAGE

The problems resulting from permanent catheterization are not only physical but also invade emotional well-being. Although this form of urinary drainage may provide increased freedom it can also severely interfere with self-esteem and dignity. However, when the alternative is the constant need for pads to control incontinence, a UDS can be a very positive form of management. Attending to individual needs and lifestyle will go a long way to ensuring optimum quality of life for the catheterized person.

Many able-bodied people have complexes about how their partners view them and so it is perfectly natural for catheterized patients to have anxieties about whether or not their partner still finds them sexually attractive. Involving the partner in the management of the UDS may not only be necessary but can also help the partner demonstrate that it does not affect a deep and loving relationship.

It is a common misconception that the presence of a urethral catheter precludes sexual intercourse. If the bladder dysfunction coexists with a physical disability, the feeling that sex is no longer possible is likely to be enhanced. This belief has been compounded by the fact that little, if any, sexual advice is given to patients with urethral catheters. A study of 36 catheterized men and women found that no professional carer had voluntarily discussed sex with any of the patients fitted with a catheter, and the patients did not know that intercourse was possible with a catheter in situ (Roe and Brocklehurst, 1987). Fifty per cent of the men questioned stated that they no longer experienced erections, and in those who did, pain was a common experience.

Sexual behaviour encompasses a range of activities from caressing, kissing and masturbation to penetration of the vagina by the penis. Therefore, it should be remembered that many people enjoy active and fulfilling sex lives without penetration taking place.

It is possible for the patient or the partner to be taught to remove the catheter and replace it after intercourse has taken place. Women can tape the catheter onto the abdomen where it will come to no harm. Men can tape the catheter along the erect penis and secure it under a condom. The drainage bag, once emptied, can be positioned out of the way in the bed, although care should be taken that the drainage tubing does not become compressed, preventing urine from draining from the bladder. Alternatively, the drainage bag can be disconnected from the catheter and a spigot attached during intercourse. A water-based lubricant can be used to facilitate insertion. Oil-based lubricants should not be used as these will rot the rubber condom and may damage the catheter. Whenever possible, a suprapubic catheter rather than a urethral catheter should be used.

The patient should be counselled about position during intercourse. While a comfortable position, in which the patient can relax, should be sought, some positions can cause increased traction on the catheter in females. An example of this is a face to face position with the male on top. Traction can be reduced by placing a pillow under the woman's bottom to raise the pelvis. Alternatively, a lateral rear entry position, where the man lies facing the woman's back, may be preferable.

These intimate problems need to be addressed in the early stages of catheterization before relationship problems have a chance to develop. Some health authorities have a sexual counsellor who will be able to offer advice and practical suggestions. In the UK, the patient's general practitioner or local Relate branch should be able to suggest other local facilities that offer this type of service.

Reading books such as *Treat Yourself to Sex – A Guide to Good Loving* by Paul Brown and Carolyn Faulder or *Sex: How to Make it Better for Both of You* by Dr Martin Cole and Professor Windy Dryden can help patients and their partners to establish sexual needs and promote discussion. The Association to Aid the Sexual and Personal Relationships of People with a Disability (SPOD: Sexual Problems of the Disabled, 286 Camden Road, London N7 0BJ) is a useful educational and informative resource for carers and clients.

CLEAN INTERMITTENT SELF-CATHETERIZATION

Clean intermittent self-catheterization (CISC) is an alternative method of bladder drainage whereby a catheter is passed into the bladder by the patient and removed once drainage is complete. It is a relatively simple procedure which can easily be taught by a nurse.

The increasing popularity of CISC is largely due to the work carried out by Lapides and his colleagues in the USA. They suggested that 'most cases of urinary tract infections are caused by some structural or functional abnormality of the urogenital tract, which leads to a decreased resistance of tissue to bacterial invasion' (Lapides *et al.*, 1974). They postulated that high intravesical pressures caused by a build-up of residual urine would compromise the vascular supply to the bladder and render the patient more vulnerable to infection. Thus they emphasized the importance of regular bladder drainage.

Lapides' studies have shown that intermittent catheterization markedly reduces the complications associated with permanent indwelling catheterization and that there is no advantage to be gained from the use of sterile intermittent self-catheterization over the clean technique in terms of increased urinary tract infection or renal damage. These findings have been based on follow-up over a number of years and have been corroborated by a number of researchers (Lapides *et al.*, 1972, 1974, 1976; Champion, 1976; Webb *et al.*, 1990).

Indications for CISC

The CISC technique is suitable for the drainage of residual urine resulting from most causes. It is most commonly used in the presence of an upper or lower motor neurone lesion, but is also appropriate in cases of diabetic neuropathy and mechanical outflow obstruction if surgery is not indicated or does not relieve the retention completely. It may be used for postoperative retention and can be used on a temporary or permanent basis.

The technique is equally suitable for males and females of all ages although location of the urethra is generally easier for males. Children of 4 years and older can be taught the procedure with parental supervision (Eckstein, 1979) and it is a technique widely used in children with spina bifida. It can also be taught to elderly people (Lawrence and MacDonagh, 1988) who may develop urinary symptoms from a build-up of residual urine due to decreased contractility of the detrusor muscle with increasing age.

Types of catheter

Because CISC does not require the catheter to be retained in the bladder, it need not have a retention balloon. Two types of catheter are commonly used, the Nelaton and Scott catheters (see Figure 5.1). The Nelaton catheter is made from soft plastic with two drainage eyes at one end and a funnel at the other and comes in two different lengths for males and females. Females, particularly those using wheelchairs, may prefer to use the length intended for males, to facilitate the drainage of urine directly into the toilet (Winder, 1995). The Scott catheter is made of harder plastic which provides increased rigidity to aid insertion and does not have a funnelled end. It is not unknown for patients to cut off the funnelled end of a Nelaton catheter to speed up drainage. However, this has resulted in the catheter disappearing into the bladder (Morgan and Weston, 1990) and thus cannot be recommended. The Scott catheter is only suitable for negotiating the female urethra and thus is only manufactured in the shorter length. Silver and stainless steel catheters are also available. The manufacturer's recommendations on cleaning are that the silver catheters should be washed in soapy water followed by boiling for 10–20 minutes daily, and the stainless steel catheters should similarly be washed and then baked in a preheated oven at 180°C (350°F) for 10 minutes. It has also been suggested that any deposits that build up in the bore of the catheter and are resistant to normal cleansing procedures can be removed ultrasonically (personal communication with S. & G. Payne, 1996).

The smallest size of catheter that will drain the urine at an acceptable speed should be used. It is important in the 'normalization' of bladder emptying for patients using CISC that they do not have to spend excessive time in the toilet, and thus slightly larger Charrière catheters, for example 14 CH or 16 CH, can be used.

Lubrication

Most catheters require lubrication to aid insertion. However, there is now available a range of self-lubricating, hydrophilic catheters which, when dipped into water, become extremely slippery. These catheters are recommended for single use only by the manufacturers since the lubricant effect may be reduced with subsequent use. Such low-friction, disposable catheters have been shown to cause less urethral trauma than PVC catheters (Hellstrom *et al.*, 1991; Vaidyanathan *et al.*, 1994) and to be more acceptable, convenient and easier to handle for both new and existing users (Diokno et al, 1995).

Patients learning CISC with an uncoated catheter are usually taught to use an anaesthetic lubricant initially, although many will then prefer to use water instead. If a tube of jelly is to be used for a number of catheterizations, it is recommended that the first squirt of gel is discarded. Excessive use of gel has been reported as being a factor in increased infection rates (Winder, 1993).

Criteria for successful use of CISC

Probably the most important criteria for the success of CISC are motivation, cognitive skills and manual dexterity. If the patient is unwilling to perform the procedure or does not understand the importance of regular bladder drainage, then the complications of urinary tract infection and upper tract dilatation are likely. For disabled females in particular, the ability to achieve a position which allows access to the urethra is vital, and in both sexes a level of dexterity to enable handling of the catheter is essential. Partners or relatives may be required to assist and therefore need to be supportive of the procedure.

Frequency of catheterization

One of the aims of CISC is to allow increased freedom and the chance to return to a more normal lifestyle than that offered by permanent catheterization. Therefore, it is important that CISC should not need to be performed at an unacceptable frequency, or take an unacceptable length of time. Assessment of the functional capacity of the bladder either by cystometry or through the use of a frequency chart will help to determine the frequency with which catheterization may be required. Too infrequent catheterization can lead to hydronephrosis which can be resolved by increasing the frequency of catheterizations. It is usually felt that every 2 hours is the maximum frequency which is acceptable during waking hours, and that sleep should be undisturbed.

It is commonly believed that intermittent catheterization should be carried out at a frequency that maintains the sum of the voided volume plus the residual volume at below 400–500 ml (Alderman, 1988). However, many patients catheterize only once or twice a day without any apparent harmful effects. In practice, CISC is a means by which the patient can control bladder emptying and symptoms, thus regimens should be encouraged to suit individual needs. For example, an extra catheterization before a period in which reaching a toilet would be impossible or prior to sexual intercourse is perfectly acceptable.

If the patient is also experiencing symptoms of a hyperreflexic bladder, such as frequency of micturition, urgency, urge incontinence, nocturia and nocturnal enuresis, anticholinergic drugs can be used. In some cases, high bladder pressures or a small bladder capacity can be remedied using the surgical procedure known as clam cystoplasty.

Learning CISC

Manual dexterity may prohibit some people from learning CISC, although most people can learn if sufficiently motivated, making use of a range of devices designed to assist in the procedure. Plastic 'handles' have been found to be a popular aid to CISC amongst a group of female users (Norton, 1993).

Poor eyesight or even complete blindness do not preclude this form of management. Providing the patient is able to identify the urethral meatus without contamination of the catheter tip and is able to clean the catheter afterwards, deficient eyesight should not present any problems.

Some people find it easier to learn CISC by touch from the outset, thus giving them an advantage when catheterizing over the toilet. This method of learning is useful when teaching elderly females with reduced spinal flexion coupled with poor eyesight which prevents them identifying the meatus using a mirror. However, many women learn CISC by lying or sitting in a comfortable position either on the bed or floor, with legs apart; a magnifying mirror and a good light source will allow identification of the meatus and passage of the catheter. Gentian violet may be used to highlight the meatus. A small dish or bowl can be used to collect the urine drained. Alternatively, there are catheters manufactured with an integral collecting bag to prevent the problem of spillage.

For some people, the effort of getting into a suitable position for CISC will be impossible or impracticable on a regular basis (Henderson, 1989), and the Deavin–Hunt device has been specifically designed to enable identification of the meatus using a mirror while in a wheelchair (Hunt and Whitaker, 1990).

Whichever technique is used for learning CISC, it is always important that the patient is as relaxed as possible and has had plenty of time to discuss with the nurse or doctor the advantages and disadvantages of the technique. Women should be shown a diagram of female genitalia and given an opportunity to familiarize themselves with their own genitalia as well as the equipment to be used. The nurse should observe the patient in all aspects of the procedure including preparation, passage of the catheter and cleaning and storage of the catheter afterwards. The nurse should ensure that the patient is familiar with potential problems, and knows how to recognize and respond to them. Written information should be provided to cover all the aspects mentioned above, as well as prescription details. There are also videos available aimed at the patient learning CISC which can be a useful teaching aid.

All questions should be answered as comprehensively as possible using terminology appropriate to the individual. Patients catheterizing at home should have easy access to their nurse and doctor and should receive as much support as they require. This will vary widely according to individual patient circumstances, but listening to the patient's needs will minimize the number of people who abandon the technique because of problems to which there is often a simple solution. If the procedure is being taught in hospital, thought should be given to how the patient will manage at home and whether adequate support can be given.

Hygiene

Hands should be thoroughly washed before and after catheterization, preferably with soap and water, although wet wipes may be used as an alternative when hand-washing facilities are unavailable. After the catheter has been withdrawn it should be washed using soapy water and the outside dried. Care should be taken to ensure that globules of lubricating jelly are flushed out from around the tip of the catheter. Hunt and Oakeshott (1993) recommended that catheters should be stored in sodium hypochlorite solution or boiled for 30 seconds after use. However, these recommendations are not backed up by other authors or recommended by manufacturers of PVC catheters. The catheter can be kept in a small plastic bag which is stored in an appropriate receptacle; as discretion and normality are so important, such receptacles may include pencil cases, make-up bags or knitting-needle holders. When the patient is at home, keeping the catheter in the refrigerator helps to maintain its rigidity and may reduce bacterial multiplication. Most uncoated Nelaton catheters can be reused for up to a week, although this practice must be based on the manufacturer's recommendations. Moore *et al.* (1993) found no advantage in using a sterile catheter for each insertion over reusing catheters.

Treatment of urethral strictures

The first of the hydrophilic catheters to be produced has been extensively used in the treatment of urethral strictures, both as a conservative method alone and as a follow-up procedure to urethrotomy. Regular urethral dilation using a low-friction catheter has been recommended as reducing the number of patients with strictures who will require urethroplasty or delaying the need for surgery, and is an acceptable method to men (Robertson *et al.*, 1991). The use of this type of catheter has been found to result in the development of fewer strictures after urethrotomy (Bodker *et al.*, 1992; Kjaergaard *et al.*, 1994). Harriss *et al.* (1994) recommended that dilation should continue for at least 1 year to ensure urethral stabilization and absence of stricture recurrence over 5 years.

Potential problems with CISC

Urinary tract infections

A reduction in the incidence of UTI associated with CISC has been reported by Lapides *et al.* (1976) and Wyndaele and Maes (1990). However, Bakke and Digranes (1991) in one series found that over 50% of patients had bacteriuria, mostly due to *E. coli* infection. Thus it is important that the patient should be able to identify the onset of a UTI, recognizing the signs and symptoms of cloudy, offensive or bloodstained urine, a sudden increase in bladder symptoms, for example urinary urgency, pain on passing urine and feeling generally unwell, with an associated fever. Most bacteriuria has been found to be asymptomatic (Bakke *et al.*, 1993) and treatment with antibiotics is not recommended unless the patient develops systemic symptoms, owing to the risk of developing resistant strains of organisms (Chawla *et al.*, 1988). The emergence of bacteria in the urine may result from increasing residual urine volumes due to poor technique in draining the bladder (Wyndaele and Maes, 1990), which should be observed and residual urine measurements checked. During periods of treatment with antibiotics, it is important that CISC continues to ensure that residual urine does not further contribute to urine infection.

Bleeding

Blood may be evident on the outside of the catheter after initial catheterization and is usually due to slight trauma during insertion. Insertion can be made easier by using a water-based lubricant jelly or a self-lubricating catheter. Haematuria also occurrs in association with UTI (Bakke *et al.*, 1993). If the bleeding becomes heavy or is persistent, a urological opinion should be sought as a matter of urgency and the patient advised to cease catheterization until the bleeding has been investigated.

Pain

Pain is often experienced during early catheterization and can be worsened by tension and anxiety. Good lubrication and the use of an anaesthetic jelly for men and women can reduce the discomfort. Men should be shown how to position the penis during insertion of the catheter to minimize trauma caused as the catheter passes through the curved portions of the urethra. Postmenopausal women may experience discomfort from trauma to de-oestrogenized tissue, particularly when they are not skilled at identifying the urethral meatus. Hormone replacement therapy can improve the quality of the urethral tissue, and reassurance that it often takes much practice to be able to insert the catheter easily can help to relax the patient.

Why should CISC be considered?

Lapides *et al.* (1976) cited CISC as a technique that offers the patient many benefits including improved renal function, a reduction in incontinence, improved bladder emptying, a reduction in UTIs and enhanced mental and emotional well-being, as well as an improved quality of life for patients and their relatives. Being able to dispense with the burden of a catheter or the need to wear incontinence pads has revolutionized the lives of many people:

'Words cannot express how different I feel. No more pads, it is marvellous. Nobody knew what I was going through. I was too ashamed and embarrassed to talk to anybody about it, not even my own mother.'

'I now feel far more confident in myself. I look forward to going out and getting dressed up. I wish I had known about self-catheterization two and a half years ago, then I wouldn't have had two and a half years of utter misery' (Sibley, 1988).

Using CISC has enabled many patients to regain control of their bladder rather than their bladder controlling their lives.

Intermittent catheterization

There are a number of people for whom self-catheterization is impossible. This may be due to physical disability such as quadriplegia, or a psychological inability to accept the technique. In these instances, intermittent catheterization (IC) can be performed by a carer who may be a friend, relative or nurse. Nurses should use an aseptic technique because of the risk of cross-infection whether in the hospital or the patient's home, and a fresh catheter should be used for each catheterization.

When embarking on a programme of IC or CISC in hospital, it is extremely important to consider whether it will be practical in the home situation. It is often useful to teach another person IC as a back-up during times of reduced ability.

CONCLUSION

This chapter aimed to provide nurses with the information required to safely establish and manage a method for urinary drainage using either indwelling or intermittent catheterization. The wide range of equipment and factors to be taken into account when establishing such a system have been presented alongside arguments for and against different types of drainage. This area of nursing care remains predominantly that of the nurse, who thus has an obligation to use this knowledge in the best interests of patients to enhance their well-being and to assist them towards acceptance of the need for an alternative method of urinary drainage.

REFERENCES

ALDERMAN C (1988) DIY catheters freedom. *Nursing Standard* **2**: 25-26.
ASSOCIATION OF CONTINENCE ADVISORS (1988) *Directory of Continence and Toiletting Aids*, 3rd edn. London: ACA.
AVORN J, Monane M, Gurwitz J H et al (1994) Reduction of bacteriuria and pyuria after ingestion of cranberry juice. *Journal of the American Medical Association* **271**: 751–754.
BAILEY S (1991) Using bladder washouts. *Nursing Times* **87**(24): 75–76.
BAKKE A and Digranes A (1991) Bacteriuria in patients treated with clean intermittent catheterisation. *Scandinavian Journal of Infectious Diseases* **23**, 577–582.
BAKKE A, Vollset S E, Hoisaeter P A and Irgens L M (1993) Physical complications in patients treated with clean intermittent catheterisation. *Scandinavian Journal of Urology* **27**: 55–61.
BARNES K and Malone-Lee J (1986) Long-term catheter management: minimising the problem of premature replacement due to balloon deflation. *Journal of Advanced Nursing* **11**: 303–307.
BARNES D G, Shaw P J R, Timoney A G and Tsokos N (1993) Management of the neuropathic bladder by supra-pubic catheterisation. *British Journal of Urology* **72**: 169–172.
BARNETT J (1991) Preventive procedures. *Nursing Times* **87**(10): 66–68.
BEARMAN E (1985) I'll never take bladder catheters for granted again. *Registered Nurse* December: 30–32.
BLACKLOCK N J (1986) Catheters and urethral strictures. *British Journal of Urology* **58**: 475–478.
BLANDY J P and Moors J (1989) *Urology for Nurses*. London: Blackwell.
BLANNIN J P and Hobden J (1980) The catheter of choice. *Nursing Times* **76**: 2092–2093.
BODKER A, Ostri P, Rye-Anderson J et al (1992) Treatment of recurrent urethral stricture by

internal urethrotomy and intermittent self-catheterisation: a controlled study of a new therapy. *Journal of Urology* **48**: 308–310.

BRADLEY C, Babb J, Davies J and Ayliffe G (1986) Taking precautions. *Nursing Times* 5 March: 70–73.

BROCKLEHURST J C, Hickey D, Davies I et al (1988) A new urethral catheter. *British Medical Journal* **296**: 1691–1693.

BRUCE A W, Sira S S, Clark A F and Awad S A (1974) The problem of catheter encrustation. *Canadian Medical Journal* **111**: 238–241.

BULL E, Chilton C P, Gould C A L and Sutton T M (1991) Single-blind, randomised parallel group study of the Bard Biocath and a silicone-elastomer coated catheter. *British Journal of Urology* **68**: 394–399.

BURKE J P, Garibaldi R A, Britt M R et al (1981) Prevention of catheter-associated urinary tract infections. *American Journal of Medicine* **70**: 655–658.

BURKITT D and Randall J (1987) Catheterisation: Urethral trauma. *Nursing Times* **83**(43): 59–63.

CHAMPION V L (1976) Clean technique for intermittent self-catheterisation. *Nursing Research* **25**(1): 13–18.

CHAWLA J C, Clayton C L and Stickler D J (1988) Antiseptics in the long-term urological management of patients by intermittent catheterisation. *British Journal of Urology* **62**: 289–294.

CHILLINGTON B (1992) Early removal advances discharge home. *Professional Nurse* November: 84–89.

CHRISP J M and Nacey J N (1990) Foley catheter balloon puncture and the risk of free fragment formation. *British Journal of Urology* **66**: 500–502.

COLLEY W (1994) Indwelling urinary catheters. *Nursing Times* **90**(43): 70.

COX A J (1990) Comparison of catheter surface morphologies. *British Journal of Urology* **65**: 55–60.

COX A J, Hukins D W L and Sutton T M (1988) Comparison of in vitro encrustation on silicone and hydrogel-coated latex catheters. *British Journal of Urology* **61**: 156–161.

CROW R, Chapman R, Roe B and Wilson J (1986) *A Study of Patients with an Indwelling Catheter and Related Nursing Practice*. Guildford: University of Surrey Nursing Practice Research Unit.

CROW R, Mulhall A and Chapman R (1988) Indwelling catheterisation and related nursing practice. *Journal of Advanced Nursing* **13**: 489–495.

CRUMMEY V (1989) Ignorance can hurt. *Nursing Times* **85**(21): 67–68.

DANCE D A B, Pearson A D, Seal D V and Lowes J A (1987) A hospital outbreak caused by a chlorhexidine and antibiotic resistant strain of *Proteus mirabilis*. *Journal of Hospital Infection* **10**: 10–16.

DAVIES A J, Desai H N, Turton S and Dyas A (1987) Does instillation of Chlorhexidine into the bladder of catheterised patients help reduce bacteriuria? *Journal of Hospital Infection* **9**: 72–75.

DIOKNO A C, Mitchell B A, Nash A J and Kimbrough J A (1995) Patient satisfaction and the Lofric catheter for clean intermittent catheterisation. *Journal of Urology* **153: 349–351.**

DoH (1993) *Urinary Drainage Leg Bags: an Evaluation*. Medical Devices Directorate, June. London: Department of Health.

DUDLEY M N and Barriere S L (1981) Anti-microbial irrigations in the prevention and treatment of catheter-related urinary tract infections. *American Journal of Hospital Pharmacy* **38**: 59–65.

ECKSTEIN H B (1979) Intermittent catheterisation of the bladder in patients with neuropathic incontinence of urine. *Zeitschrift fur Kinderchirurgie und Grenzgebiete* **28**(4): 408–412.

EDWARDS L E, Lock R, Powell C and Jones P (1983) Post-catheterisation urethral strictures: a clinical and experimental study. *British Journal of Urology* **55**: 53–56.

EKELUND P, Anderstrom C, Johansson S L and Larsson P (1983) The reversibility of catheter-associated polypoid cystitis. *Journal of Urology* **130**: 456–459.

ELLIOT T S J, Gopal Rao G, Rigby R G and Woodhouse K (1989) Bladder irrigation or irritation? *British Journal of Urology* **64**(4): 391–394.

FALKINER F R (1993) The insertion and management of indwelling catheters – minimising the risk of infection. *Journal of Hospital Infection* **25**: 79–90.

FENELEY R C L (1983) The management of female incontinence by supra-pubic catheterisation, with or without urethral closure. *British Journal of Urology* **55**: 203–207.

FLACK S (1993) Finding the best solution. *Nursing Times* **89**(11): 68–74.

GETLIFFE K A (1993) Freeing the system. *Nursing Standard* **8**(7): 16–18.

GETLIFFE K A (1994) The characteristics and management of patients with recurrent blockage of long-term urinary catheters. *Journal of Advanced Nursing* **20**: 140–149.

GETLIFFE K A (1995) Long-term catheter use in the community. *Nursing Standard* **9**(31): 25–27.

GETLIFFE K A and Mulhall A B (1991) The encrustation of catheters. *British Journal of Urology* **67**: 337–341.

GIBBS H (1986) Catheter toilet and urinary tract infections. *Nursing Times* 4 June: 75–76.

GILLESPIE W A, Lennon G G, Linton K B and Phippen G A (1967) Prevention of urinary infection by means of closed drainage into a sterile plastic bag. *British Medical Journal* **3**: 90–92.

GIVENS C D and Wenzel R P (1980) Catheter-associated urinary tract infections in surgical patients: a controlled study on the excess morbidity and costs. *Journal of Urology* **124**: 646–648.

GLENISTER H (1987) The passage of infection. *Nursing Times* **83**(22): 68–73.

GRIFFITHS G (1985) Urinary drainage in patients with spinal injuries. *Nursing Times* December 4: 63–67.

HAMMARSTEN J and Lindqvist K (1992) Supra-pubic catheter following transurethral resection of the prostate: a way to decrease the number of urethral strictures and improve the outcome of operations. *Journal of Urology* **147**: 648–652.

HARRISS D R, Beckingham I J, Lemberger R J and Lawrence W T (1994) Long-term results of intermittent low-friction self-catheterisation in patients with recurrent urethral strictures. *British Journal of Urology* **74**: 790–792.

HASHISAKI P, Swenson J, Mooney B et al (1984) Decontamination of urinary bags for rehabilitation patients. *Archives of Physical and Medical Rehabilitation* **65**: 474–476.

HEDELIN H, Bratt C G, Eckerdal G and Lincoln K (1991) Relationship between urease-producing bacteria, urinary pH and encrustation on indwelling urinary catheters. *British Journal of Urology* **67**: 527–531.

HELLSTROM P, Tammela T, Lukkarinen O and Kontturi M (1991) Efficacy and safety of clean intermittent self-catheterisation in adults. *European Urology* **20**: 117–121.

HENDERSON J S (1989) Intermittent clean self-catheterisation in clients with neurogenic bladder resulting from multiple sclerosis. *Journal of Neuroscience Nursing* **21**(3): 160–164.

HENRY M (1992) Catheter confusion. *Nursing Times* **88**(42): 65–72.

HILTON P and Stanton S L (1980) Procedures in practice: supra-pubic catheterisation. *British Medical Journal* **281**: 1261–1263.

HUNT G and Oakeshott P (1993) Self-catheterisation: worth a trial. *Geriatric Medicine* April: 17–18.

HUNT G M and Whitaker R H (1990) A new device for self-catheterisation in wheelchair bound women. *British Journal of Urology* **66**: 162–163.

KASS E H (1957) Bacteriuria and the diagnosis of infections of the urinary tract. *Archives of Internal Medicine* **100**: 709–714.

KENNEDY A (1983a) Incontinence advice: long-term catheterisation. *Nursing Times* **79**(17): 41–45.

KENNEDY A (1983b) Care of the elderly catheterised. *British Journal of Geriatric Nursing* **2**(6): 10–15.

KENNEDY A (1984a) Catheter concepts. *Nursing Mirror* **159**(15): 42–44.

KENNEDY A (1984b) An extra hot water bottle? *Nursing Times* **80**(17): 57–61.

KENNEDY A (1984c) Trial of a new bladder washout system. *Nursing Times* **14**: 48–51.

KENNEDY A, Brocklehurst J C and Lye M D W (1983) Factors related to the problems of long-term catheterisation. *Journal of Advanced Nursing* **8**: 207–212.

KJAERGAARD B, Walter S, Bartholin J et al (1994) Prevention of urethral stricture occurrence using clean intermittent self-catheterisation. *British Journal of Urology* **73**: 692–695.

KOHLER-OCKMORE J (1992) Urinary catheter complications. *Journal of District Nursing* February: 18–20.

KUNIN C M (1989) *Detection, Prevention and Management of Urinary Tract Infection*, 3rd edn. Philadelphia: Lea & Febiger.

KUNIN C M, Chin Q F and Chambers S (1987) Formation of encrustations on indwelling urinary catheters in the elderly: a comparison of different types of material in blockers and non-blockers. *Journal of Urology* **138**: 899–902.

KUNIN C M, Douthitt S, Dancing J et al (1992) The association between the use of urinary catheters and morbidity and mortality among elderly patients in nursing homes. *American Journal of Epidemiology* **135**(3): 291–301.

LAPIDES J, Diokno A C, Silber S J and Lowe B S (1972) Clean intermittent self-catheterisation in the treatment of urinary tract disease. *Journal of Urology* **107**: 458–461.

LAPIDES J, Diokno A C, Lowe B S and Kalish M D (1974) Follow-up on unsterile intermittent self-catheterisation. *Journal of Urology* **111**: 184–187.

LAPIDES J, Diokno A C, Gould F R and Lowe B S (1976) Further observation on self-catheterisation. *Journal of Urology* **116**: 116–119.

LAWRENCE W T and MacDonagh R P (1988) Treatment of urethral stricture disease by internal urethrotomy followed by intermittent 'low-friction' self-catheterisation preliminary communication. *Journal of the Royal Society of Medicine* **81**: 136–139.

LOWTHIAN P (1989) Preventing trauma. *Nursing Times* **85**(21): 73–75.

McCULLOUGH J (1989) Catheter care at home. *Community Outlook: Nursing Times* **85**: 4–8.

MEERS P D, Ayliffe G A J, Emmerson A M et al (1981) Report on the national survey of infection in hospitals: 1981. *Journal of Hospital Infection* **2** (suppl.): 25–28.

MOISEY C U and Williams L A (1980) Self-retained balloon catheters: a safe method for removal. *British Journal of Urology* **52**: 67.

MOORE K N, Kelm M, Sinclair O and Cadrain G (1993) Bacteriuria in intermittent catheterisation users: the effect of sterile versus clean re-used catheters. *Rehabilitation Nursing* **18**(5): 306–309.

MORGAN J D T and Weston P M T (1990) The disappearing catheter – a complication of intermittent catheterisation. *British Journal of Urology* **65**(1): 113–114.

MOTIWALA H G, Amlani J C, Visana K N and Patel P C (1992) Migration of supra-pubic catheter to anterior urethra. *British Journal of Urology* **69**(2): 211–212.

MULHALL A (1991) Biofilms and urethral catheter infections. *Nursing Standard* **5**(18): 26–29.

NACEY J N and Delahunt B (1991) Toxicity study of first and second generation hydrogel-coated latex urinary catheters. *British Journal of Urology* **57**: 314–316.

NACEY J N, Tulloch A G S, Ferguson A F (1985) Catheter induced urethritis: a comparison between latex and silicone catheters in a prospective clinical trial. *British Journal of Urology* **57**: 325–328.

NOBLE J G, Menzies D, Cox P J and Edwards L (1990) Midnight removal: an improved approach to removal of catheters. *British Journal of Urology* **65**: 615–617.

NORTON C (1986) *Nursing for Continence.* Beaconsfield: Beaconsfield Publishers.

NORTON C (1993) A helping handle. *Nursing Times* **89**(16): 76–78.

PARSONS C L, Mulholland S G and Anwar H (1970) Antibacterial activity of bladder surface mucin duplicated by exogenous glycosaminoglycan (heparin). *Infection and Immunity* **25**: 552–554.

PLATT R, Polk B F, Murdock B and Rosner B (1989) Prevention of catheter-associated urinary tract infection: a cost benefit analysis. *Infection Control Hospital Epidemiology* **10**(2): 60–64.

POMFRET I (1991) The catheter debate. *Nursing Times* **87**(37): 67–68.

POMFRET I (1992) Conformacath update. *Journal of Community Nursing* November: 14–16.

REID R I, Pead P J, Webster O and Maskell R (1982) Comparison of urine bag changing regimens in elderly catheterised patients. *Lancet* **ii**: 754–756.

ROBERTS J B M, Linton K B, Pollard B R et al (1965) Long-term catheter drainage in the male. *British Journal of Urology* **37**: 63–72.

ROBERTSON G S M, Everitt N, Lamprecht J R et al (1991) Treatment of recurrent urethral strictures using clean intermittent self-catheterisation. *British Journal of Urology* **68**: 89–92.

ROE B (1989a) Long-term catheter care in the community. *Nursing Times* **85**(36): 43–44.

ROE B (1989b) Use of bladder washouts: A study of nurses' recommendations. *Journal of Advanced Nursing* **14**: 494–500.

ROE B (1990) Do we need to clamp catheters? *Nursing Times* **86**(43): 66–67.

ROE B (1992a) The use of indwelling catheters. In *Clinical Nursing Practice: The Promotion and Management of Continence.* London: Prentice-Hall.

ROE B (1992b) From Pompeii to the present. *Nursing Times* **88**(31): 57–60.

ROE B (1993) Catheter-associated urinary tract infection: a review. *Journal of Clinical Nursing* **2**: 97–203.

ROE B and Brocklehurst J C (1987) Study of patients with indwelling catheters. *Journal of Advanced Nursing* **12**: 713–718.

ROE B, Reid F J and Brocklehurst J C (1988) A comparison of four drainage systems. *Journal of Advanced Nursing* **13**: 374–382.

ROGERS J (1991) Pass the cranberry juice. *Nursing Times* **87**(48): 36–37.

RUUTU M, Alfthan O, Talja M and Andersson L C (1985) Cytotoxicity of latex urinary catheters. *British Journal of Urology* **57**: 82–87.

RYAN-WOOLLEY B (1987) *Aids for the Management of Incontinence.* London: King's Fund.

SABOTA A E (1984) Inhibition of bacterial adherence by cranberry juice: potential use for the treatment of urinary tract infection. *Journal of Urology* **131**: 1013–1016.

SIBLEY L (1988) Confidence with incontinence. *Nursing Times* **84**(46): 42–43.

SLADE N and Gillespie W A (1985) *The Urinary Tract and the Catheter: Infection and Other Related Problems.* Chichester: John Wiley.

STICKLER D J, Clayton C L and Chawla J C (1987) The resistance of urinary tract pathogens to chlorhexidine bladder washouts. *Journal of Hospital Infection* **10**: 28–39.

STUDER U E, Bishop M C and Zing E J (1983) How to fill a silicone catheter balloon. *Urology* **22**(3): 300–302.

VAIDYANATHAN S, Soni B M, Dundas S and Krishnan K R (1994) Urethral cytology in spinal cord injury patients performing intermittent catheterisation. *Paraplegia* **32**: 493–500.

WEBB R J, Lawson A L and Neal D E (1990) Clean intermittent self-catheterisation in 172 adults. *British Journal of Urology* **65**(1): 20–23.

WILKSCH J, Vernon-Roberts B, Garrett R and Smith K (1983) The role of catheter surface morphology and extractable cytotoxic material in tissue reactions to urethral catheters. *British Journal of Urology* **55**: 48–52.

WINDER A (1993) Intermittent self-catheterisation. In B Roe (ed.), *Clinical Nursing Practice: The Promotion and Management of Continence,* p. 163. London: Prentice Hall.

WINDER A (1994) Supra-pubic catheterisation. *Community Outlook* December: 25.

WINDER A (1995) Intermittent self-catheterisation. *Journal of Community Nursing* February: 24–28.

WRIGHT E (1989) Teaching patients to cope with catheters at home. *Professional Nurse* **4**(19): 191–194.

WYNDAELE J and Maes D (1990) Clean intermittent self-catheterisation: a 12-year follow up. *Journal of Urology* **143**: 906–908.

FURTHER READING

BROWN P and Faulder C (1989) *Treat Yourself to Sex – A Guide to Good Loving,* 2nd edn. Penguin.

COLE M and Dryden W (1993) *Sex: How to Make it Better for Both of You.* 2nd edn. Vermillion.

URINARY TRACT STONES

6

Contents

Urinary calculi are among the most common of urological problems. It is estimated that 2–5% of the UK population suffer with stones in the urinary tract, with 20–40% of these sufferers requiring hospitalization owing to pain, urinary tract obstruction or infection (Lingeman et al, 1990a). Relics of Egyptian skeletons dating back to 4800 BC offer the earliest evidence of urinary calculi, and some of the earliest surgical procedures described are operations for stone removal. Particularly in recent years, enormous advances have been made in the treatment and removal of urinary calculi. However, urinary calculi continue to cause problems, particularly for those living in Europe, North America and Japan. This is believed to be due to an affluent diet rich in refined foods and protein (Fellström et al, 1989).

CAUSES OF RENAL STONE FORMATION

Many patients with a stone-forming tendency have abnormal crystallization in the urine. Diseases that result in excessive urinary excretion of solutes such as calcium, oxalates, amino acids (e.g. cystine) or urates exacerbate this tendency to crystallization. If there is any nucleus on which the crystals can grow, for example another fragment of stone, sloughed renal papillae, or a foreign body such as a stent, a suture or a urinary catheter, then they may precipitate to form stones. This is especially true if there is some urinary obstruction, stagnant pockets of urine (as found in medullary sponge kidneys, for example) or if the patient has reduced mobility.

Many renal calculi have a nucleus made up of microcrystals of precipitated solute embedded in a substance known as the matrix, which is a mucoprotein/protein complex probably secreted by renal tubular cells. Eighty-five per cent of stone-forming patients have matrix substance A which develops calcium-binding properties in the urine. As substance A is not found in the urine of patients free from renal stone disease, it is thought that matrix deposition may be the precursor of stone formation.

All patients having treatment for renal stones, either surgical or medical, should undergo evaluation to identify specific metabolic abnormalities that can sometimes be corrected and thus prevent or minimize further stone formation.

On admission to the ward, the patient with urinary stones needs a full nursing assessment using the appropriate nursing model. This provides a valuable opportunity for the nurse to establish a rapport with the patient and to commence an education programme regarding the prevention of renal stones. The assessment should include:

◆ Present state of health: is the patient suffering from pain? If so, assess for the type, locality and severity of the pain, and how it is best relieved. (The pain that occurs when a kidney stone passes into the ureter is mild at first, but quickly increases to an intensity that many patients find unbearable, requiring pethidine or diclofenac injections for pain relief.) Enquire as to how well the patient actually feels. Enquire into any medication the patient may be taking, prescribed or otherwise, and assess its effects; for example, a patient with a propensity for calcium stones should not be taking phosphate-binding antacids.

◆ Breathing and circulatory state: signs of hypertension may accompany idiopathic hypercalciuria or hyperparathyroidism. A raised blood pressure may also be indicative of deteriorating renal function which could be due to the presence of calculi in the urinary tract.

◆ Maintaining fluid and electrolyte balance: particular attention should be given to the patient's usual daily fluid intake and urine output. Advice should be offered as appropriate to maintain a fluid intake of 3 litres per day. Dipstick urinalysis should be performed and the specific gravity, presence of blood, pH (a urinary pH less than 5.5 is suggestive of a tendency to form uric acid stones), presence of protein and any other abnormalities are recorded. If a 24-hour urine collection for metabolic studies has not been recorded within the last 6 months, then one should be commenced. Blood should be tested for urea, calcium, phosphorus, uric acid, creatinine, etc.

◆ Nutritional status: the nurse should be aware of any present dietary restrictions or requirements; for example an excessive intake of vitamin C can be a cause of hyperoxaluria, as can excessive consumption of calcium or foods high in oxalates. It is important to assess what the patient normally eats at home, and the dietician should be consulted as necessary. Any signs or history of nausea and vomiting, which could be secondary to renal colic, should be noted.

◆ Eliminating body waste: observations should be made for signs of urinary frequency, dysuria, haematuria or urgency of micturition. The nurse should assess urinary stream and check for signs of urinary incontinence. The patient should be assessed for signs of urinary tract infection, and a mid-stream urine specimen sent for microscopy and culture. Enquiries should be made concerning whether the patient has passed any gravel or stone fragments, and if possible these should be obtained for analysis. Bowel actions should also be assessed, as chronic diarrhoea and malabsorption syndrome can both be causes of hyperoxaluria.

◆ Level of independence: observations should be made for signs of mobility impairment, as individuals who have difficulties in moving are more at risk of developing renal stones. In addition, immobilization and skeletal disease can be signs of gout. It should be noted that urinary calculi are more common in professional groups and those working in raised environmental temperatures than in those with active physical employment.

◆ Attitudes to hospitalization: the assessment should also consider the patient's psychological needs. The nurse should look for signs of anxiety and stress, which could arise from the patient feeling powerless and out of control; fear of loss of identity or loss of independence; financial worries, particularly if the patient has had previous hospital admissions; or the patient's anxiety could be related to insufficient knowledge about the reason for admission.

The patient will be assessed by the urologist, and radiological investigations such as a kidney, ureter and bladder X-ray (KUB) will be performed. An intravenous urogram or ultrasound scan may be carried out to identify urinary obstruction. If the patient is pyrexial, blood cultures may be taken and the patient given a course of antibiotics. Any inherited metabolic disorder will be discussed, as will risk factors for recurrence, and if stones have been passed or retrieved, a stone analysis will be performed. If surgical removal of stones is required, then preparations will be made as described below.

TYPES OF RENAL STONE

There are four major types of renal stone:

◆ Struvite or infection stones
◆ Uric acid stones

◆ Calcium-containing stones – mainly calcium oxalate, but also calcium phosphate
◆ Cystine stones

Figure 6.1 illustrates the likely areas of stone formation within the urinary tract.

Struvite stones

Struvite stones are composed of calcium, magnesium and ammonium phosphate, known as 'triple phosphate'. They occur only when the urinary pH is above 7.5 and form only in the presence of chronic urinary tract infection. They are more common in women than in men. Patients with neuropathic bladder are particularly at risk of developing struvite stones (Wasserstein, 1986). They are formed by the action of urease-producing pathogens, espe-

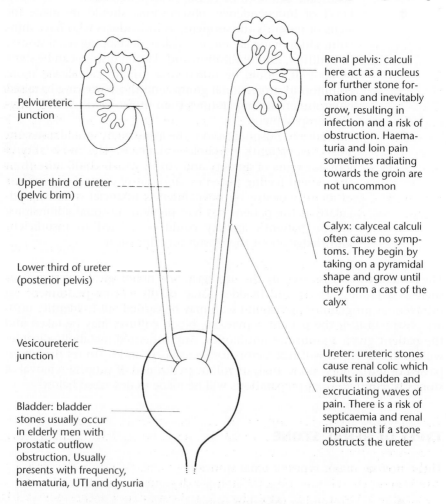

Figure 6.1 *Likely areas of stone formation within the urinary tract*

cially *Proteus mirabilis*, but also *Pseudomonas aeruginosa*, *Klebsiella* and *Enterobacter*, which produce the enzyme urease which hydrolyses urea to form ammonium ions; with the result that the urine becomes intensely alkaline (Lingeman *et al.*, 1990a). The phosphates normally present in urine are insoluble in alkaline urine, resulting in the precipitation of struvite. Struvite stones continue to grow as the bacteria multiply. These stones tend to be soft and crumbly, and grow very rapidly, often forming large, irregular staghorn calculi. They can grow to fill each calyx and the renal pelvis, causing obstruction and damage to the kidney, and can lead to renal failure.

Once formed, struvite stones cannot be dissolved and require lithotripsy or surgical removal. All the fragments must be removed, otherwise any that are remaining will regrow. Following complete removal of the struvite stone, antibiotics such as trimethoprim 200 mg twice daily must be administered for 2–4 weeks, to prevent recurrence of infection in the urinary tract. In order to maintain sterile urine, patients who suffer from recurrent urinary tract infections are often treated with a long-term low-dosage antibiotic, such as trimethoprim 100 mg at night.

Uric acid stones

Uric acid is a normal urinary solute, but is almost insoluble in acid urine; therefore those patients who habitually produce acid urine are at increased risk of developing uric acid stones. These types of stones can grow very large and fill the whole of the collecting system, forming staghorn calculi. It is believed that a raised urinary concentration of uric acid may be a factor in the formation of these stones, but it appears that overall persistent acidity of urine is the most likely cause (Lingeman *et al.*, 1990a). Dehydration resulting in low urinary volume can also result in an increased urinary uric acid concentration. Additional predisposing factors other than a urinary pH persistently less than 5.5 are:

- Hyperuricosuria (up to 40% of patients with uric acid stones have this condition)
- Excessive purine in the diet – derived from foods such as meats (liver, sweetbreads etc.), fish (anchovies), seafood, poultry and yeast
- Gout
- Malignancy
- Obesity
- Metabolic errors such as Lesch–Nyhan syndrome
- Alcohol ingestion

Patients with ileostomies suffer from alkaline losses in the upper gastrointestinal tract which result in a persistently acid and concentrated urine that also predisposes to the formation of uric acid stones.

The normal range of urate present in urine varies with age, diet and sex, and is between 250 mg and 1,000 mg per day. About two-thirds of urate is excreted in urine and the remainder is lost via bile and intestinal and gastric secretion.

Uric acid stones are radiolucent and are only seen on X-ray if they also contain calcium. However, they are echogenic and can be identified by ultrasound, and show up as filling defects on an intravenous urogram (Coe and Parks, 1988).

Initial treatment consists of advising patients to restrict purine in their diets, and limit their meat and fish ingestion to 150–200 g daily. If this fails, allopurinol is indicated for patients with hyperuricosuria. Patients without hyperuricosuria but who have persistently acid urine are advised to increase their urine volumes by drinking at least 3 litres of fluid daily and by taking sodium bicarbonate 10–20 mg daily as prescribed or potassium citrate tablets, in order to maintain a constant urinary pH of 6.5. A urinary pH greater than 7 should be avoided, because of the risk of calcium stone formation due to precipitation of calcium phosphate (Lingeman *et al.*, 1990b). Patients should be taught to check their urinary pH at home.

Calcium-containing stones

Hypercalciuria

The most common type of stones are those that contain calcium, with about 70% of all kidney stones consisting of calcium oxalate or calcium phosphate (Wasserstein, 1986). Hypercalciuria is the most common abnormality in patients with calcium-containing renal calculi and has many causes, including:

- Idiopathic hypercalciuria
- Hyperparathyroidism
- Malignancy, associated with bony metastases or multiple myeloma
- Sarcoid
- Excessive dietary ingestion of calcium and vitamin D (can exacerbate hypercalciuria)
- Renal tubular acidosis
- Medullary sponge kidney
- Prolonged recumbency

Hypercalciuria is identified by urinary calcium excretion of more than 300 mg per day in men and 250 mg per day in women. Known causes of stone development should be treated appropriately, for example patients with distal renal tubular acidosis should be treated with bicarbonate, and those with primary hyperparathyroidism require surgical intervention. However, such a specific diagnosis is not reached with many patients, and therefore efforts should be made to inhibit stone-forming conditions.

A fluid intake of over 3 litres daily is recommended to reduce the chance of calcium precipitating in the urinary tract. Patients should be advised to check their domestic water supply; for example, in London tap water is 'hard', containing about 2.5 mmol l^{-1} (10 mg per 100 ml) of calcium. Sugary drinks which can increase urine calcium excretion should be discouraged, as should orange and cranberry juice which are high in oxalates. Use of antacids and vitamins A, D and C should be kept to a minimum. A moderate intake of calcium of two or three servings daily should be maintained to keep the daily calcium intake to 800 mg. If calcium consumption is too restricted an increased urinary excretion of oxalate results and this leads to a negative calcium balance which can cause osteoporosis (Wasserstein, 1986).

If hypercalciuria persists despite a calcium restriction of 800 mg maximum daily, normal levels are often achieved by the administration of sodium cellulose phosphate 5 g three times daily, half an hour before meals. Sodium cellulose phosphate is an agent that binds intestinal calcium. Thiazide diuretics are often beneficial, as they work by lowering urinary calcium excretion by increasing calcium reabsorption in the renal tubules (Coe and Parks, 1988). For an effective response, patients should also be advised to reduce their dietary sodium intake (Wasserstein, 1986). Bendrofluazide is the drug of choice, and a dosage of 5–10 mg is usually effective.

Hyperoxaluria

Oxalate salts are extremely insoluble and even mild hyperoxaluria may significantly increase the rate of calcium oxalate stone formation. The underlying cause in most hyperoxaluric patients is acquired enteric hyperoxaluria, which occurs as a secondary abnormality in conditions associated with fat malabsorption, for example inflammatory bowel disease, small bowel resection and intestinal bypass.

Primary hyperoxaluria has a poor outlook, and end-stage renal failure is common by the teenage years. At postmortem, oxalate crystals are often found in the renal parenchyma, blood vessels, epiphyses, the heart and the testes. Primary hyperoxaluria is a hereditary condition and often causes more than 100 mg of oxalate excretion daily.

Mild to moderate hyperoxaluria (40–80 mg per day) can be caused by an excessively high intake of foods rich in oxalates, such as grapefruit, cola, tea, strawberries, raspberries, nuts, chocolate, tomatoes, rhubarb and spinach. As ascorbic acid is metabolized to oxalate, the foods rich in vitamin C are therefore also contributory factors to the formation of oxalate stones.

Treatment consists of the patient consuming a low-oxalate, low-fat diet with an increased consumption of foods rich in calcium. If this is unsuccessful, calcium supplements 1–4 g daily in divided doses with meals are prescribed. This does result in increased urinary calcium, but apparently the benefits far exceed the risks. Cholestyramine is sometimes used as it binds both bile salts and oxalates so that they do not injure the colon. It is effective, but most patients do not like it because of its odour and the bulky stools it causes. It also causes vitamin K depletion which must be treated prophylactically.

Cystine stones

Cystine stones are exclusively synonymous with cystinuria. Cystinuria is a rare autosomal recessive disorder of the proximal tubules. A defect of amino acid transportation by the brush border membranes of the proximal tubule results in a failure of tubular reabsorption of the amino acids cystine, ornithine, arginine and lysine (can be remembered using the mnemonic

COAL). In cystinuria, urinary lysine excretion is twice that of cystine but lysine stones do not form, as cystine is much less soluble than lysine in urine. Cystine stones therefore form in the urinary tract while lysine remains inconspicuously in solution.

Cystinuria is frequently diagnosed in the late teenage years and early twenties. It is diagnosed by either a nitroprusside test of the urine which is used as a qualitative screen, or by demonstration of the typical hexagonal shape of cystine crystals in urine. A cystinuric patient may excrete over 200 mg of cystine daily, compared with a normal urinary excretion of up to 40 mg daily.

Cystine stones have a low radio-opacity, but they can be detected on a plain abdominal X-ray, especially when coated with calcium phosphate which serves to increase their radiodensity. Cystine sometimes forms a sludge-like substance in the renal tract, while cystine stones can grow large enough to form staghorn calculi.

Large volumes of fluid decrease the cystine concentration in the urine and increase its solubility; therefore, the first line of treatment is fluid therapy. If urine volumes can be consistently maintained at over 3 litres in 24 hours, cystine stores can be either dissolved or their formation discouraged. Total cystine excretion is measured by testing a 24-hour urine collection, and a urine volume is then aimed for which is high enough to maintain the final cystine excretion below 250 mg per day. For example, a patient with a cystine excretion of 1,000 mg per day should produce a daily urine volume of at least 4,000 ml. The fluid intake should be spread out over 24 hours, and it is particularly important that the patient drinks at night when the urine is more concentrated and the volume generally decreased. Ideally the patient should drink 800 ml of fluid before going to bed, and on waking in the night to pass urine, a further 800 ml should be consumed. This pattern should be continued throughout the night. It is not surprising that many patients are reluctant to follow this advice, but nevertheless it should be encouraged.

In cases where cystine excretion is persistently too high for an increased fluid intake to be effective (for example, if the 24-hour urinary cystine were 2,000 mg, the urine volume would need to be at least 8 litres per day!), then an alternative form of treatment is necessary. Alkali can be used to raise the urinary pH above 7.4 which enhances cystine solubility, but patients usually find the large doses needed very difficult to take (Coe and Parks, 1988). The drug D-penicillamine is effective in reducing the concentration of cystine, but it is reserved for use as a last resort owing to its many potential side-effects. Penicillamine is nephrotoxic, can cause Goodpasture's syndrome, haemolytic anaemia, systemic lupus erythematosus, rheumatoid-like disorders, thrombocytopenia and myasthenia gravis, and is known to be teratogenic in rats. Because of these severe side-effects, the patient taking penicillamine should be carefully monitored, particularly for signs of nephrotic syndrome.

WHERE DO CALCULI FORM?

Although renal calculi can form in any part of the renal tract, in practice they form mainly in the kidney and bladder. Ureteric calculi are in transit from the kidney to the bladder. Calculi tend to lodge at the natural narrowings in the renal tract:

- Renal calyces and pelvis
- Pelviureteric junction
- Where the ureter passes over the pelvic brim
- Vesicoureteric orifice
- Bladder
- Urethra

Patients therefore present with stones at these points (NB – on a KUB a lower ureter stone is low down in the pelvis).

SIGNS AND SYMPTOMS

Renal calculi can be diagnosed from the following findings:

- Pain – ureteric colic is described by Whitfield (1985) as severe, intermittent pain and tenderness radiating from loin to groin and the labia or scrotum, associated with nausea and vomiting, haematuria and tachycardia. Stones in other parts of the renal tract cause localized pain.
- Haematuria.
- Impaired renal function.
- Opacity on KUB.
- Positive intravenous urogram (IVU).
- Positive midstream urine (MSU) sample.
- Altered pH of urine.

PERCUTANEOUS NEPHROLITHOTOMY

Percutaneous nephrolithotomy (PCNL) is a renal surgical procedure whereby calculi are removed through a narrow tract under X-ray vision. The tract is established by gradual dilation following an initial needle puncture of the kidney. The tract, passing through the skin, muscle and parenchyma, is dilated to a size of 26–30 Charrière, large enough to allow the introduction of a nephroscope enabling inspection of the interior of the kidney. The procedure requires the close co-operation of the radiologist and urologist.

Using this technique it is possible to extract renal stones by various methods. Intact renal stones with a diameter of up to approximately 1 cm may be removed via a nephrostomy tract using alligator forceps or other pronged grasping forceps. Alternatively the stone may be disintegrated by:

- Ultrasonic lithotripsy
- Electrohydraulic lithotripsy
- Lithoclast treatment

In ultrasonic lithotripsy, high-frequency ultrasound vibrations via a steel probe in direct contact with the stone cause a 'jackhammer' effect which reduces the stone to sand.

Electrohydraulic lithotripsy uses electrohydraulic shock waves in repeated bursts to disrupt the stone. Although there is a risk of damage to surrounding tissue within 5 mm of the stone which also receives the full strength of the emission, such as oedema or 'shrapnel' effects from stone fragments, this technique is widely regarded as the most efficient means of stone disruption available.

Originally developed for the mechanical disintegration of bladder stones in 1976 by Mauermayer and Hartung, the lithoclast has been adapted for use in the more confined space of a nephrostomy track. This instrument uses a trigger mechanism to effect the shearing off of the portions of stone with which it is in contact.

In all these procedures the resulting stone fragments and debris are flushed out continuously through the nephroscope or passed spontaneously down the ureter. During the procedure the patient is intubated under general anaesthesia and fluid is given intravenously to replace intraoperative blood loss. In most cases a urethral catheter is inserted at the outset of the procedure as haematuria with blood clots may occur. Following the extraction of the stone the kidney is screened to ensure that no fragments remain in the collecting system. A whistle-tipped nephrostomy tube is left in the track to facilitate drainage of blood and urine and reduce the risk of formation of an intrarenal haematoma. Stone fragments are sent for biochemical analysis and in certain cases advice may be given to the patient to reduce the risk of stones re-forming postoperatively.

History

The percutaneous route was first used in 1941 when Rupel and Brown (1976) used a cystoscope and forceps to remove a stone which was obstructing a single kidney. A number of similar procedures were performed in the following years but the most significant development took place in 1976 in Sweden when Fernstrom and Johansen (1976) combined the use of a percutaneous tract and the extraction of stones under X-ray guidance using stone-grabbing forceps.

In 1981 Wickham reported the successful removal of stones via the percutaneous route at the Institute of Urology in London (Wickham and Kellett, 1981). He was the first to use the procedure in Britain in association with radiologist Dr M J Kellett.

Indications

The indications for PCNL are the same as for open renal surgery and are as follows:

- ◆ Persistent or intermittent loin pain
- ◆ Haematuria
- ◆ Recurrent urinary tract infection
- ◆ Obstruction of a kidney by a stone
- ◆ Rapid growth of an existing stone
- ◆ Asymptomatic patients found to have stones on routine screening whose profession precludes the presence of stones, e.g. airline pilots, owing to the risk of renal colic

Contraindications

There are only two major contraindications to PCNL:

- Renovascular abnormality, e.g. arterial aneurysm identified by preoperative ultrasonography of the kidney
- Blood clotting disorders, which preclude surgery unless remedial treatment is undertaken

Preoperative investigations

Preoperative investigations are shown in Table 6.1.

Advantages of the percutaneous route

Advantages of PCNL are as follows:

1. It allows direct access to the renal pelvis with clear vision of stones, particularly those in the pelvis and upper part of the ureter; removal is therefore simpler.
2. The procedure may be carried out under light general anaesthesia, thus enabling patients who would be at risk during a long procedure under general anaesthesia (e.g. patients with spinal injuries, cardiac arrhythmias, obstructive airways disease, spina bifida) to undergo PCNL and be relieved of painful symptoms.
3. Reduced trauma at the time of operation: a small wound and reduced postoperative hospital stay result in early recovery and resumption of work. This in turn has economic benefits, i.e. savings on payment of sickness benefits, faster turnover of hospital inpatients.
4. Reduced risk of wound infection – the nephrostomy drain site does not require sutures and is healed within 48 hours.
5. Reduced postoperative pain following minimally invasive surgery, generally managed with oral analgesia.

PROCEDURE	RATIONALE
Midstream urine samples (MSU)	To exclude urinary tract infection/ commence appropriate antibiotic therapy
Plain abdominal X-ray (KUB)	To show current position of stone
Serum urea and electrolytes	To establish status of renal function
Serum full blood count	To exclude anaemia
Serum clotting screen	To exclude clotting abnormalities
Intravenous urography (IVU)	To show anatomy of kidney
Cross-match 2 units of blood	In case of haemorrhage

Table 6.1   *Preoperative investigations for PCNL*

6. Low patient morbidity.
7. Reduced risk of postoperative complications associated with prolonged immobility following open surgery (e.g. chest infection, thromboembolic problems).

Complications of surgery

Haemorrhage

The risk of haemorrhage increases with the longer operation time required to remove large or multiple stones. Intravenous fluids are increased to maintain the blood pressure, the nephrostomy tube is spigoted to tamponade the track.

In rare cases persistent bleeding may need to be investigated by arteriogram to identify and embolize the vessels involved.

If haematuria persists the urethral catheter remains in situ until the urine clears; a bladder washout may be required to remove clots. The patient is asked to maintain a high intake of oral fluids, at least 3 litres every 24 hours.

Bacteraemia

Postoperative pyrexia is not uncommon although less than 5% of patients have been found to have developed bacteraemia, caused by the presence of infective stones. Intravenous antibiotics are given prophylactically on induction of anaesthesia in all cases (e.g. cefuroxime 750 mg and at 8-hourly intervals thereafter for 24-48 hours postoperatively).

Paralytic ileus

Paralytic ileus has been noted in 4% of patients and is managed conservatively with intravenous fluid replacement. The patient is given nil by mouth and a nasogastric tube is passed if nausea and vomiting persist.

Pneumothorax

The risk of pneumothorax increases if the kidney lies high and puncture is above the level of the twelfth rib. A chest drain may have to be inserted.

Nursing management

Preoperative

Nursing management on admission and preoperatively is shown in Table 6.2.

PROCEDURE	RATIONALE
Record temperature, pulse, respirations and blood pressure	Establishes baseline observations, identifies abnormalities
Routine urine test	Excludes diabetes and other underlying disease
MSU for microbiological assessment	Excludes infection, ensures results are current, determines appropriate antibiotic cover is prescribed
Record patient's weight	Enables accurate dosage of premedication, antibiotic and anaesthetic to be prescribed
Complete nursing assessment document (current health status, activities of daily living)	Ensures patient details are correct, identifies special needs and ensures they are met
Complete preoperative care plan	Provides opportunity for patient to receive information about pre- and postoperative care
Patient has nil by mouth for 2 hours preoperatively and no solid food for 6 hours preoperatively. Patient may drink up to a maximum of 1 litre of water between 6 and 2 hours preoperatively	Reduces risk of aspiration of vomit
Premedication is given as prescribed	Reduces patient's anxiety

Table 6.2 *Preoperative nursing management*

On return to the ward

The patient returns with an intravenous infusion in progress. This is maintained until oral intake of fluid can be resumed.

In most cases a nephrostomy drain is left in the track. The volume of drainage is recorded on the fluid balance chart along with bladder urine and fluid intake. It is not a cause for concern if the nephrostomy does not drain a significant amount as long as the patient remains comfortable. The drain may have slipped out of the collecting system; this is confirmed by X-ray.

A urethral catheter may remain in situ if urine drainage is heavily blood-stained. Drainage is observed closely and the urine bag tubing may be gently 'milked' manually to encourage the passage of blood clots or debris.

The patient's pulse and blood pressure are recorded on return and at half-hourly intervals for a period of 2 hours. The temperature may be recorded less frequently, e.g. 2–4 hourly, unless the patient shows signs of pyrexia. The nurse should also be aware of the respiratory rate and record any abnormalities. The frequency of observations may be increased or decreased as the patient's condition dictates.

Following the operation day little is generally required in the way of nursing care as the patient is able to get up on recovery from the anaesthesia. The patient may need assistance with manoeuvring the catheter and nephrostomy tube if they are present but they do not greatly impede mobility.

First postoperative day

The intravenous infusion is discontinued if:

◆ normal diet and fluid have been resumed with no nausea or vomiting
◆ patient is apyrexial; if low-grade pyrexia is present, an intravenous cannula may be left in situ for administration of antibiotics

Temperature, pulse, respiration and blood pressure are recorded 4-hourly unless:

◆ heavy haematuria persists
◆ pyrexia persists
◆ recovery has not been straightforward

A KUB X-ray is performed. If no stone fragments remain the nephrostomy tube may be clamped (on the surgeon's instructions).

Second postoperative day

The nephrostomy tube is removed if:

◆ no pain has been experienced since clamping
◆ no leakage has occurred at the nephrostomy site

Possible problems

Leakage of urine from nephrostomy site

Leakage can persist if oedema is present in the kidney or ureter following the trauma of surgical intervention. It may also indicate the presence of stone fragments not seen on X-ray which obstruct the normal flow of urine. The nephrostomy site will normally close within 24 hours with a firmly applied pressure dressing.

If persistent leakage causes distress to the patient and the skin becomes sore, a urostomy bag can provide accurate measurement of drainage and also help prevent excoriation. This measure should only be taken as a last resort, however, as some urologists believe that the bag encourages the track to continue draining. However, in practice, as the internal oedema decreases, urine drainage via the track diminishes and the bag can usually be removed 24–48 hours later and a light dressing is applied.

Pain

Patients generally experience little pain postoperatively. Pain is managed with oral analgesics and more severe pain can be managed effectively with diclofenac suppositories 100 mg once daily (a non-steroidal anti-inflammatory drug).

Infection

The nephrostomy site itself rarely becomes infected, but urinary tract infections can persist. Oral antibiotics are prescribed according to the sensitivities obtained with the MSU result.

Discharge from hospital

Patients may be discharged from hospital on the third postoperative day if they:

- ◆ are afebrile
- ◆ have a normal urine output, i.e. colour and volume
- ◆ have a dry nephrostomy site

Advice on discharge

Rest and activity

Patients who have a sedentary occupation may return to work as soon as they feel well enough. Patients involved in more active or manual labour should allow 1–2 weeks to convalesce. Any patient with children or a household to look after may find it useful to arrange for help in the home to be available for the first week or so.

Sexual relations

This is very much up to the individual but there are no contraindications to resuming usual relations after recovering from PCNL. Women using the contraceptive pill should seek medical advice about when to start taking it again.

Eating and drinking

Normal diet can be taken unless advice to the contrary is given. An increased intake of fluid is advised to 'flush' the kidneys and help prevent recurrence of stones; 2.5–3 litres per 24 hours is the aim. A moderate amount of alcohol can improve the appetite and is not thought to be harmful, though it may be contraindicated by certain drugs and this should be ascertained before discharge.

Bowels

Irregular bowel habits may follow a period in hospital after surgery but this usually corrects itself with the resumption of normal diet and exercise. A mild laxative may be required in the short term.

Urine

Patients should be advised that they may continue to have blood in the urine after being discharged home. This is not a cause for concern as long as it is possible to pass urine without difficulty and no blood clots are present. However, if the bleeding is heavy and persists with accompanying discomfort the patient should contact his or her general practitioner who may refer the patient back to the hospital for investigations. Any urinary symptoms, e.g. frequency, burning pain on micturition and urgency, should not be ignored as they may indicate the presence of a urinary tract infection which should be treated with the appropriate antibiotic.

Wound healing

The nephrostomy site should be kept covered with a light sealed-edge dressing until a dry scab forms over it. The scab should form by the third or fourth day after removal of the tube. The dressing need only be changed in the unlikely event that oozing or bleeding occurs once the patient is at home. Dressings should be provided for a further two changes or information should be given on purchasing a suitable alternative.

The patient should be advised that itching, tingling or numbness may be experienced at the nephrostomy site, and that the tissue may feel hard and lumpy as the healing process progresses. Help should be sought if:

- pain in the wound increases
- redness or swelling in the wound increases
- any discharge occurs

Driving

All patients should ensure that their insurance policy covers them to drive after a general anaesthesia; a time limit to allow for full recovery may apply. Patients must then decide when they feel strong enough to cope with the various traffic conditions likely to be encountered, e.g. emergency stops.

Follow-up

The patient should attend the outpatient clinic for review by the urologist 6 weeks after discharge. At this time a KUB X-ray will be performed, an MSU is sent for microbiological assessment and a blood sample is sent for biochemical assessment to ascertain that renal function has not been impaired. The results of the stone analysis should be available and advice is given on what measures should be taken to reduce the risk of recurrence. In the majority of cases the simple step of increasing fluid intake to 2.5–3 litres per 24 hours may be all that is required.

Persistent stone-formers with underlying metabolic causes should be kept under review every 3–6 months to monitor renal function.

NEPHROSTOMY TUBES

Insertion of a nephrostomy tube is a temporary method of draining the renal pelvis. There are two types of tube:

◆   A needle nephrostomy tube is very fine, is inserted under local anaesthesia and is used to relieve hydronephrosis caused by ureteric obstruction.

◆   A 28 French gauge nephrostomy tube is used as a drainage tube following percutaneous nephrolithotomy and laparoscopic nephrectomy, and can be very uncomfortable (Figure 6.2).

Care of the nephrostomy tube

Nephrostomy tubes are deeply invasive, linking the pelvis of the kidney directly to the outside of the body. There is a high risk of infection occurring

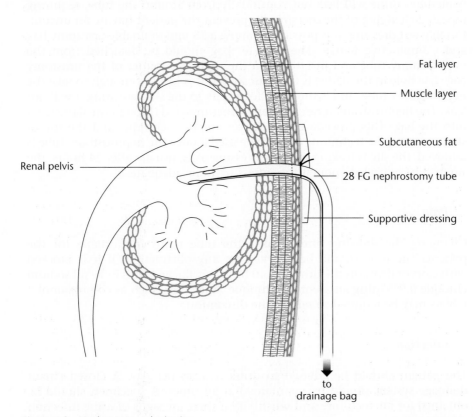

Fat layer

Muscle layer

Subcutaneous fat

Renal pelvis

28 FG nephrostomy tube

Supportive dressing

to
drainage bag

Figure 6.2   *Nephrostomy tube in situ*

so the tube must have an occlusive dressing at all times which should be changed if it is soiled, becomes detached, or if the patient complains of discomfort. With a needle nephrostomy tube, it is important that the tube is coiled around and taped securely as they can kink very easily and the suture can come out. For large nephrostomy tubes, the tube should be taped to the patient's side, so that it does not become occluded while sitting.

The patient should be advised to drink 3 litres a day.

Night catheter bags can be attached to the nephrostomy tube and a closed circuit drainage system should be maintained at all times. Leg bags with long tubing can be used if the patient is mobile during the day.

Complications

Haemorrhage

If used postoperatively, the tube may drain large amounts of blood (500–1,000 ml) immediately after the procedure. If this occurs, the tube can be clamped for 1 hour and then released.

Leakage around the tube

Sometimes urine will leak out continually from around the tube, requiring repeated changing of the dressing. To prevent the patient having an uncomfortable wet dressing, it is possible to apply a 28 mm drainable urostomy bag and Combihesive flange. The catheter bag should be detached from the nephrostomy tube and inserted into the night bag outlet of the urostomy bag. The hole in the flange is then cut so that it is just big enough to take the nephrostomy tube, and is then applied firmly to the skin ensuring it will not leak. The nephrostomy tube can then be manipulated through the flange and into the bag. This procedure requires an aseptic technique and the use of sterile gloves. The technique can also be used if once the nephrostomy tube is removed, the site is leaking through dressing pads; usually after 24 hours, the site will have healed enough for a dressing to be adequate.

Pain

Changing the dressing often makes the tube more comfortable for the patient. The tube should be checked for any obstruction; if it is blocked with clots or debris in the urine, it can be gently flushed with 5–10 ml sodium chloride 0.9% using an aseptic technique. Analgesics such as co-proxamol 2 tablets may be required to relieve the discomfort.

Infection

The patient should be advised to drink 3 litres per day. A closed circuit drainage system should be maintained at all times. A specimen should be obtained for microculture and sensitivity if there are signs of urine infection present.

ADVICE FOR PATIENTS FOLLOWING INSERTION OF A NEPHROSTOMY TUBE

THIS ADVICE SHEET WILL BE GIVEN TO YOU BEFORE YOU LEAVE HOSPITAL. THIS SHEET IS IN ADDITION TO ANY VERBAL ADVICE YOU MAY BE GIVEN BY MEDICAL AND NURSING STAFF. KEEP THIS SHEET AND READ IT FROM TIME TO TIME.

A nephrostomy tube is a hollow tube which goes through your back and into the kidney. The tube is stitched to your skin to hold it in place and is attached to a drainage bag.

Nephrostomy tubes are used to drain the kidney when there is obstruction and the urine cannot drain freely down the ureter and into the bladder.

Drainage bags

During the day you will be able to wear a leg bag strapped to your waist or thigh. However, at night you may need a night drainage bag attached to the bottom of the leg bag to maintain drainage. You will be taught how to attach and detach the bag and how to empty it. The leg bags hold 500–750 ml (1–1½ pints) of urine and need to be emptied every few hours. The night bag holds 2,000 ml (4 pints) and will not require emptying overnight.

Care of the nephrostomy tube

1. The dressing will need changing if it gets wet, becomes soiled or starts to come off. If the tube is a fine one, it must be kept coiled under the dressing and will be secured by tape so that it does not become kinked. Before you leave hospital, the ward staff will make arrangements for the dressings to be changed.
2. We advise you to drink 2–3 litres (4–6 pints) a day to reduce the risk of infection.
3. If any signs of infection occur, i.e.
    the urine in the bag becomes cloudy or contains blood
    the urine is offensive smelling
    you have a fever
    you should drink 3 litres (6 pints) a day and contact your general practitioner who may take a specimen of urine to confirm if you have an infection.
4. If your bag does not drain any urine for more than an hour, you should check for any kinks in the tubing, ensure the tap at any

connection is switched on, and drink 500 ml (1 pint) of water. If it still does not drain after a further hour, you should contact your general practitioner.

5. If you develop severe pain or have blood in your urine, you should contact your general practitioner.

LASERTRIPSY

Lasertripsy is a method for the fragmentation of ureteric calculi using a laser (light amplification by stimulated emission of radiation).

Procedure

The patient is positioned in the lithotomy position (on the back with legs apart and feet held up in stirrups). A ureteroscope is passed along the urethra into the bladder, through the vesicoureteric opening and into the ureter. When the calculus is visualized, the Q-switched dye laser is fired using 100 to 1,000 shocks. This type of laser causes minimal soft-tissue damage. The calculus is broken into tiny fragments which the patient can then pass urethrally. The procedure can take from 30 minutes to 2 hours.

Lasertripsy is usually a retrograde procedure; however, if the calculus is at the top of the ureter, the procedure can be antegrade. For the antegrade approach, a needle nephrostomy tube is inserted under local anaesthesia 5 days preoperatively. The patient is then discharged and readmitted 1 day preoperatively.

Preoperative preparation

A midstream specimen of urine (MSU) is obtained. The patient is prepared for general anaesthesia; however, premedications are only given if necessary so that an X-ray of the kidneys, ureter and bladder (KUB) can be performed immediately preoperatively (ideally). The patient is then asked to rest quietly before going to theatre.

Postoperative complications

Obstruction of the urinary tract

- Monitor urinary output.
- Assess the patient for pain on the treated side.
- Sieve urine for calculi and send for chemical analysis.
- KUB to check fragments have been passed.

Haematuria

- Observe and record the degree of haematuria in urine and

warn patients so they are not alarmed by it. Haematuria is usually present for 1–2 days postoperatively.

◆ Once the patient has recovered from the anaesthesia, ensure that he or she is encouraged to drink 3 litres of fluid per 24 h.

Pain

◆ Co-proxamol is usually adequate; however, if the calculus was stuck in the ureteric wall, diclofenac 100 mg per rectum or orally twice daily may be required.

◆ If a double-J stent is present, the patient may experience discomfort, and will be reassured if the cause is explained.

◆ Encouraging the patient to drink 3 litres of fluid per day will also ease the pain.

Infection

◆ Prophylactic antibiotics are given on induction of anaesthesia, e.g. gentamicin 80 mg IV.

◆ The patient's temperature is monitored and the doctor informed of any pyrexia as this may be indicative of an infection which needs treating with antibiotics; it may also be a sign of obstruction.

Perforation of the ureter

There is a risk of perforation of the ureter causing extravasation of urine. This is characterized by severe pain and tenderness. An ultrasound scan is required to confirm a perforation and a double-J stent may be required to allow the perforation time to heal.

Failure of the procedure

If the stone cannot be fragmented by the laser, the alternatives are:

◆ The calculus is flushed up into the renal pelvis with saline and a double-J stent is inserted. The patient is then treated with extracorporeal piezoelectric lithotripsy (EPL).

◆ If the stone is in the lower third of the ureter, it is retrieved using a Dormia basket (Figure 6.3).

Discharge from hospital

The patient is usually discharged the day after the operation. Follow-up depends on whether there are any remaining stones: e.g. EPL may be required. Otherwise, the patient will be seen again after 6 weeks for a KUB radiograph to check that no fragments are present and that no further stone formation has occurred.

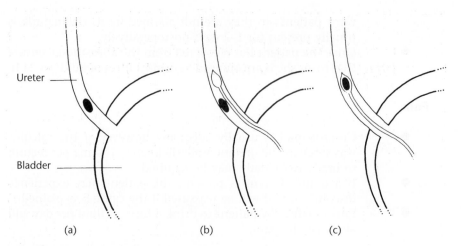

Figure 6.3 *Use of the Dormia basket: (a) stone in lower ureter; (b) Dormia basket in situ; (c) stone trapped in basket*

OPEN NEPHRECTOMY

Open nephrectomy is still used to treat renal calculi. Stones are sometimes discovered so late that the kidney is virtually destroyed (providing less than 10% of total renal function) and there is no option but to remove it.

PYELOLITHOTOMY AND NEPHROLITHOTOMY

Open removal of stones is required when minimally invasive procedures have failed or the stones are large and multiple. There are two approaches used. If the stone is in the renal pelvis a pyelolithotomy is performed, and if the kidney tissue is incised it is called a nephrolithotomy. A combination of the two is often required to remove the stone.

Procedure

The patient is prepared as for any major open surgery.

The incision is made along the bed of the twelfth rib. After removal of all the stones the calices are flushed. An X-ray is taken to check that no fragments remain before the incision is closed.

For nephrolithotomy, the renal artery must be clamped and if ischaemia is to last longer than 30 minutes, the kidney needs to be cooled to 20°C to prevent damage.

Postoperative care

Following recovery from the anaesthesia the patient must be taught to breathe deeply and cough while supporting the wound. Physiotherapy and early mobilization are very important in preventing chest infection.

ADVICE FOR PATIENTS FOLLOWING TREATMENT FOR STONES IN THE URETER

THIS ADVICE SHEET WILL BE GIVEN TO YOU BEFORE YOU LEAVE HOSPITAL. THIS SHEET IS IN ADDITION TO ANY VERBAL ADVICE YOU MAY BE GIVEN BY MEDICAL AND NURSING STAFF. KEEP THIS SHEET AND READ IT FROM TIME TO TIME.

On discharge from hospital

1. You may feel a little tired owing to the anaesthetic and should allow yourself time to rest if necessary. You can resume your normal activities and should take gentle exercise to help the stone fragments to pass.
2. If you work, staff can discuss with you whether you need to take time off after the operation. The Sister or staff nurse will give you a sickness certificate to cover the time you are in hospital and your GP will provide a certificate for any convalescence you have at home.
3. You may be given a follow-up appointment by the ward staff. This is to check that you have recovered from the operation and to arrange any further investigations that may be necessary.
4. The ward staff will arrange for any tablets you need and explain them to you. It is important that you take the medications as directed.
5. You should drink 3 litres of fluid per 24 h (6 pints, 15 cups or 10 mugs) to flush out the kidney.

What to look out for

1. If any signs of infection occur, i.e. a burning sensation when you pass urine, offensive-smelling urine, you should drink 3 litres each day (15 cups or 12 mugs) and contact your general practitioner, who may ask you to provide a specimen of urine for examination to confirm whether or not you have an infection.
2. If you start to shiver and think you have a temperature, telephone the ward you were on or the urology doctor on call promptly.
3. If your urine is slightly stained with blood or you pass small clots, this should clear if you drink more. However, if you have prolonged bleeding or pass large clots, contact the nurse in charge of the ward you were on or the urology doctor on call.

> 4. You may pass some fragments of stone in your urine which may cause discomfort. If it is painful contact your general practitioner who will be able to prescribe painkillers.
> 5. It may have been necessary to insert a stent during the operation. You may find this uncomfortable, especially when you pass urine. You will be informed when the stent needs to be removed – this must be within 6 months.

Haemorrhage

The patient must be observed for signs of haemorrhage, especially following a nephrolithotomy. A nephrostomy tube is left in situ for about 48 hours or until there is minimal drainage. The drainage should be observed for quantity and consistency.

Temperature

The patient may be hypothermic on return to the ward and require a space blanket for a few hours. The patient's temperature must be carefully monitored throughout the postoperative period and any pyrexia reported to the doctor.

Risk of infection

Three litres of fluid per day are required, at first intravenously and then orally so that the patient produces enough urine to keep the renal tract flushed and reduce the risk of infection. Intravenous antibiotics, e.g. cefuroxime 750 mg twice daily and then cefadroxil 500 mg twice daily are given.

The dressing over the incision should be changed as required using an aseptic technique, and the dressing around the nephrostomy tube must be changed when wet to prevent infection of the incision site.

Pain

Strong analgesics are required initially, e.g. intramuscular diclofenac 75 mg or pethidine 50–100 mg to keep the pain under control so that the patient is able to perform deep breathing and leg exercises. The patient will require assistance in adopting the most comfortable position with the incision and nephrostomy tube supported.

Urine output

Urine output should be measured to assess the patient's hydrational state. The concentration and consistency should also be noted.

Discharge

The patient is discharged 7–10 days postoperatively. The sutures are removed 10 days postoperatively and a practice or district nurse appointment may need to be arranged for this. The patient should be seen again after 6 weeks.

LAPAROSCOPIC SURGERY

Laparoscopic surgery is one of the latest advances in urology. Laparoscopic varicocele repairs can now be performed as day-case surgery. Major laparoscopic surgery (e.g. nephrectomies and reimplantation of ureters into the bladder) is also being performed, although these procedures remain innovations and it is common for the operation to proceed to open surgery.

Laparoscopic nephrectomy

Nephrectomy generally involves a large, painful incision, close to or involving the twelfth rib pair. This is the reason behind the development of percutaneous (or laparoscopic) nephrectomy, which uses essentially the same method as that employed for percutaneous nephrolithotomy. To be considered for the technique, patients must be non-obese and fit to withstand a long anaesthesia, and the kidney to be removed must be both small and free of malignancy.

Patient preparation is similar to that for percutaneous nephrolithotomy, and the postoperative care also involves the same priorities. Prior to the procedure, angiographic embolization of the kidney is performed. Some 24–36 hours later, three laparoscopic tracks are made into the lumbar region. Laparoscopes are inserted and the kidney is freed from its blood vessels and surrounding tissues. A modified surgical liquidizer/blender is inserted down one of the laparoscopes. This is used to liquefy the renal substance, and each liquidized segment in turn is then removed by aspiration or forceps. As the method is still experimental the procedure can be prolonged (4–6 hours is not uncommon) when compared with conventional nephrectomy.

Postoperative problems

Breathing

At present the procedure entails a long period of anaesthesia; however, this will become less of a problem as the procedure is perfected.

Haemorrhage

The patient should be monitored closely for signs of haemorrhage. A wound drain is left in situ for 24–48 hours or until there is minimal drainage, both to allow adequate wound drainage and to observe for any signs of significant postoperative haemorrhage.

Pain

Pain is mainly due to abdominal gas which is relieved by movement. The patient should be encouraged to move about in bed as much as possible, and at the earliest opportunity should be assisted out of bed.

The patient is more critically ill during the first 24 hours postoperatively; however, after this initial period recovery is rapid and the patient is discharged after 4–5 days. This procedure is advantageous from a cosmetic point of view, the tracks heal very quickly and the possible complications of chronic wound pain associated with open nephrectomy are eliminated.

PERCUTANEOUS PYELOLYSIS

Percutaneous pyelolysis is a treatment for pelviureteric junction (PUJ) stenosis, and is particularly effective in secondary PUJ obstruction following scarring from calculous disease.

Preoperative preparation

Prepare the patient for major surgery, as for PCNL.

Procedure

A guidewire is passed in a retrograde direction up the ureter. A percutaneous puncture to the kidney is then made and the track dilated to 24 FG. Through this, the ureteric guidewire is grasped and pulled through the PUJ to the surface.

From the top, a urethrotome is passed alongside the guidewire to the PUJ. A 5 cm length of the ureteric wall is incised in a posterolateral direction (this direction is important so as not to transect the lower pole vessels).

A 16 FG Payne drain (a tapered splint nephrostomy tube which has holes that lie in the renal pelvis) is passed down the ureter over the guidewire, and urine drains to the surface and into a nephrostomy tube drainage bag.

Postoperative care

A nephrostogram is performed 48 hours postoperatively, to check that the Payne drain is in a good position. If so, it is spigoted and strapped down under a dressing. The tube is left in situ for 4–6 weeks when a further nephrostogram is performed; and if this shows good drainage, the tube can then be removed.

A care plan is shown in Table 6.3.

PATIENT'S PROBLEM	AIM OF NURSING ACTION	NURSING ACTION
Pain following surgery and due to presence of Payne drain	Patient will state that the pain is relieved or reduced to a tolerable level so the patient can move around freely	1. Ensure that Payne drain is taped securely and not pulling 2. Ensure that Payne drain is not blocked and is draining freely 3. Assist patient to adopt a comfortable position supported by pillows 4. Give analgesics as prescribed and required and monitor effect
Potential infection following operation and presence of Payne drain	Patient's temperature will be 36–37°C Patient's wound will not be red and swollen Patient will state that he or she does not feel feverish	1. Monitor temperature 4-hourly and report to doctor if above 38°C 2. Give antibiotics as prescribed 3. Re-dress Payne drain as required, i.e. if dressing is soiled, has come loose or if painful 4. Ensure patient is aware of the need to drink 3 litres per day
Potential obstruction of Payne drain	Maintain free flow of urine through Payne drain, i.e. continuous urine drainage	1. Empty Payne drain 4-hourly and record on fluid balance chart 2. Ensure drain is not kinked, and re-dress if necessary 3. Flush drain with 5–10 ml sodium chloride 0.9% using an aseptic technique if drain is blocked
Knowledge deficit regarding care of Payne drain at home	By date of discharge, patient will state that he or she feels competent regarding care of Payne drain	1. Teach patient to redress Payne drain 2. Refer to district nurse and arrange visit 3. Teach patient to recognize problems that require further advice

Table 6.3 *Care plan for specific problems following percutaneous pyelolysis*

EXTRACORPOREAL LITHOTRIPSY

Extracorporeal shock-wave lithotripsy

History

The 'first-generation' Dornier lithotriptor was developed at the University of Munich, Germany by Professor E. Schmidt and Professor Eisenberg and came into use in 1981. The Dornier aircraft company had observed that shock waves induced by high-speed aircraft flying in stormy weather conditions had caused damage to internal equipment while the exterior of the craft remained intact. As a consequence, research was carried out into the effects of focusing shock waves onto hard objects, e.g. renal calculi, to bring about their destruction. Since this machine has now been superseded by the 'second generation' the treatment is only briefly described below.

Outline of treatment

Shock waves are generated by underwater discharge of a high-voltage spark. The shock waves are transmitted to the stone through de-ionized, de-gassed water heated to 37°C (the efficiency of shock waves is adversely affected by air bubbles). The stone is located by two diagonally directed X-ray beams. The patient is supported in the water in a computer-controlled hydraulic chair. The chair is positioned so that the stone is at the focus of the shock waves.

Up to 4,000 shocks may be required to disintegrate a stone. Treatment is painful; therefore, the patient needs general or epidural anaesthesia with its attendant risk.

Temporary haematuria is caused by the shocks and a urethral catheter is inserted in case of clot retention. It is removed when the urine is clear.

Cardiac arrhythmias can occur. The heart beat is monitored throughout the treatment and the shock waves are synchronized to the refractory phase of the cardiac cycle on the R wave.

The patient is observed as usual following general anaesthesia. Oral fluids (3 litres per 24 hours) are encouraged to promote the passage of stone fragments out of the system. This can take anything from 24 hours to 2 weeks. Radiography (KUB) confirms the position of remaining fragments 2 days after treatment. Patients can then be discharged if they are:

- apyrexial
- pain-free
- taking normal diet and increased fluids without nausea or vomiting
- passing clear urine without difficulty

Extracorporeal piezoelectric lithotripsy

The 'second-generation' lithotriptors such as the Wolf lithotriptor are now in use. With this system the stone is disintegrated by shock waves generated by the piezoelectric effect – this is the vibration which results from a high voltage passing across the piezoelectric ceramic crystals. Approximately 2,000 crystals form a mosaic in a concave dish and the shock waves produced from each crystal are collected at the focus, i.e. the kidney stone. This focus is much more accurate than in the Dornier machine and this results in more efficient delivery of shocks to the stone in a shorter time. Consequently the treatment is not so painful and the patient does not need anaesthesia, although children and anxious adults may need sedation. The shock wave is transmitted through de-gassed, preheated water which is contained in a closed bath. The patient lies over the bath with only the loin area in contact with the water. The stone is located by ultrasound probe which is fixed within the dish; an image of the stone's position can be seen on the ultra-sound monitor.

Up to 4,000 shocks can be given in one session and this lasts 45 minutes on average. There is no risk of induction of cardiac arrhythmias so cardiac monitoring is not necessary.

The majority of patients may be treated as outpatients but hospital admission is necessary if the patient needs to be observed closely after treatment, e.g. where there is a single kidney, renal impairment, ileal conduit or other urinary diversion, and in cases of obstruction or deterioration of renal function. Hypertensive patients may experience raised blood pressure, which should be monitored, as should patients with cardiac or respiratory problems. Such problems may be exacerbated by stress rather than the treatment itself. Patients with reduced mobility as a result of spinal injury, spina bifida, multiple sclerosis, etc. are admitted, as repeated journeys to hospital are time-consuming and difficult. To avoid inconvenience and possible financial hardship, hostel accommodation may need to be provided for those travelling long distances for treatment.

The introduction of the Wolf lithotriptor has significantly reduced the medical and nursing needs of patients with renal stones as 85% are now treatable by lithotripsy.

Pretreatment investigations

The patient attends a pretreatment clinic where a detailed clinical history is taken; the following investigations are carried out routinely:

1. Blood pressure is recorded.
2. Blood is screened for clotting abnormalities.
3. Blood urea and electrolytes are checked to assess renal function.
4. MSU is microbiologically screened.
5. Urine is tested for glucose, ketones, blood, protein, etc.
6. KUB X-ray and IVU are performed if indicated.
7. 24-hour urine collection is made for 'stone screen'.
8. Suitability for treatment as an outpatient is assessed.
9. Special needs are identified, arrangements made for admission to ward or hostel after treatment.

Advantages of treatment

The advantages of treatment by extracorporeal piezoelectric lithotripsy (EPL) include the following:

1. EPL reduces in-patient stay. Only those who meet previously mentioned criteria need be admitted.
2. Most patients can resume normal activities the next day and can return to work within 1 week.
3. There is minimal morbidity – worldwide 80,000 patients had been treated up to 1986 with no deaths.
4. There is minimal pain following treatment, most patients being treated with oral analgesics.
5. Eighty-five per cent of renal stones can be treated by EPL, including those in patients previously considered unsuitable for open or minimally invasive surgery, e.g. spinal injury patients, and patients with cardiac and obstructive airway conditions.
6. Repeated treatments may be carried out with no ill-effects discerned as yet. It is possible to keep those with metabolic calculous disease free from stones, thus preserving their renal function.
7. There is reduced exposure to X-rays – ultrasound is used to monitor progress during treatment.
8. Although the initial cost of the lithotripsy machine is high, the procedure is more cost-effective than open or minimally invasive surgery. One patient can be treated every hour, allowing high patient turnover.

Disadvantages of treatment

Disadvantages of EPL include the following:

1. The technique cannot be used initially on staghorn calculi.
2. The technique cannot be used on cystine stones as they are too hard.
3. Large stones (more than 2 cm in diameter) need repeat treatments and patients incur travelling expenses for repeated journeys to hospital. It can also prove inconvenient for those who have to arrange time off work.
4. Admission to hospital has to be arranged for insertion of a ureteric stent prior to treatment of large stones and removal of the stent on completion of treatment.

Lithotripsy treatment

The introduction of the Wolf lithotriptor (Figure 6.4) has significantly reduced the medical and nursing needs of patients with renal stones. No special preparation is required for the treatment.

The patient attends the radiography department for a KUB film to check the stone's position 30 minutes prior to treatment except on the first visit as an X-ray would have been taken at the pretreatment clinic attendance. The patient is introduced to the lithotriptor staff who will explain the procedure. After the patient has undressed and put on an open-backed gown (and

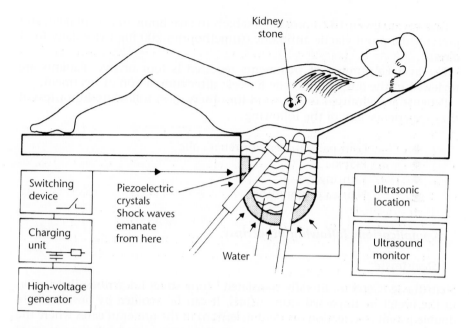

Figure 6.4 *The patient's position on the Wolf lithotriptor*

disposable paper pants if desired), the renal stone is located manually by ultrasound probe and its position is marked on the patient's back.

The patient is helped on to the lithotriptor, and lies in a supine position with the marked loin sagging into the water close to the ultrasound probe. The dish and probe are moved electrically until the stone is aligned in two planes at the focus of the shock waves. Shock waves are then generated, building up to the maximum rate and intensity that can be tolerated by the patient. These levels are reduced if the patient experiences pain.

The position of the stone is monitored throughout on the ultrasound screen and the patient may be repositioned as required during the procedure (position may be changed if pain is experienced).

On completion of the treatment, the patient is helped down from the lithotriptor, given a towel and allowed to dress.

A recovery area is provided where patients may sit and relax before their journey home. Patients are encouraged to begin their increased fluid intake at this stage. If they are to remain in hospital, they may return to the ward with or without an escort as their condition dictates. There is no reason why patients may not leave for home as soon as the treatment is over if they feel able.

Patients are advised to drink large amounts of fluid to encourage diuresis and flushing out of stone fragments from the kidney. A minimum of 3 litres every 24 hours is recommended.

Initially two appointments for treatment are given with dates approximately a week apart, with an X-ray prior to treatment. Further sessions are booked as necessary and progress is reviewed after four treatments to evaluate the effectiveness of the treatment. If the stone is broken into fragments of less than 2 mm no further treatment is necessary as these should pass spontaneously.

Patients are given 10 co-proxamol tablets to take home in case of pain, and prescribed a prophylactic antibiotic (trimethoprim 200 mg twice daily for 3 days).

The average number of treatments required is four or five. Patients are reviewed in the outpatient clinic 6 weeks after completion of treatment.

Patients are admitted to the ward for observation following lithotripsy if they experience any of the following:

- Loin pain, ureteric or renal colic
- Pyrexia
- Fainting
- Nausea or vomiting

Complications following lithotripsy

Steinstrasse

Steinstrasse (German: literally translated 'stone street') describes obstruction of the ureter by impacted stone debris. It can be avoided by positioning a double-J stent (see section on stent insertion) in the ureter in cases where the stone is over 2–3 cm in diameter prior to the commencement of a course of treatment.

Signs of steinstrasse are:

- Severe loin pain
- Pyrexia
- Nausea and vomiting

Treatment of steinstrasse involves the use of analgesia: an opioid if pain is severe, otherwise oral analgesics or non-steroid anti-inflammatory suppositories (e.g. diclofenac 100 mg) are prescribed.

Antibiotics are prescribed prophylactically or as appropriate to urine cultures. Intravenous fluid replacement is commenced if indicated and an antiemetic given.

Renal ultrasonography is performed to determine the degree of obstruction. If the tract is dilated a percutaneous nephrostomy drain is inserted and attached to a drainage bag to relieve hydronephrosis. The gradual dispersal of debris is effected by continued ureteric peristalsis. The patient is kept under X-ray review and the nephrostomy is removed when the steinstrasse has dispersed.

Dispersal of debris may be achieved more speedily if the patient undergoes endoscopic insertion of a ureteric stent, as the ureter dilates around the stent, allowing stone fragments to pass down more easily.

Ureteric colic

There is reduced incidence of colic after treatment on the Wolf lithotriptor as the stones are broken into small pieces. However, if it does occur the patient may have to be admitted to hospital for observation and administration of analgesics parenterally, orally or rectally as dictated by the degree of discomfort.

ADVICE TO PATIENTS FOLLOWING LITHOTRIPSY

Treatment is generally carried out on an outpatient basis but sometimes a patient may need to be admitted overnight. This is usually planned before treatment.

Lithotripsy is a comparatively painless procedure; however, occasionally patients have experienced some discomfort or pain during treatment. If you experience pain during treatment, inform the surgeon who will adjust the shockwave.

Instructions to patients after treatment

1. Some patients experience pain after treatment. This is mostly caused when stone fragments pass from the kidney to bladder.
2. You will be given painkilling tablets, with instructions how to take them.
3. Most stones are infected. In order to prevent infection spreading you will be given a course of antibiotics to take for 3 days. It is important that you complete this course even if you feel quite well.
4. If you develop a temperature, feel generally unwell or are having a lot of pain, you should contact your local doctor who will have been informed about your treatment.
5. After treatment you may pass bloodstained urine. You should not worry as this is normal after the treatment. However, if the urine remains heavily bloodstained on the day following treatment contact your local doctor.
6. After treatment you should drink plenty of fluid – about 3 litres (6 pints, 15 cups, 10 mugs) in the first 24 hours after treatment. This will help to clear the urine of stone fragments and blood.

If you have further queries ask the surgeon or the nurse in the Lithotriptor Centre.

Pyrexia

Pyrexia may indicate a urinary tract infection. An MSU is taken for microbiological assessment and the patient commences a suitable antibiotic, e.g. trimethoprim 200 mg twice daily, until the laboratory report indicates the appropriate drug. If the pyrexia persists blood should be sent for culture and antibiotics given intravenously.

Inadequate fragmentation

Inadequate fragmentation is confirmed by X-ray after treatment. If the ureter is not obstructed repeat treatments can be arranged.

Haematuria

Patients are warned before treatment that this may occur and it is not a cause for alarm as long as they are able to void urine without difficulty. An increased intake of fluids is recommended as mentioned previously.

Combined techniques

Staghorn calculi

A combined approach is used for large staghorn calculi; the stone is 'de-bulked' by percutaneous nephrolithotomy, and EPL is used to disintegrate residual stone fragments when the patient has recovered from the initial procedure.

'Push-bang' or 'push-pull' procedure

These procedures are used for stones in the middle and upper third of the ureter which are not accessible to ureteroscopic removal or lasertripsy. During ureteroscopy, a narrow catheter is passed into the ureter through which saline is flushed rapidly, dislodging the stone back into the kidney where it can be treated with EPL or nephrolithotomy. Stent insertion is often carried out at this time to prevent the stone from falling back into the ureter.

An antegrade approach can also be used to retrieve stones in the upper third of the ureter. A nephroscope is introduced into the ureter via a percutaneous tract and the stone is disintegrated with a flexible lithotripsy probe. The laser may also be used via this route.

Stent insertion

Indications

Indications for the insertion of a stent are:

- ◆ prelithotripsy, where the stone is larger than 2 cm in diameter
- ◆ to relieve ureteric obstruction or stricture, e.g. calculi, tumour, retroperitoneal fibrosis
- ◆ to facilitate drainage of urine when ureteric trauma has occurred, e.g. oedema or perforation of ureter during endoscopic removal of stone

Stent insertion takes place under general anaesthesia and the patient may be treated as a day-case. A cystoscopy is performed, the appropriate ureteric orifice is identified and the stent is inserted into the ureter as shown in Figure 6.5. When the guidewire is removed the stent remains positioned between the kidney and bladder. Patients are warned that they may experience some disturbances to their normal voiding pattern but these should resolve within 24–48 hours.

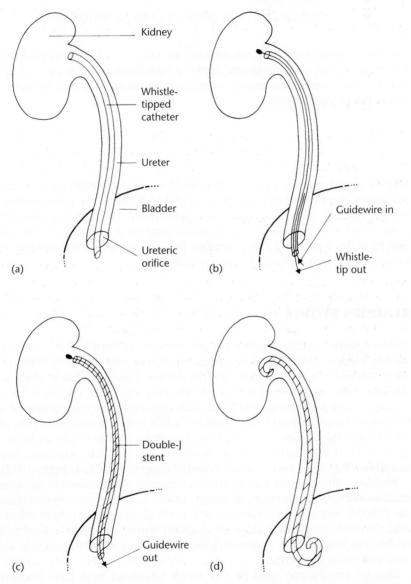

Figure 6.5 *Double-J stent insertion: (a) whistle-tipped ureteric catheter is introduced via the ureter into the renal pelvis cystoscopically; (b) a guidewire is introduced through the lumen of the ureteric catheter which is then withdrawn leaving the tip of the guidewire in the renal pelvis; (c) the double-J stent is inserted over the guidewire and positioned correctly; the guidewire is then removed; (d) when the guidewire is out, both ends of the stent curl into a 'J' shape in the kidney and bladder, thus securing it in place*

Possible problems

Possible problems following stent insertion include:

- frequency of micturition
- urgency of micturition
- haematuria
- suprapubic pain, particularly on finishing voiding

These symptoms resolve spontaneously in most cases but some patients may have to be given oral analgesics. Again, a high fluid intake is advised to flush out the haematuria and relieve suprapubic discomfort, which is more acute when the bladder is empty.

Stent removal

Stent removal can be done under general or local anaesthesia as a day-case procedure if a flexible cystoscope is available. Cystoscopy is performed, and the end of the stent is grasped and withdrawn through the bladder and urethra. If local anaesthesia is used, lignocaine gel is inserted into the urethra and in males a penile clamp is applied for 20 minutes. Oral analgesia should be used, as the procedure can be uncomfortable.

BLADDER STONES

Primary stones of the bladder are uncommon in both children and adults within Europe. However, it is commonplace to find children with bladder stones in parts of India, Indonesia, the Middle East and China. These stones usually occur in urine which is sterile, and are more common in males (Tanagho and McAninch, 1992). In such countries, the mechanism of stone formation would appear to be related to a diet low in protein and phosphate, which may then be compounded by dehydration (due to the ambient temperature) and also diarrhoea. In areas where such stones are endemic, they are usually ammonium and/or urate based (Tanagho and McAninch, 1992).

Bladder stones among Europeans, in contrast, are commonly the result of bladder outflow obstruction, although stones can form within diverticula of the bladder mucosa (especially if the diverticulum does not drain effectively, and therefore contains a pool of stagnant urine), or upon a foreign body within the bladder (e.g. a catheter), which acts as a nidus for calcium deposition and stone formation.

Bladder calculi may also be the result of stones that have successfully passed down the ureter, but then lodged and subsequently enlarged within the bladder lumen. Bladder stones, within a European context, are nearly always seen in men, and are frequently associated with urinary stasis and/or chronic urinary tract infection. The exact composition of these stones varies, according to the urinary pH and also the concentration of stone-forming elements within the urine. In the USA, calcium oxalate is the most common stone constituent, whereas in European populations, uric acid and urate stones predominate (Tanagho and McAninch, 1992).

Presenting problems

The typical presentation is the sudden loss of urinary stream during voiding, along with the acute onset of pain radiating into the penis or perineum. Small amounts of blood may also be passed.

Pain radiating down and along the penis may be present when the stone intermittently obstructs the bladder neck, acting in much the same way as a ball-valve. Pain resulting from bladder calculi is relieved when the patient lies down, as the stone will then fall backwards away from the trigone, thus relieving the obstruction.

Urinary infection is also common when bladder stones and outflow obstruction coexist, particularly as bacteria can lodge within the stone matrix, which then serves to partially (or completely) protect such pathogens from antibiotic agents within the urine. Thus patients with bladder stones frequently give a history of hesitancy, frequency, dysuria, haematuria, dribbling and poor urinary stream, or of a chronic urinary tract infection unresponsive to antibiotic therapy.

Treatment

Bladder stones can be removed endoscopically or via an open procedure, or can be treated with lithotripsy (EHL or ultrasound) or laser. Small bladder stones may be removed via transurethral irrigation, under either general or local anaesthesia.

Larger stones need to be broken into fragments, to facilitate their removal. This fragmentation can be achieved using either lithotripsy or laser (which is more recent). Lasertripsy requires the passage of an endoscope, and is thus performed under general or local anaesthesia, with appropriate precautions (e.g. eye protection).

Patient care

The nursing management of these patients is the same as that of any patient undergoing lithotripsy or lasertripsy, although haematuria is less likely as the stone is not tightly held within the substance of the bladder.

The patient must be reassured that the passage of small stone fragments is normal, following the procedure, and encouraged to drink an adequate amount of fluid to facilitate removal of such fragments (at least 3 litres a day, if there is no medical contraindication).

Litholapaxy

The historical and still commonly employed method for bladder stone removal is litholapaxy. A manual lithotrite is used. This is an instrument which resembles an adjustable set of 'jaws' which can be controlled from the exterior. Once inside the patient's bladder the jaws of the lithotrite are closed, with the stone between them, resulting in fragmentation of the stone.

The lithotrite is introduced via the urethra, and the stone gripped. It is then crushed into pieces small enough to be evacuated from the bladder via cystoscopy and irrigation. Originally the procedure was performed 'blind', but nowadays the optical lithotrite is used (incorporating a fibreoptic light source and telescope), which allows the stone to be crushed under direct vision, reducing the risk of bladder damage. Stone fragments are removed via irrigation, and the bladder lumen rechecked. The procedure is usually performed under general or spinal anaesthesia and the postoperative care centres upon observing for excessive haematuria, and ensuring that the patient maintains an adequate oral fluid intake, to facilitate the removal of any small stone fragments that remain. Advice and reassurance for the patient are important.

Cystolithotomy

Stones that cannot be crushed safely (e.g. stones that are very large) may need to be removed surgically, via a suprapubic incision. The bladder wall is opened, and the stone removed.

Patient care

Patients will return from theatre with a urinary catheter in situ. Some units will use both a suprapubic catheter and a urethral catheter, especially if the patient has a history of outflow obstruction. There will also be an intravenous infusion. Some form of wound drainage may also be present.

The patients may eat and drink as soon as they feel able, and some form of analgesia will be required.

The catheter remains in situ until the bladder wall has healed (7–10 days) and a cystogram may then be performed to check that there is no leakage from the bladder wall. The catheter will then be removed.

If the bladder stone has resulted from chronic outflow obstruction, this will also need to be treated. An open removal of the stone may be combined with either retropubic or transvesical prostatectomy. Some units prefer, on the basis of safety, to resect the prostate first, via a transurethral approach, and then to open the bladder simply to remove the stone.

Occasionally longstanding bladder calculi may cause sufficient urothelial irritation or inflammation as to induce squamous metaplasia and then carcinoma of the bladder. In such cases, the stone is removed, any outflow obstruction relieved and the tumour managed according to its staging and histology.

URETHRAL STONES

Urethral stones are rare; they are usually stones that have formed elsewhere and then lodged in the urethral lumen.

Most small stones (less than 1 cm in diameter) will pass down the urethra (though often with pain), but larger stones can impact, causing pain, bleeding and actual retention.

Primary urethral stones are usually found in association with lower tract abnormalities that may then induce urinary stasis or chronic urinary tract infection. Patients with urethral diverticula, strictures, urethral foreign bodies, chronic fistulae and meatal stenosis, as well as benign prostatic hyperplasia, are all more prone to urethral stone development.

Most urethral calculi (about 60%) are located in the anterior urethra and up to 10% at the fossa navicularis. However, up to 40% impact at the membranous urethra or external urinary sphincter (Tanagho and McAninch, 1992).

In females, such stones can often be seen in the urethra, or are evident on transvaginal urethral palpation. In males, retrograde urethrography will identify the presence and location of the stone.

Treatment

In females, urethral stones can be removed directly, or pushed back into the bladder and then evacuated (e.g. by litholapaxy). In males, the stones can usually be pushed back into the bladder via a cystoscope (i.e. under direct vision) and then evacuated. However, in some male patients, impaction of the stone may be so severe as to rule out any attempt to push the stone back up into the bladder. In this situation, the stone is retrieved via a direct incision into the urethra, via the underside of the penis. The incision is then closed, and a urethral catheter left in situ for at least 7 days, to allow closure of the incision line.

Patient care

Patients may return from theatre fitted with both a suprapubic and a urethral stent catheter (though this may vary with individual units), which remain for 7–10 days. Patients may, however, resume both diet and fluids and begin to mobilize as soon as they are able.

Urethrography will be performed prior to the removal of the catheters, to ensure that healing has occurred. If any underlying pathology is present (e.g. a diverticulum) then this may also need to be repaired at the time of surgery.

Prostatic calculi

Prostatic calculi are common. They usually form just within the prostatic capsule in cases of benign prostatic hypertrophy and are unable to migrate into the urethra. During prostatectomy such stones will usually be removed, to prevent them from subsequently impacting in the urethra.

REFERENCES

COE F L and Parks J H (1988) Pathophysiology of kidney stones and strategies for treatment. *Hospital Practice* March: 185–207.

FELLSTRÖM B, Danielson B G, Karlstrom B, Lithell H and Ljunghall S (1989) Dietary habits in renal stone patients compared with healthy subjects. *British Journal of Urology* **63**, 575–580.

FERNSTROM I and Johansen B (1976) Percutaneous pyelolithotomy. *Scandinavian Journal of Urology and Nephrology* **10**: 257–259.

IKARO O, Netto N Jr, Palma P C and D'Ancona C A (1990) Percutaneous nephrectomy in non-functioning kidneys: a preliminary report. *Journal of Urology* **144**(4): 966–968.

ISON K T, Copcoat M J, Timoney A and Wickham J E (1989) The development and application of a new surgical device – the endoscopic liquidiser and surgical aspirator (ELSA). *Journal of Medical Engineering and Technology* **13**(6): 285–289.

LINGEMAN J E, Preminger G M and Wilson D M (1990a) Kidney stones: identifying the cause. *Patient Care* September: 31–46.

LINGEMAN J E, Preminger G M and Wilson D M (1990b) Kidney stones: acute management. *Patient Care* August: 20–37.

RUPEL E and Brown R (1976) Nephroscopy with removal of stone following nephrostomy for obstructive calculus. *Journal of Urology* **46**: 177–182.

TANAGHO E A and McAninch J W (eds) (1992) *Smith's General Urology*, 12 edn. London: Prentice-Hall.

WASSERSTEIN A G (1986) Kidney stones: advice on preventing first episodes and recurrences. *Consultant* May: 81–102.

WHITFIELD H N (1985) *Pocket Consultant Urology.* Oxford: Blackwell Scientific.

WICKHAM J E A and Buck A C (1990a) *Renal Tract Stone: Metabolic Basis and Clinical Practice*, p. 521. Edinburgh: Churchill Livingstone.

WICKHAM J E A and Kellet M K (1981) Percutaneous nephrolithotomy. *British Journal of Urology* **53**: 297–299.

FURTHER READING

HUTCHINSON A, Maltby J R, Reid C R G (1988) Gastric fluid volume and pH in elective inpatients. Part I: coffee or orange juice versus overnight fast. *Can J Anaes* **35**: 12–15.

MARBERGER M, Fitzpatrick J M, Jenkins A D and Pak C Y C (1991) *Stone Surgery*, Chapters 3 and 5. Edinburgh: Churchill Livingstone.

MENDELSON C L (1946) The aspiration of stomach contents into the lungs during obstetric anaesthesia. *American Journal of Obstetrics and Gynaecology* **52**: 191–205

OLSSON G L, Hallen B, Hambraeus-Jonzon K (1986) Aspiration during anaesthesia: a computer-aided study of 185358 anaesthetics. *Acta Anaesthesiologica Scandinavica* **30**: 84–92

PHILLIPS S, Hutchinson S, Davidson T (1993) Preoperative drinking does not affect gastric contents. *British Journal of Anaesthetics* **70**: 6–9.

WARNER M A, Warner M E, Weber J G (1993) Clinical significance of pulmonary aspiration during the perioperative period. *Anaesthesiology* 1993; **78**: 56–62.

WATSON G M and Wickham J E A (1989) The development of a laser and a miniaturised ureteroscope system for ureteric stone management. *World Journal of Urology* **7**: 147–150.

WICKHAM J E A and Buck A C (1990b) *Renal Tract Stone: Metabolic Basis and Clinical Practice*, pp. 633–639. Edinburgh: Churchill Livingstone.

RECONSTRUCTIVE SURGERY FOR URINARY TRACT DEFECTS

7

Contents

This surgical subspeciality has been developed in order to repair anatomical defects in the urinary tract that result from congenital deformity, trauma or tissue damage. Surgery of this type requires not only a skilled surgeon, but also nursing care delivered by nurses who are able to empathize with the patients and their families, as many of these patients have already had protracted hospital stays.

Damage can occur to any area of the urinary tract. This chapter looks at the treatment and nursing care for repairing defects in the kidney, the ureters, the bladder and the urethra.

THE KIDNEY

Trauma

The kidney, by virtue of its anatomical position, surrounded by the ribs, the vertebral column and the paravertebral musculature, is relatively well protected from trauma. However, certain events can cause damage to the kidney, and when this occurs it is often serious. Depending on the nature of the injury, different types of damage will occur. A penetrating wound, such as that resulting from a gunshot wound or a stabbing, will result in severe blood loss and damage to the kidney. A non-penetrating wound may occur as a result of a sports injury or following a direct blow to the loin. A severe injury of this type may cause the kidney to shatter within its capsule. Owing to the highly vascular nature of the kidney any injury is always associated with some degree of haematuria; more severe damage will be accompanied by hypotension and loin swelling.

Diagnosis

The following considerations form the basis for diagnosis:

- history of injury to loin area
- haematuria
- loin pain
- swelling in the loin area
- hypotension and tachycardia

Confirming diagnosis

To assess the extent of the damage the following investigations will be performed:

  intravenous urography (IVU)
  a renal ultrasound scan
  a renal arteriogram

Treatment

If the damage is major and accompanied by severe hypotension, emergency surgery is indicated. If attempts to repair the kidney fail then either partial or total nephrectomy is performed. The damage may also extend to the renal artery. If the injury is more minor then conservative management is indicated. This consists of the following:

1. Bed rest.
2. Observations in order to detect shock – half-hourly measurements of blood pressure and pulse, observations of urine volume.
3. Observation of urine colour.
4. Pain relief.
5. Measurement of abdominal girth, an increase in which will indicate continued bleeding.
6. Replacement of lost fluid either by an increased oral input or by intravenous replacement. Blood products may be required to replace lost blood volume.
7. Antibiotic therapy to prevent infection as a result of the extravasation of urine.
8. The patient must continue to rest for at least 2 weeks following the injury as the risk of secondary haemorrhage is high. The patient should be warned to look for renewed bleeding at 10–14 days after the injury.

The patient should be seen in the outpatient department and a repeat IVU performed after 6 weeks.

Nephrectomy

Nephrectomy refers to the surgical removal of a kidney. This is performed for a variety of reasons, including the arrest of uncontrollable haemorrhage following renal trauma. Other common reasons for removing a kidney are:

- renal cancer (see Chapter 10)
- chronic infection, which has led to renal scarring and loss of function
- renal calculi, which have destroyed most of the viable renal substance, and which continue to cause recurrent urinary infection
- live donor renal transplant

The kidney is removed via one of three approaches: flank approach, lumbar approach, or thoracoabdominal approach. Traditionally, the thoracoabdominal approach has been reserved for cases of renal cancer, as it would appear to allow earlier clamping of the major renal blood vessels, prior to mobilization of the kidney (thereby reducing the risk of systemic, tumour dissemination). However, this is not universal, and some centres may only consider a thoracoabdominal approach in cases where the tumour mass is very large. However, such an incision may cause signficant postoperative problems relating to both respiration and also possible involvement of the peritoneal cavity.

The loin incision is most commonly employed, as it offers a retroperitoneal approach.

Unfortunately, the operative incision (whichever 'open' approach is used) is usually large and extremely painful postoperatively. For this reason, and because of the risk of possible complications, some centres are now experimenting with endoscopic nephrectomy, as described in Chapter 6. However, it remains an experimental procedure.

Preoperative care

The preoperative care of patients undergoing nephrectomy centres upon the following considerations:

- *Safety aspects* – as for any patient undergoing surgery.
- *Adequate explanation and information*: postoperative pain relief should be discussed, and the available options explained. Postoperative breathing exercises should be taught by the physiotherapy department. The elective patient should also be encouraged to give up smoking.
- *Routine blood assay*: cross-match at least two units of blood.
- *Assay (and/or culture) of urine* – to ensure that no preoperative urinary infection is present.

Prior to the removal of a kidney, it is essential to ascertain that there is a contralateral, functional kidney present. In emergency cases, this would usually be done by a single film IVU (see Chapter 2), taken at 20 minutes, which would display both the size and number of kidneys present.

In cases where nephrectomy is an elective procedure, more detailed estimation of renal function will be performed. This will usually involve isotopic study of the kidneys using some form of renogram. In addition, in cases where the kidney is being removed because of cancer, renal arteriography may also be used to display the nature and extent of the blood supply to the tumour mass.

Postoperative care

The nursing management of patients undergoing nephrectomy, owing to the nature of the incision, centres upon the following priorities:

◆ *Effective pain management*: aggressive pain control after nephrectomy is crucial, as the patient will not breathe effectively (or cough) if pain control is neglected. The use of patient-controlled analgesia is to be encouraged (*Drugs and Therapeutics Bulletin*, 1993); an intravenous or subcutaneous opioid infusion, via a pump, is also an excellent management option. Epidural infusions can be used as long as the level of the block is not too high. An intercostal catheter may be sited into the line of the incision (during wound closure) and analgesic agents such as bupivacaine then injected into this. Other alternative strategies may be used as required (e.g. localized heat, transcutaneous electrical nerve stimulation, appropriate relaxation methods, etc.).

◆ *Positioning of the patient* – to enhance comfort and maximize chest expansion on the affected side. This will usually involve either a semirecumbent position, well supported with pillows, or a side-lying position (on the unaffected side), with the patient's head and chest elevated by pillows, to maximize chest expansion on the side where the operative incision has been made.

◆ *Observation for signs of possible haemorrhage*: at least two suction drains are normally inserted during the operation, because of the risk of bleeding postoperatively. Any blood loss from the wound site is observed, and marked if appropriate.

◆ *Observation of postoperative urine output*: this is important, and some units may catheterize the patient in order to measure urine volumes more accurately.

◆ *Assisting the patient with deep breathing and coughing*: to minimize the risk of postoperative chest infection, all patients will receive physiotherapy. This aspect of care will only be effective if the patient's pain is adequately controlled.

◆ *Effective wound management*: wound dressings are usually removed after approximately 48 hours (or sooner if they are heavily bloodstained) and an appropriate dry dressing then applied.

◆ *Intravenous fluids* are given until bowel sounds are present and the patient is tolerating small amounts of fluid without adverse effect. The exact time scale for reintroducing the patient to food and fluids will vary with individual patients.

◆ *Early ambulation* is only realistic if pain control is effective. Also, the use of antiembolism stockings, in association with subcutaneous heparin, forms a common postoperative strategy to help reduce the risk of deep vein thrombosis or pulmonary embolism.

◆ *Adequate information and explanation* should aim to reinforce preoperative teaching.

◆ *Suture removal, if appropriate*: the suture may be subdermal, traditional skin sutures or clips. If removal is required, this will normally be performed approximately 10 days after surgery, when the wound edges are healed.

If the patient has undergone removal of a kidney because of cancer, the ureter is also likely to be removed, along with surrounding perinephric fat, the adrenal gland and associated lymph nodes (radical nephrectomy). As this will require the wall of the bladder to be sutured (at the previous point of ureteric entry) these patients may return from theatre with a urethral catheter in situ, which aims to prevent pressure being placed on the anastomosis by bladder filling. The catheter is then removed 48–72 hours following surgery. This practice is not, however, universal.

Possible complications

Shock

Shock can be caused by loss of circulating volume.

Chest infection

Chest infection may occur as a result of poor chest expansion postoperatively (often as a result of inadequate pain control).

Pneumothorax

Pneumothorax is a possible complication because the loin incision is very close to the twelfth rib. Further, in cases where it is difficult to mobilize the kidney (e.g. if there has been previous renal infection with subsequent fibrosis and scarring) it may be necessary actually to remove the twelfth rib, in which case pneumothorax becomes more likely. Patients may therefore return from theatre with underwater seal chest drainage in situ.

Pulmonary embolism

Pulmonary embolism may result from compression on the venae cavae and other large vessels during surgery. It is, however, a very rare occurrence.

Wound infection

Wound infection is more common in cases where renal infection has been present.

Subphrenic abscess

Subphrenic abscess is more likely if pre-existing renal infection has been present.

Urinary tract infection

Urinary tract infection is more likely to occur if a urinary catheter is present or if the patient's mobility is poor postoperatively.

Pyeloplasty

A structural defect of the pelvis of the kidney can exist at its junction with the ureter, resulting in obstruction (pelviureteric junction obstruction). This may be a congenital problem, or may result from repeated infection or injury (either from surgery or external trauma). There is a narrowing of the ureter, causing an obstruction to the free flow of urine. Pyeloplasty involves altering the structure of the renal pelvis.

Diagnosis

There is a history of colicky pain, which may be accompanied by vomiting, especially after the consumption of large volumes of fluid.

Confirming diagnosis

The following investigations may be performed:

- ◆ An IVU; this may be performed with a diuretic challenge
- ◆ A renogram
- ◆ A Whitaker's test

Preoperative care

In addition to basic preoperative needs the patient should be protected from postoperative infection. A midstream specimen of urine should be obtained at the time of admission, in order that any pre-existing infection can be treated appropriately. Prophylactic antibiotics are usually given at the time of surgery. The risk of postoperative chest infection is high owing to the location of the surgical incision, the pain from which can inhibit deep breathing. The patient should be discouraged from smoking and be seen by the physiotherapist for instruction in deep breathing techniques.

Postoperative care

In addition to the basic postoperative needs the patient should be observed for potential chest infection and difficulties with breathing. The patient should be positioned in such a way as to promote deep breathing (this is usually the position that the patient finds most comfortable) and should be well supported with pillows. The physiotherapist should be involved and regular physiotherapy given. In order to help facilitate deep breathing, early mobilization should occur.

Postoperative pain

The successful relief of pain is of paramount importance in the prevention of complications, i.e. chest infection and deep vein thrombosis. Patient-controlled analgesia is indicated; alternatively, high doses of opiate analgesia are given in regular doses intramuscularly or continuously subcutaneously or intravenously via a pump, with careful observation being made for signs of respiratory depression. When the patient is tolerating food oral analgesia should be given regularly, and the dose of opiate analgesia gradually reduced. Patients should also be taught how to support themselves when moving or coughing.

Potential haemorrhage

Owing to the highly vascular nature of the kidney the risk of haemorrhage is high. Blood pressure and pulse should be recorded in order to detect shock; initially this is usually at half-hourly intervals. This frequency can be reduced as the patient's condition allows. The wound site should be observed for blood loss and the wound drainage measured. Excessive blood loss should be reported. Urine output should be measured and the degree of haematuria assessed.

Prevention of potential blockage to urinary output

In order to protect the surgical anastomosis and prevent extravasation of urine the patient will either have a double-J stent from the kidney to the bladder or have external drainage of urine via a nephrostomy tube. If there is a nephrostomy tube it is important that it is kept patent; if it becomes blocked the patient will experience increased pain and the resultant collection of urine will damage the repair. If the tube becomes blocked it should be gently flushed using 10–20 ml of sterile normal saline. The tube should be dressed in such a way as to avoid any kinking of the tube, maximizing patient comfort and preventing accidental dislodgement.

At 10–14 days after surgery a nephrostogram may be performed in order to establish the patency of both the repair and of the ureter. If all appears to have healed then the tube can be removed. Some units do not perform a nephrostogram but simply clamp the tube, and if the patient experiences no pain or increase in temperature then the tube is removed. Following removal of the tube the patient can be warned to expect some leakage of urine from the site for up to 24 hours. If this is troublesome a stoma bag can be used in order to promote comfort. If the patient has a double-J stent this should be removed in the outpatient department after 2–3 months, under local anaesthesia.

Potential inability to take normal diet and fluids owing to nausea and possible paralytic ileus

On return from theatre if bowel sounds are absent the patient should only be allowed 15–20 ml of fluid orally per hour. As bowel sounds return fluids and diet can be gradually reintroduced. Initially fluid will need to be given intravenously as directed. Nausea should be controlled using an appropriate entiemetic, since vomiting will be painful.

Prevention of possible wound infection

The wound should be kept clean and re-dressed as necessary. The clips or sutures should be removed 10–12 days after surgery.

Advice on discharge

Patients should be advised not to return to work for 2–6 weeks depending on their occupation, in order to allow for repair of the muscular tissue.

THE URETERS

Trauma

Injury to the ureters from external violence or from penetrating wounds seldom occurs. Most commonly any injury to the ureter occurs as a result of iatrogenic damage during abdominal surgery.

Diagnosis

Extravasation of urine will occur. This may be either intraperitoneal or extraperitoneal. It often remains unrecognized for some time. If the urine is sterile at the time of injury its presence in the peritoneal cavity will cause few symptoms, apart from increasing abdominal distension as a result of it collecting. Eventually urine may begin to drain either via a wound or from the vagina. If the urine is infected at the time of injury, peritonitis will occur and the patient will complain of abdominal pain in the lower abdominal quadrant. Vomiting may also occur due to paralytic ileus.

Injury may also occur as a result of accidental ligation of the ureter during surgery. This results in complete blockage to the passage of urine from the kidney on that side, resulting in hydronephrosis. The presence of the ligature will also cause local tissue necrosis and possible formation of a fistula which leads to delayed extravasation.

The diagnostic signs can be summarized as follows:

- ◆ Pain in lower abdominal quadrant
- ◆ Vomiting and paralytic ileus
- ◆ Peritonitis
- ◆ Leakage of urine from wound or vagina

Confirming diagnosis

A specimen of any leaking fluid should be sent for urea and electrolyte analysis to confirm the diagnosis. If complete occlusion is present serum creatinine levels will be raised. A plain abdominal X-ray may show the presence of extravasated urine. An intravenous urogram and isotope scanning tests should be done.

Treatment

At time of operation

1. *End-to-end anastomosis*. The ends of the severed ureter are rejoined, and a double-J stent inserted.
2. *Transureteroureterostomy*. The damaged ureter is anastomosed to the other ureter.
3. *Implantation of ureter into bladder (ureteroneocystostomy)*. If the upper part of the ureter is long enough to reach the bladder without undue tension, it can be implanted directly into the bladder wall. The anastomosis at the bladder must be tunnelled, in order to prevent reflux. A double-J stent is inserted to splint the ureter and to promote healing, and the patient should have a urethral catheter.
4. *Boari flap procedure*. If the upper length of the ureter is not sufficiently long to reach the bladder a Boari flap can be created. A rectangular flap is cut into the bladder wall and rolled to create a tube into which the ureter can be secured. A double-J stent should be inserted and the patient should have a urethral catheter.
5. If a bladder flap cannot be made long enough a segment of ileum with its blood supply can be used to replace it.

Conservative management

If the patient is unfit for major surgery, a nephrostomy tube can be inserted into the affected kidney to provide external drainage and maintain renal function.

Nursing care

Preoperative

In addition to basic preoperative nursing, it is necessary to establish the correct diagnosis. The nurse should observe for leakage of urine via the wound, wound drainage system or vagina, sending a specimen if possible for estimation of urea and electrolyte levels. The nurse should also check for possible septicaemia and shock. Blood pressure, pulse and temperature should be recorded, observing for shock.

Postoperative

The postoperative care depends on the procedure employed. In addition to basic postoperative needs the patient has the following requirements.

1. *Maintain urinary drainage.* Depending on the surgical technique used, either double-J stents or ureteric splints will be used to facilitate healing of the anastomosis. Ureteric splints are commonly brought out through the abdominal wall. This enables the drainage from each kidney to be assessed. The patient should also be observed for the development of loin pain, indicating obstruction. If a blockage occurs it may be gently flushed out using 10-20 ml of sterile normal saline. The bladder may be drained by catheterization and this should be kept patent. Fluid input should be maintained at a level of 2–3 litres per day in order to maintain urine output. Splints and catheters are normally removed 10 days postoperatively. Double-J stents can be retained in place for up to 3 months and removed under local anaesthesia.

2. *Observations for haemorrhage.* Urine should be observed for the presence and degree of haematuria. The wound site should be observed for blood loss and wound drainage measured. Excessive blood loss should be reported.

3. *Control of discomfort and pain.* Relief of pain should be achieved by the administration of suitable analgesia to allow mobility.

4. *Prevent wound infection.* The wound should be kept clean and re-dressed as necessary. Prophylactic antibiotics may be given in order to render sterile any urine that leaks through the anastomosis.

5. *Possible nausea and paralytic ileus resulting in inability to take normal diet and fluids.* On return from theatre if bowel sounds are absent the patient should be allowed no more than 15–30 ml of fluid per hour orally. Fluids should be given intravenously and reintroduced orally when bowel sounds return. Nausea should be controlled using appropriate antiemetics.

THE BLADDER

Trauma

The bladder can be injured in a number of different ways:

1. *External force* – this is commonly seen as a result of a road traffic accident, especially if the bladder was distended with urine.
2. *Perforation* – this can occur as a result of a fractured pelvis in 10% of cases. It may also occur during surgery as a result of accidental incision, e.g. during laparoscopy or cystoscopy.
3. *Penetrating wounds* – these may occur as a result of stabbing, etc.
4. *Following radiotherapy of the pelvic organs.*

Diagnosis

The diagnosis may be difficult to make as often the patient presents with multiple injuries. Injury to the bladder will result in leakage of urine. This may be extraperitoneal or intraperitoneal.

Extraperitoneal rupture

Extravasation of urine occurs into the perivesical space:

- there will be increasing abdominal tenderness
- the pulse will rise
- only small quantities of urine will be passed

Intraperitoneal rupture

Signs of intraperitoneal rupture are:

- abdominal distension occurs
- bowel sounds decrease
- peritonitis may occur if urine is infected or if diagnosis is delayed
- there is failure to pass urine

Confirming diagnosis

The following tests are used:

- cystoscopy
- cystogram
- IVU

Treatment

Extraperitoneal rupture

Catheterization over a period of 7–10 days will normally be sufficient to allow the rupture to heal.

If the defect results from damage due to radiotherapy, tissue damage may be widespread. Defects are normally excised and a substitution cystoplasty performed (see Chapter 8).

THE URETHRA

Damage to the urethra can occur in a number of ways:

1. *Trauma* – due to a direct blow or straddle injury, or by passage of a stone.
2. *Iatrogenic* – injury to the urethra is a complication of many treatments, including catheterization and instrumentation of the urinary tract, and can also follow prostatectomy.
3. *Infection*, e.g. non-specific urethritis.
4. *Childbirth and gynaecological procedures.*

Trauma

Damage to the male urethra by trauma usually affects the bulbar and membranous portions of the urethra. The anterior urethra is rarely affected.

Bulbar urethra

Bulbar injuries normally result from direct trauma, for example falling astride a crossbar.

Diagnosis

Diagnosis is based on the following:

- history of injury
- bruising of the external genitalia
- blood at the urethral meatus

Treatment

The patient should be given the opportunity to void normally. If he fails to do so a suprapubic catheter should be inserted. A urethral catheter should not be passed because this may aggravate the injury and increase the risk of infection. Prophylactic antibiotic treatment should be given. A urethrogram should be performed on those who fail to void to assess the degree of the injury, so that future treatment can be planned. All patients should have urological follow-up, as progression to stricture is common.

Membranous urethra

Injury to the membranous urethra occurs in approximately 10% of men with a pelvic fracture. Injuries to this area have a high morbidity rate associated with stricture formation, incontinence and impotence. This area is surrounded by sphincter-active tissue and held in place by the pubovesical and pubourethral ligaments. The dislocation of the symphysis pubis can lead to a complete rupture of the urethra, resulting in extravasation of urine, haematoma formation, and the upward dislocation of the bladder and prostate.

Diagnosis

Diagnosis is based on the following:

- history of injury
- bruising of the external genitalia
- blood at the meatus
- retention of urine
- signs of extravasation
- high-riding prostate with bladder displacement

Treatment

Associated injuries often require life-saving treatment and therefore must take precedence over the urethral injury. However, catheterization is generally required for the monitoring of fluid balance. Urethral catheterization should only be attempted if there is no blood at the meatus. A small catheter may be gently introduced without the use of force. If urethral catheterization fails or there is blood at the meatus, a suprapubic catheter should be passed.

An IVU should be performed with an ascending urethrogram when the patient's condition allows, in order to assess the degree of damage, which may be partial or complete rupture of the urethra.

1. *Partial rupture.* Urethroscopy should be performed with suprapubic exploration undertaken in order to drain any haematoma or extravasated urine. A small catheter should also be passed.
2. *Complete rupture.* Suprapubic exploration should be performed in order to drain any haematoma or extravasated urine and under direct vision a urethral catheter passed to act as a splint to keep the urethra in alignment. Fixation of the prostate should be performed along with fixation of the fracture. These patients usually require reconstruction in the long term.

Urethral stricture

Damage to the urethra by whatever cause invariably results in stricture formation. The management of strictures is very variable from centre to centre. Treatment options will depend on the following factors: the patient's general condition; the location of the stricture; the length of the stricture; previous treatment given; the patient's wishes; and the surgeon's skill.

Diagnosis

Diagnosis is based on the following:

- history of predisposing factor
- thin or forked stream
- postmicturition dribble
- incontinence of urine
- frequent infections
- retention of urine

Confirming diagnosis

- urinary flow rate
- urethrogram
- cystourethroscopy
- midstream specimen of urine for culture

Treatment

Urethrotomy

Urethrotomy is a technique used in both the primary and long-term management of urethral strictures. It involves cutting the stricture along its length under direct vision, commonly with an Otis urethroscope. Ideally, following this, new epithelial tissue grows to fill the deficit, widening the narrowed urethra. The complications of this technique are the high incidence of stricture recurrence and the possible damage to the sphincter mechanism, resulting in incontinence.

Preoperative care of the patient should include obtaining a urinary flow rate.

Postoperatively, urinary drainage should be maintained. Catheterization is normally performed at the time of surgery. The length of time that the catheter is retained is dictated by the surgeon.

There is a risk of haemorrhage. Haematuria commonly occurs in the postoperative period and may persist for up to 10 days. Initially the patient will have a urethral catheter which will act as a splint. The colour of the urine should be assessed to determine the degree of haematuria. On removal of the catheter the patient may experience fresh bleeding due to the disturbance of the healing tissues.

There should be adequate pain control. The patient usually experiences minimal pain, but mild to moderate analgesia may be needed. The pain may be more apparent when the patient starts voiding urethrally, owing to the irritation of the urine on the healing tissues.

Dilation

Dilation is used in the long-term management of strictures, and may be performed on an outpatient basis. The treatment aims to stretch the urethral scar tissue by the introduction of a series of urethral dilators (bougies), increasing in size until the urethra has been adequately dilated. Prior to treatment a local anaesthetic is inserted into the urethra and a penile clamp applied, in order to produce local anaesthesia.

Following the procedure the patient will require a mild analgesic. A urinary flow rate should be taken in order to monitor the effectiveness of treatment.

Complications of this procedure include:

1. *Bacteraemia*, possibly due to poor aseptic technique, or introduction of bacteria into the circulation from a pre-existing urinary tract infection.
2. *Haemorrhage*, due to trauma. The patient's urine should be observed prior to discharge, and a high fluid intake advised.
3. *Urethral rupture*: the membranous urethra is particularly vulnerable to rupture following instrumentation.
4. *Restricturing* of the affected area is common.

Self-dilation

The introduction of self-dilation of strictures has led to a decrease in the number of patients requiring regular surgery (Harriss *et al.*, 1994). Meatal strictures can be treated by teaching the patient to self-dilate by the introduction of a well-lubricated catheter tip into the meatus. Dilation should be performed on a twice-weekly basis. Other strictures have successfully been treated by urethrotomy followed by dilation using a low-friction hydrophilized disposable catheter, twice weekly for at least 1 year (Harriss *et al.*, 1994).

Stenting

A stent suitable for use in the urethra was developed in the 1980s. It is made of an inert metal mesh which is placed over the site of the stricture using an introducer, then released. It then springs into position holding open the stricture. The stent is gradually covered by epithelial tissue, rendering it continuous with the urethral tissue. The advantage of this procedure is that it can be performed under local anaesthesia, offering a curative therapy to the medically unfit. It has been found to be very beneficial in the treatment of recurrent bulbar strictures (Milroy *et al.*, 1988).

Infection should be eliminated before the operation is performed. Urine should be sent for culture, and broad-spectrum antibiotics given at the time of operation.

Infection should also be prevented postoperatively. The patient's temperature should be monitored and a course of antibiotics given. Pain or discomfort should be controlled. Perineal pain may be a problem initially, particularly associated with nocturnal erections (Oesterling, 1995). Suitable analgesia should be given.

Complications of this procedure include:

1. *Stenosis.* The overgrowth of epithelial tissue has been reported, particularly following placement for strictures caused by trauma. This leads to the stent being removed.
2. *Misplacement of the stent.* Incorrect placement may lead to the development of incontinence.
3. *Encrustation* can also occur if the stent protrudes above the bladder neck.
4. *Perineal pain* may persist after the initial postoperative period. If this cannot be controlled, removal may be necessary.

The patient with a stent should not undergo urethral catheterization as this may lead to displacement, and should therefore be encouraged to carry a card indicating the presence of a stent.

Long-term catheterization

Catheterization, usually suprapubic, can be considered for the management of a stricture in the severely debilitated patient and in those not wanting further surgery.

Urethroplasty

The type of surgery undertaken to reconstruct the male urethra is dependent upon the following factors:

- length of the defect
- location of the injury within the urethra

A defect of up to 1.5 cm in length can be repaired by excising the strictured tissue and creating an end-to-end anastomosis. Any stricture longer than this will require a 'substitution' urethroplasty, where the defect is repaired by grafting.

The location of the injury will affect the choice of treatment, as follows:

1. *The glans meatus* (see Chapter 8).
2. *The penile urethra* – this area is amenable to the whole variety of treatment methods.
3. *The bulbar urethra* is best repaired by skin grafting, as end-to-end anastomosis can result in chordee of the penis.
4. *The prostatic, membranous urethra* is sphincter-active, and surgery normally consists of grafting by an experienced surgeon.

Surgical techniques

End-to-end anastomosis

The strictured part of the urethra is excised and the continuity of the urethra restored by the anastomosis of the ends.

Substitution urethroplasty

Substitution urethroplasty can be performed in either one or two stages (Figure 7.1). The urethra is exposed via a midline perineal incision and if the stricture occurs high in the urethra an abdominal incision is sometimes also required. Once the strictured area is exposed it is excised and replaced by grafted skin.

If the procedure is complex and hair-bearing skin is used for the graft, it may be decided not to close the wound but to have a two-stage procedure. This allows for inspection of the graft prior to closure, and an opportunity for epilation of the graft. If this is the case the patient will void via a perineal urethrostomy.

The second stage of the urethroplasty involves closure of the new urethra. If the procedure can be done in one stage the graft is closed and a urethral catheter inserted.

Skin grafting

Types of skin

There has been much debate over the merits of different types of skin used for urethral grafting, both in the short and long term (Blandy, 1986; Turner-Warwick, 1988; Mundy, 1995).

1. *Wet* – epidermal skin, which is adapted for a moist environment such as urethra, oral mucosa, vagina, labia.
2. *Dry* – scrotum, thigh, abdominal skin, which in a moist environment becomes inflamed.
3. *Penile* – moisture-resistant skin, which is relatively hairless.

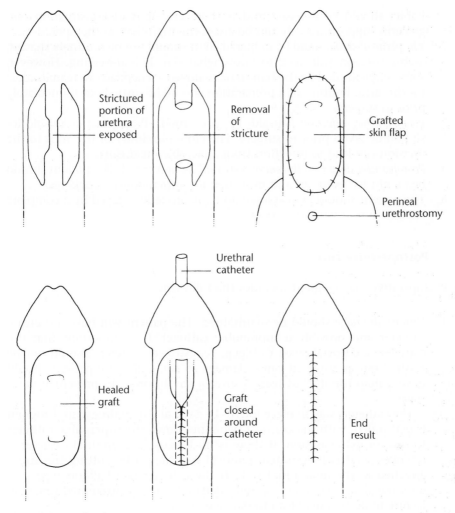

Figure 7.1   *Urethroplasty*

Types of grafting

The grafts may be:

- ◆   *Free grafts* (use full-thickness skin)
- ◆   *Mesh grafts* (skin is perforated prior to grafting)

Free grafts and mesh grafting are dependent upon survival of the whole graft. In pedicle grafting the skin is taken along with its blood supply.

Preoperative care

Preoperative nursing care should encompass the following:

1. *Postoperative constipation* should be prevented to avoid straining and painful evacuation of the bowels postoperatively. The patient's bowel

habits should be assessed and if there are signs of constipation two glycerin suppositories should be given the night before the operation.

2. *The perineal skin* should be prepared. Skin should not be routinely shaved, as the surgeon will need to know what skin is hair-bearing. However, some surgeons do like the hair to be removed – a depilatory cream is ideal for this area. Routine skin preparation should be carried out immediately prior to surgery.

3. *Postoperative infection* should be prevented. Prophylactic antibiotics should be given prior to surgery. The close proximity of the anus to the incision can lead to infection from anaerobic organisms.

4. *Postoperative deep vein thrombosis* should be prevented. The patient should be taught leg exercises and measured for antiembolism stockings.

5. The patient should be reassured and any anxieties allayed by a complete explanation of what to expect.

Postoperative care

Postoperative management includes the following:

1. *Urinary drainage* should be maintained. The patient will have a urethral catheter and possibly a suprapubic catheter. It is important that the catheters are not allowed to block. Fenestrated catheters should not be washed out as this will cause damage to the graft. The patient should have a fluid input of at least 3 litres a day in order to prevent urinary stasis.

   The catheters stay in place for 10–14 days, at which time a urethrogram is performed, with the contrast being put down the suprapubic catheter to test for extravasation. If there is no leakage, the urethral catheter is removed. If it is fenestrated, removal is achieved by cutting the stitch attached to the abdominal wall. If the catheter is a balloon type it is essential that the balloon is fully deflated prior to attempted removal. Failure to do this may lead to damage of the graft.

2. *Haematoma formation and excessive swelling of the scrotal or penile area* should be prevented. This is not only a source of discomfort but also can lead to failure of the graft. There is often some form of compression applied to the penis. This may be a foam dressing or a semiconstricting piece of tape applied around the shaft of the penis. The whole of the scrotal area should be well supported with bulky padding secured with Elastonet pants.

   There may also be some type of wound drainage, via either a corrugated drain or a vacuum system. It is usual to leave the initial dressing in place for 3 days until the incidence of swelling is reduced. However, padding should be changed if it is bloodsoaked. The drain is normally removed 2–3 days postoperatively.

   In the initial postoperative period the patient's activity should be limited to moving from bed to chair, as greater exertion could lead to further swelling.

3. *The perineal wound* should be protected from infection. Owing to the close proximity of the incision to the anus, the wound is at risk of infection from anaerobic microbes.

After a one-stage procedure the patient should be allowed to bathe as soon as the wound drain has been removed, and should be encouraged to do so daily and after any bowel motion. If the procedure is the first of a two-stage repair, bathing should not be permitted until 4–5 days postoperatively. After a bath the wound should be cleaned with sterile saline and a supportive dressing applied. The urethral catheter should be taped in such a way as to elevate the penis on the abdominal wall. This helps to reduce swelling. Care must be taken not to put too much traction on this catheter. Antibiotic therapy is usually given until the catheters are removed. Initially this will be intravenously.

4. *Deep vein thrombosis* must be prevented. This is achieved by the wearing of antiembolism stockings, leg exercises while the patient is immobile, early mobilization, and by giving heparin subcutaneously as prescribed.

5. *Straining* will result in pain and discomfort to the patient and so constipation should be prevented as far as possible. If the patient is usually constipated a gentle laxative should be given prophylactically.

6. The patient will experience discomfort in the early postoperative period and opioid analgesia should be given. An anti-inflammatory drug should also be given regularly, either rectally or orally, as this will help to reduce pain from the oedema. A supportive wound dressing does much to relieve discomfort.

The patient may also suffer from bladder spasm resulting from the catheterization. If this is troublesome an anticholinergic drug such as oxybutynin should be given regularly. After a satisfactory urethrogram, the urethral catheter is removed. The suprapubic catheter can be clamped and the patient should void normally.

Residual urine volumes can be measured via the suprapubic catheter and if these are low the suprapubic catheter can be removed. A flow rate should be obtained.

Postoperative advice

The patient should be told never to allow an inexperienced person to catheterize him urethrally – a suprapubic catheter is preferable. The patient should continue to rest for a further month. Prolonged sitting and driving should be avoided. Sexual intercourse should not be resumed for 6 weeks.

REFERENCES

BLANDY J (1986) *Operative Urology*, 2nd edn, pp 206–207. Oxford: Blackwell Scientific.

Consumers Association (1993) *Drug and Therapeutics Bulletin* **31**(3): 11–12.

HARRISS D R, Beckingham I J, Lemberger R J and Lawrence W T (1994) Long term results of intermittent low-friction self-catheterisation in patients with recurrent urethral strictures. *British Journal of Urology* **74**(6): 790–792.

MILROY E J G, Cooper J E, Wallsten H *et al.* (1988) A new treatment of urethral strictures. *Lancet* **i**: 1424–1427.

MUNDY A R (1995) The long-term results of skin inlay urethroplasty. *British Journal of Urology* **75**: 59–61.

OESTERING J (1995) Use of intraluminal stents in the management of intravesical obstruction. *Journal of Urological Nursing* **13**(3): 787–804.

TURNER-WARWICK R (1988) Urethral stricture surgery. In: Mundy A R (ed.) *Current Operative Surgery – Urology*, pp 160–218. London: Baillière Tindall.

8 RECONSTRUCTIVE SURGERY FOR THE PROMOTION OF CONTINENCE

Contents

It is commonly supposed that incontinence is a problem that is exclusive to the elderly. Few people realize that it can affect almost anyone. It is not confined to the elderly or disabled, but is common in people of all ages, fit or disabled. Incontinence can be defined as the involuntary passing of urine and/or faeces in a socially unacceptable place. The International Continence Society defines urinary incontinence as 'a condition where involuntary loss of urine is a social or hygienic problem'.

This distressing and socially disabling condition affects 5% of the population, with women affected more than men – 8% of all women in the population are affected as opposed to only 3% of men (Bullock *et al.*, 1989). Many people see incontinence as an inevitable discomfort and embarrassment. The general public's interpretation of the term 'incontinence' is often different from its medical interpretation. Many people use the term to describe a total lack of control and deny being incontinent even though they may admit to 'wetting' or 'leakage' (Norton, 1986). Many sufferers hide their problem from society, their family, friends and even from themselves. Children are teased by their schoolmates, leading to a dread of going to school, absences, deterioration in schoolwork and a growing sense of isolation. Hiding the problem – even denying its existence – may be their coping mechanism to deal with the ridicule, and help them feel less ostracized.

Older sufferers also show these feelings. The embarrassment and shame of being wet, the risk of leakage, and having to wear incontinence aids can drive them to cut themselves off from others, with grave repercussions on their educational, working and social lives. Loss of self-esteem and confidence, the conviction that the condition is discernible by and obvious to all those around them, the belief that they smell and that this cannot be hidden, no matter how much washing or perfume is used, all contribute to the negative self-image of the incontinent. These people will not feel attractive to the opposite (or same) sex, and existing relationships may suffer and founder as a consequence. It is an unsurmountable obstacle for the unattached sufferer who wants to establish a relationship, as the fear of rejection is powerful and restricting.

Incontinence does become more common as one becomes older, though it is not an inevitable part of the ageing process. Older people may find talking about the problem impossible, because it relates to a very personal and 'taboo' area of their bodies. It is also a sign of their loss of 'control' and may indicate that hospitalization or institutionalization may result.

The cost of incontinence, both in the practical sense (i.e. the money to buy aids, replace bedding, furniture, laundry bills, etc.) and in the emotional sense (i.e. the guilt, and feelings of inadequacy and hopelessness experienced by the carers), is almost incalculable. Ignorance about the way the body functions, and the conviction that nothing can be done to improve the condition, lead to the sufferer becoming pessimistic about the prospect of any improvement.

Incontinence creates psychosocial problems for all sufferers, and causes disruptions, big and small, to their lifestyles, depending on their ability to cope. It is important that sufferers become aware that help is available, and that if a cure is not possible, then considerable help and support is, and should be offered (Norton, 1986).

THE INCONTINENT PATIENT IN HOSPITAL

A patient suffering from incontinence, when admitted to a specialist unit, arrives with a mixture of apprehension, hope and relief. Many have endured their condition for some time, and may have consulted (unsuccessfully) their general practitioner or other specialists for help. Having finally been referred to a specialist unit and undergone tests which show the cause of their problem, the fact that something is finally going to happen which may cure them seems hardly possible. It is always wise to be completely honest with these patients and explain all that they should expect as a result of the surgery they are to have. The idea is not to discourage them, but to give a realistic picture of the positive and negative aspects of the treatment. Many patients may have to undergo more than one surgical intervention until the result is deemed acceptable by themselves and their consultants. A greater understanding of their condition, the expected outcome of the surgery, the possible setbacks which may occur and what they are expected to contribute to their care and recovery, helps give these patients a sense of control and aids in ensuring compliance with the treatment.

When admitted to the ward, patients often feel that they have found a place where it is no longer 'taboo' to talk about the problem, because all the staff are experienced in the treatment of incontinence. It may be the first time that many details of the condition have been revealed, and the reassurance the patient receives may alleviate feelings of guilt or disgust at the problem. In the author's unit, this care starts in the outpatient and urodynamics departments and is continued on the ward. The patients are involved in their own care from the very start.

WHAT IS INCONTINENCE?

Urinary incontinence is the involuntary loss of urine. It is often a symptom of an underlying problem. This loss of urine may occur via the urethra or from an abnormal extraurethral route.

Classification of incontinence

Incontinence is classified as follows:

- ◆ stress incontinence
- ◆ urge incontinence
- ◆ neurogenic bladder
- ◆ outflow incontinence
- ◆ incontinence secondary to fistulae or congenital anomalies (Sokeland, 1989 – according to the International Continence Society)

STRESS INCONTINENCE

The term 'stress incontinence' refers to either a symptom or a medical diagnosis. Genuine stress incontinence refers to incontinence caused by a weak or incompetent sphincter. A rise in intra-abdominal pressure, transmitted to the bladder, exceeds urethral closure pressure in the absence of detrusor activity (Bullock *et al.*, 1989). Stress incontinence as a 'symptom' describes the experience of leaking urine upon physical exertion, such as in patients with cough or strain-induced detrusor instability, where leakage is due to the abnormal detrusor activity and not sphincter weakness. A patient in urinary retention can experience overflow incontinence on exertion. Urodynamic investigations are required to determine the true cause of the leakage.

Sphincter weakness is more common in women than in men. Some of the causes include obesity, multiparity and childbirth. Men may also suffer sphincter weakness following pelvic fracture injuries or prostatectomy. In postmenopausal women a loss of tone in the urethral mucosa and muscle is the result of an oestrogen deficiency.

Surgical treatment

Before surgery is attempted, the patient will be encouraged to try non-invasive treatment. It is only after trying a whole range of such treatments that surgery is contemplated. The aim of the surgery is to elevate and support the bladder neck so that this will be repositioned correctly above the pelvic floor muscles. The repairs can be done vaginally together with repair to any existing cystocele. Repairs also can be done via a suprapubic approach.

There is no special preoperative physical care for anyone undergoing these types of operation. The important thing is to explain that sometimes the results can vary, and the chances of total cure cannot be guaranteed. However, the results may be *too* good in some cases, and the patient may not be able to pass urine urethrally at all. It is always a good idea to warn the patient of this, and to discuss and demonstrate intermittent self-catheterization as a possible solution should this happen. A woman who has not yet completed her family should be warned that vaginal delivery may be difficult, and may also undo the effects of surgery. All patients should be told that even if the surgery is successful, there is a possibility of stress incontinence recurring at a later date.

Vaginal repair

There are many variations on vaginal repair. The bladder neck and proximal urethra are displayed via the divided anterior vaginal wall. The exposed bladder neck and urethra are then mobilized upwards and held with buttress sutures.

Abdominal repairs

Abdominal repairs are usually via a bikini-line incision. The colposuspension operation is a modification of the Marshall–Marchetti–Krantz procedure where the bladder neck is hitched to the back of the symphysis pubis by sutures placed on either side of the urethra. In the colposuspension, sutures are placed in the lateral vaginal fornices, elevating and supporting the bladder neck. Either organic material (e.g. strips of fascia or muscle) or synthetic slings (e.g. polypropylene or polyethylene) can be used to support and elevate the bladder neck by attachment to ligaments or periosteum. In the Stamey operation, a long needle is passed via a small suprapubic incision and nylon sutures are placed in either side of the bladder neck.

Postoperative care

The specific postoperative care these patients require involves the care of their newly 'hitched up' bladder necks, to ensure they heal adequately and prove strong enough to give some degree of continence back to the patient. The patient returns to the ward with a vaginal pack in situ (to stem vaginal bleeding), a suprapubic catheter, and sometimes a urethral catheter. Besides the usual immediate postoperative care, it is most important that these patients' catheters are checked frequently to ensure they are patent and urine is able to drain out freely. This may involve flushing the catheters to remove debris and blood clots. The patient's fluid intake should also be monitored. An intravenous infusion is usually in progress for the first 24 hours, and the patient is allowed and encouraged to drink as soon as she can tolerate it. The patient's fluid intake over the remainder of her hospital stay is important and she should be encouraged to drink at least 3 litres of fluid a day to keep her bladder and catheters flushed and patent. The vaginal pack is removed after 24 hours, and usually so is the urethral catheter. The latter sometimes depends on the surgeon's preference.

The patient is encouraged to start mobilizing on the first postoperative day and is usually independent again by the second or third postoperative day. The rest of her stay in hospital is really a period of waiting until it is time to clamp the suprapubic catheter. For a Stamey operation this is usually within 7 days. This again depends on the individual surgeon's preference. Once the catheter is clamped, the patient should begin passing urine urethrally. It is at this point that the patient needs maximum support. Sometimes the patient is able to pass good amounts (200–300 ml) of urine every 2–3 hours with no leaking urethrally between visits to the toilet. Some patients, however, find that they pass small amounts (20–60 ml) every 10–60 minutes. This does sometimes improve over the following few days, and patients should be reassured and supported through this time.

Once the patient has passed urine two or three times after clamping, the catheter can be released and any residual urine in the bladder drained out and measured. This is usually measured two or three times a day. The residual volume aimed for is an amount between 0 ml and 50 ml. Again, if the bladder is holding more than this, the amount may also improve after a day or two.

Once the residual volume is 50 ml or less, the catheter is removed and the patient discharged home. There may be some leakage via the suprapubic catheter site. The patient should be reassured that this usually stops after a day or two, and if the leakage is severe, a stoma bag can be worn over the site to collect the urine and keep the patient dry. If the residual volumes remain large or the patient continues to pass small frequent amounts of urine, with some leakage, then she may be discharged home with the suprapubic catheter still in place, and she will be shown how to clamp and release this herself and record her progress over a period of 2–3 weeks.

Once the residual measurements are within acceptable limits the patient is readmitted to have the catheter removed and her micturating pattern monitored. If the residual volumes remain large, the patient may have to be taught how to empty her bladder completely by using intermittent clean catheterization (see Advice Sheet).

Endoscopic treatment

Another surgical option is the endoscopic injection of Teflon paste on either side of the bladder neck to relieve stress incontinence. However, Teflon has been found to migrate from its original position of insertion, and has been found lodged in brain tissue (Kulber *et al.*, 1995; McKinney *et al.*, 1995). This makes it dangerous to use in the younger patient. A new substance has been

ADVICE FOR PATIENTS FOLLOWING BLADDER NECK SUSPENSION PROCEDURES

THIS ADVICE SHEET IS IN ADDITION TO ANY VERBAL ADVICE YOU MAY BE GIVEN BY THE MEDICAL AND NURSING STAFF ON BEING DISCHARGED: PLEASE READ THIS SHEET AND KEEP IT FOR FUTURE REFERENCE

Passing Urine

You may still be passing urine frequently, in small amounts, with some discomfort on leaving hospital. This is to be expected and should gradually improve over the following weeks. You should try to hold your urine for 5–10 minutes longer in between visits to the toilet each day, so that eventually you will be able to pass urine every 2–4 hours, and will be dry and comfortable between times. This may take some time to achieve, but please persevere. You must not strain to pass urine.

Fluid Intake

Drink at least 2 litres of fluid daily. This may help keep infection in your urine from occurring. You should reduce the amount that you drink up to 2 hours before your bedtime so that your urine output at night will be reduced too and so you may not have to pass urine too frequently at night. This frequency will also improve in time.

Work, Rest and Exercise

Allow yourself plenty of rest. Avoid lifting heavy objects (e.g. shopping, suitcases, or children) for at least 6–8 weeks, then gradually increase your level of activity. You should aim to reach your pre-operation level by the time of your first outpatient's appointment (about 6–8 weeks). It is a good idea to take some gentle exercise during this period too (e.g. a short daily walk) if you can manage it.

Returning to work will depend on the type of work you do. If your job involves lifting or standing for long periods of time, you may be advised to take at least 4–6 weeks off work. Please ask the doctor or nurse on the ward for advice if you are not certain what to do.

developed which is now being used instead of Teflon, called Bio or Macro-plastique.

Stress incontinence in men

In men, operations as described above have not been successful.

Implantable mechanical devices, such as a silicone gel prosthesis (Kauf-man), can be implanted in the perineum to provide constant urethral compression. Another option is the insertion of an artificial urinary sphincter. This is covered later in the chapter.

URGE INCONTINENCE

Urge incontinence occurs when there is an involuntary loss of urine following a strong desire to void. This urgency may be extreme, with urine being voided simultaneously with the sensation to void. Sometimes there is a short delay between the sensation and capacity, but the sufferer may still be incontinent even if the toilet is reached in time. Detrusor hyperreflexia is the result of involuntary bladder contractions while the bladder is filling. When the normal inhibiting impulses are not sent from the bladder centre in the cortex the reflex arc is completed. The bladder responds by contracting before micturition is initiated voluntarily. This causes a variety of symptoms which include frequency, urgency, urge incontinence, nocturia and possibly nocturnal enuresis. Detrusor instability may be secondary to bladder outflow obstruction or idiopathic in origin (Figures 8.1 and 8.2). Patients suffering from bladder instability may have no obvious neurological lesion causing

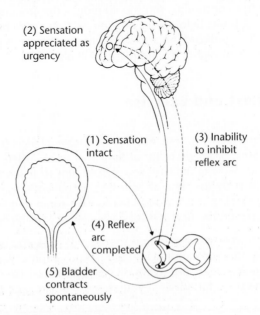

Figure 8.1 *Detrusor instability*

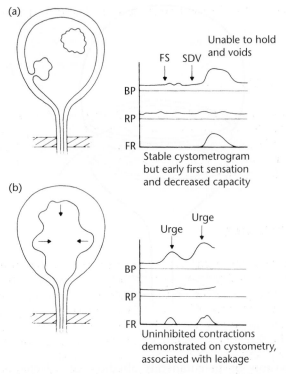

Figure 8.2   *Urge incontinence – CMG profiles: (a) sensory urge; (b) motor urge. BP, bladder pressure; FR, flow rate; FS, first sensation; RP, rectal pressure; SDV, strong desire to void*

their inability to inhibit bladder contractions. The condition often presents in the second, third or fourth decades of life, and may have no obvious cause.

Urge incontinence may also have sensory as well as motor causes. Sensory urgency may result because of intravesical pathology (e.g. urinary infection, interstitial cystitis, bladder calculi, bladder tumours); however, some patients have no demonstrable problem and pyschological factors may be involved.

Surgical treatment

Hydrostatic bladder distension is one procedure usually performed under general anaesthesia; it involves expanding the bladder with fluid and keeping it distended for 5 minutes. The patient usually stays in hospital for 24 hours after the operation and is discharged once the urine is clear and blood-free. A Helmstein distension is a more prolonged procedure where a balloon is inflated within the bladder to a pressure between the systolic and diastolic blood pressures for 2–4 hours. It is usually performed under epidural anaesthesia. Bullock *et al.* (1989) claimed that although improvement occurs in 60–80% of patients, recurrence of symptoms is common. There is also a risk of bladder rupture occurring during the procedure.

Cystoscopic subtrigonal injection of phenol has been used to cause partial denervation of the bladder. Rosenbaum et al (1990) reported that this has not been found to be as effective as hoped. This denervation can also be achieved

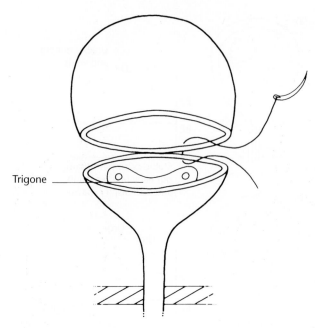

Figure 8.3 *Bladder transection*

by surgical division or percutaneous ablation of selected sacral nerves (usually S3), or by division and resuturing of the bladder just above the trigone. This is called bladder transection (Figure 8.3).

If these procedures do not help, the only alternative may be that the bladder will have to be enlarged so that bladder capacity is increased. This procedure is known as a cystoplasty. Again, any patient who is to undergo one of the above surgical procedures should be instructed in self-catheterization, as there is a possibility of not being able to empty the bladder completely afterwards. Failing a cystoplasty, the patient may have to undergo urinary diversion.

Cystoplasty

A segment of detubularized bowel (ileum is usually preferred though the colon can also be utilized) is used to increase the functional capacity of the bladder. This is known as *augmentation cystoplasty*. Alternatively, the bulk of the bladder can be removed and the bladder refashioned using caecum (Figure 8.4). This is known as *substitution cystoplasty*. The type of operation is decided following tests, and taking the individual patient's condition into consideration. The patient is warned at this stage that it is a major operation and will entail being admitted to hospital 2–3 days before surgery itself to be prepared for the operation. The patient is told to expect to be in hospital for a minimum of 2 weeks. Self-catheterization is also discussed at this point and more information about this as well as a practical demonstration may be required before the patient decides to go ahead with the procedure.

The main reason for being admitted a few days earlier is to ensure that the patient's bowel is cleared prior to a portion of it being used as part of the new

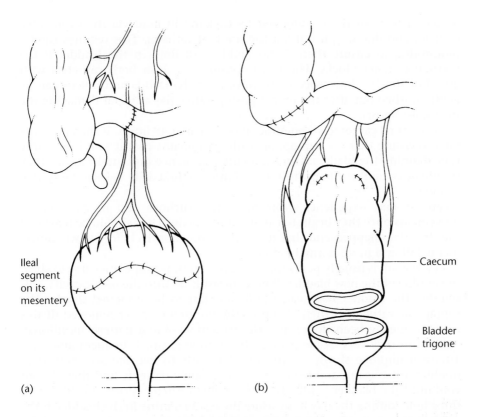

Figure 8.4   *Enterocystoplasty: (a)'clam' ileocystoplasty; (b) caecocystoplasty*

bladder. The patient is allowed to eat a low-residue diet on being admitted 3 days before the operation. The patient is then allowed to drink free fluids on the next day and given oral aperients such as sodium picosulphate (Picolax). On the day before the operation the patient is only allowed clear free fluids which will not form a residue in the bowel, and another dose of aperients. This is a difficult period for the patient. It is also embarrassing if any faecal accidents occur. Patients should be well supported and allowance made for tiredness and weakness. Visitors should be encouraged, as well as some form of entertainment or distraction to help the patient and ensure compliance with the procedure. Some surgeons favour starting intravenous fluid therapy some hours before the start of the operation to help replace fluid lost by the profuse diarrhoea.

Postoperative care

The most important part of postoperative care involves the newly formed bladder. The aim is to keep the bladder deflated so that the new anastomosis heals. The patient usually has a suprapubic and a urethral catheter in situ. It is essential that these are kept patent to allow all urine and debris to drain out. The bowel part of the bladder will also continue to form mucus which may cause obstruction. These catheters are kept patent by flushing them. Again, this depends on the surgeon's preference. Some surgeons advocate flushing only if the catheters seem blocked. Some prefer to attach continuous irrigation to flush the bladder out by trickling in fluid via the suprapubic catheter and draining it out via the urethral catheter. This requires careful monitoring to ensure there is no build-up of fluid in the bladder if the urethral catheter blocks. The third option is to flush both catheters with 20 ml of sterile saline twice or three times daily. Debris and mucus can be gently washed out after the fourth postoperative day without damaging the new anastomosis.

The urethral catheter is sometimes removed after 48 hours. It then becomes vital to ensure that the suprapubic catheter remains patent as it is the only tube draining the bladder. Once patients commence oral intake again, they should be encouraged to drink at least 3 litres of fluid daily to keep the system flushed.

Patients may experience problems with diarrhoea and irregular bowel movements once they begin to eat and drink again. They should be reassured that this does happen and that it may be some months before bowel movements follow a more normal pattern.

A cystogram is usually performed after the tenth postoperative day to show the outline of the new bladder; if no contrast leaks into the pelvic cavity, this signifies the bladder has healed and can start to be stretched slowly. The suprapubic catheter is then clamped, the urethral catheter removed (if this has not already been done) and the patient's voiding pattern monitored. Again, this may vary. Some patients begin to void small, frequent amounts. This will improve slowly, as the bladder starts to become accustomed to holding urine again, and begins to stretch. Some patients find they do not void until the bladder is full. The suprapubic catheter is unclamped two or three times during the day to measure the residual urine in the bladder. If the residual volume is 50 ml or less, the suprapubic catheter is removed and the patient discharged home. If the residual volume is large, the patient will have to empty the bladder by intermittent self-catheterization. It is vital that the possibility of this happening is made known to the patient before the operation, so that though the result of the operation may be a disappointment, it will not be completely unexpected. Some patients find that they only have to catheterize for a few months, and after a while can cut this down to once or twice a day. Some patients may have to start catheterizing some months after surgery. The bladder will have stretched to hold a large volume (at times as much as 800–1000 ml or even more) and they find they cannot empty the bladder completely when they void. They complain of feeling uncomfortable and pass urine frequently. The build-up of urine also leads to recurrent urine infections. By self-catheterizing, these patients can reverse this process.

Another complication of this operation is that some patients begin to experience spasms of pain in the bladder. These contractions usually originate in the bowel part of the new bladder (though not always) and if very intense, could lead to urine leaking out of the bladder because of the increase in pressure. Antispasmodic medication such as Colpermin or oxybutynin, which work on the smooth muscle contractions, may help. Oxybutynin, though effective, may cause severe side-effects including blurred vision and extreme thirst. Intravesical administration of this drug has been shown to minimize these side-effects and be as effective in controlling the muscle spasms (Enzelsberge *et al.*, 1995). However, some patients may need another section or patch of bowel added to the original cystoplasty to enlarge the bladder further and stop the spasm pattern.

Excess mucus production may lead to recurrent urinary tract infections and bladder stones (Woodhouse, 1994). The importance of frequent (3–4 hourly) bladder emptying and the intake of at least 3 litres of fluid daily must be reinforced to these patients. Drinking cranberry juice (200 ml) twice a day has been shown to reduce the quantity of mucus produced in some patients (Rosenbaum *et al.*, 1989). Some patients may have to resort to removing excess mucus by bladder washout via a urethral catheter.

Artificial urinary sphincters

Some patients may have both stress and urge incontinence and so will require a cystoplasty, as already described, but with a simultaneous bladder neck suspension or the insertion of an artificial urinary sphincter to keep them dry (Figure 8.5).

All compression devices such as the sphincter or the Kaufman's prosthesis (mentioned earlier) are prone to complications including urethral erosion, infection and mechanical failure. Preoperative preparation is vital to reduce the risk of these complications. The specific preparation depends on the individual surgeon's preference. However, all methods involve some form of bowel preparation to ensure the rectum is empty at operation. The patient is encouraged to have two or three baths using an antiseptic skin detergent or an iodine-based surgical skin scrub. Some units prefer patients to use the detergent on their hair also. Rectal antibiotics are given as part of the premedication and the patient's pubic area is always shaved in the operating theatre immediately before surgery. These procedures all reduce the risk of infection.

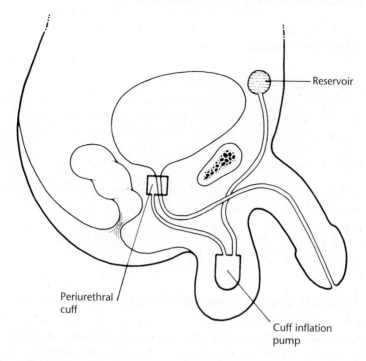

Figure 8.5 *Artificial urinary sphincter*

ADVICE FOR PATIENTS FOLLOWING BLADDER AUGMENTATION PROCEDURES

THIS ADVICE SHEET IS IN ADDITION TO ANY VERBAL ADVICE YOU MAY BE GIVEN BY THE MEDICAL AND NURSING STAFF ON BEING DISCHARGED: PLEASE READ THIS SHEET AND KEEP IT FOR FUTURE REFERENCE

Passing urine

You may find passing urine difficult at first, and it may take some time for you to establish a normal pattern. You may find that you are passing urine frequently and in small amounts. Try holding your urine for 5–10 minutes longer each time you need to pass urine. This will help expand your bladder, and in time it will be able to hold more urine.

If you find that you are passing less and less urine and feel you have a full bladder, and start to get more urine infections, please contact your doctor or the ward for advice.

Do not strain when trying to pass urine

Diet and fluids

You may find that you have irregular bowel habits when you are first discharged home. This is because some of your bowel has been used to create the new bladder. Eat a varied diet, with plenty of fruit and vegetables, which should stop you becoming constipated. Your appetite may be smaller than it used to be, so you may prefer to eat smaller, more regular meals, instead of three main meals a day.

Drink at least 3 litres of fluid a day. Drinks that are high in vitamin C and cranberry juice may help to reduce the mucus production of the bowel part of your new bladder. The fluid will dilute the mucus, making it easier to pass out of the bladder, and reduce the risk of you developing a urine infection.

Please contact your general practitioner if:

- your urine becomes thick and smells offensively, if you suffer fevers or shivering, feel unwell or your urine contains blood

> - your operation scar becomes hard, reddened or inflamed, or begins to ooze
> - you have abdominal pain which does not get better within 2–3 hours, even after taking painkillers
>
> **Please contact the ward if:**
>
> You begin to pass smaller, more frequent amounts of urine and feel your bladder is still full of urine and never completely empty.

Post operative care also varies, though a period of bed rest ranging from a few days to 3 weeks is common to all. Patients usually have a suprapubic catheter in situ to drain away urine, though this is usually removed before discharge. The sphincter is not activated until 6 weeks after the operation. The patient must be prepared to be wet during this time, and to watch out for any sign of infection so that this can be treated immediately. The patient is allowed to have a bath, but instructed to dry the area well afterwards.

The patient is usually taught to activate the device in the outpatient department. Some patients with neurogenic bladder problems may have a cystoplasty and insertion of the artificial sphincter but actually empty their bladders by self-catheterizing. This may sound complicated, but it gives the individual control and it achieves the aim of making the patient continent and improving the quality of life.

NEUROGENIC BLADDER

Continence is not something we are born with, it is a skill we acquire and retain in childhood. A baby voids in response to a sacral reflex arc. With practice, voluntary control of the bladder becomes possible, and the reflex arc response to a full bladder can be blocked, and micturition can be prevented (Figures 8.6 and 8.7). The bladder and urethra therefore act as a single functional unit, and the storage and expulsion of urine are controlled by

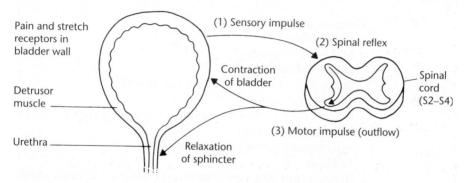

Figure 8.6 *Sacral reflex arc*

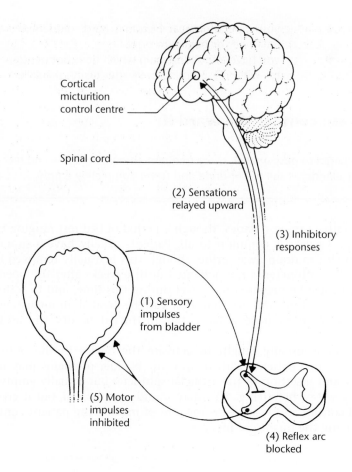

Cortical
micturition
control centre

Spinal cord

(2) Sensations
relayed upward

(3) Inhibitory
responses

(1) Sensory
impulses
from bladder

(5) Motor
impulses
inhibited

(4) Reflex arc
blocked

Figure 8.7   *Inhibition of the sacral reflex arc*

a complex neurological system. Lesions at any point in the neurological pathway can disturb the continence voiding mechanism.

Neurogenic bladder disorders resulting from central nervous system (CNS) lesions are:

◆   Congenital anomalies:
    spina bifida
    myelomeningocele
    spinal dysraphism
    dermoid cyst or fistula of the sacral cord
◆   Acquired CNS lesions:
    trauma with partial or complete damage of spinal cord or
    bladder innervation
    inflammatory process (poliomyelitis)
    tumours
    degenerative diseases (Parkinson's disease, diabetes mellitus, encephalomyelitis)

In some cases bladder function is disturbed before symptoms of the neurological disease become manifest (e.g. urinary retention can be the first symptom in multiple sclerosis). The micturition centre is located between the vertebral bodies S1 and S4. The detrusor muscle is innervated by parasympathetic nerves originating from S2–S4 and reaches the bladder wall via the pelvic nerve. Sympathetic fibres from the thoracolumbar plexus at T11–L2 reach the trigonal muscle and the bladder neck via the pelvic nerve. The pudendal nerve (S2–S4) controls the external sphincter. The sensory nerves follow the sympathetic and parasympathetic fibres (S2–S4 and T9–L2).

Since the underlying disease causing the neurogenic bladder is often incurable, medical and/or surgical treatment of the local symptoms originating from the bladder is indicated. Figure 8.8 shows common causes of neuropathic bladder dysfunction.

Lesions that affect the sacral cord or peripheral nerves can result in both the detrusor and urethra becoming underactive. Lesions of the suprasacral cord result in fewer inhibitory impulses, causing detrusor overactivity. The urethra is also overactive and unco-ordinated with detrusor contraction (dyssynergia). Lesions that occur above the pons result in the loss of cerebral inhibition; this may produce an overactive detrusor. The detrusor and urethral activity remain uncoordinated.

Besides suffering from bladder disorders, these patients may also suffer

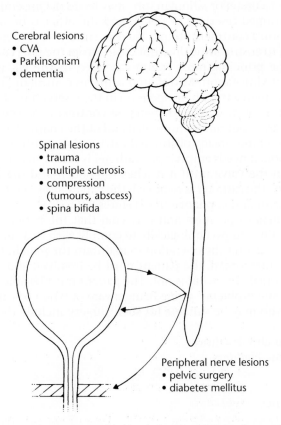

Cerebral lesions
• CVA
• Parkinsonism
• dementia

Spinal lesions
• trauma
• multiple sclerosis
• compression
  (tumours, abscess)
• spina bifida

Peripheral nerve lesions
• pelvic surgery
• diabetes mellitus

Figure 8.8 Common causes of neuropathic bladder dysfunction (CVA, cerebrovascular accident)

from upper tract dilatation as a result of high intravesical pressures caused by detrusor hyperreflexia and detrusor sphincter dyssynergia. Vesicoureteric reflex may also occur, especially in children with congenital lesions of the spinal cord.

Surgical treatment

The management of incontinence in these patients depends on an accurate diagnosis of the cause of the change in the detrusor and urethral function. Some conditions may respond to drug treatment, while in others some form of surgery may be required. Ultimately, however, the patient may have to undergo a urinary diversion. The field of urinary diversion is expanding and new procedures are constantly being developed. Some patients may have to have a conventional ileal or colonic conduit formed and collect the urine formed using external appliances (see Chapter 11). Recent developments in this field have resulted in the development of continent urinary diversions. These work on the principle of forming a reservoir for the urine which can then be drained by catheterizing a continent abdominal stoma. The 'reservoir' can be the bladder itself (with or without the urethra closed), or a bladder that has been augmented with bowel or indeed completely made of bowel. The catheterization channel can be the appendix, or made of ileum or colon. Alternatively, part of a ureter or fallopian tube may be used. One end is tunnelled into the newly formed reservoir or pouch and the other is brought to the skin's surface to form a continent stoma. There are many ways to make a continence mechanism to ensure urine does not escape from the reservoir via this tunnel. Arguably the principle most commonly used in the UK is that of French surgeon Paul Mitrofanoff. Mitrofanoff achieves continence of his channel by burying 2–3 cm in a trough he opens up in the reservoir wall. This forms a flap valve which is obstructed and therefore continent. As the pouch fills with urine, pressure is put on the tunnelled end of the channel, thereby increasing the pressure on the already obstructed valve and preventing urine leaking out. When the pouch needs emptying, a catheter is gently inserted into the tunnel and through the valve until it reaches the pouch and the urine drains out. When empty, the catheter is removed, the valve closes and the patient is once more continent and appliance-free (Figures 8.9 to 8.12).

This is a major operation and it is vital that the patient is well prepared both physically and psychologically to comply with treatment and especially the care needed after the operation to maintain the pouch. Just as in the care of a transplanted organ, the patient must be involved and aware of what to expect as normal, and what is not. The patient must be able to recognize and deal with some problems, while being aware of when to call for help.

Patients who may be suitable for such surgery include those with:

congenital abnormalities
neuropathic bladders
cancer
trauma
incontinence
fistulae
other diversions, e.g. ureterosigmoidostomies and ileal conduits

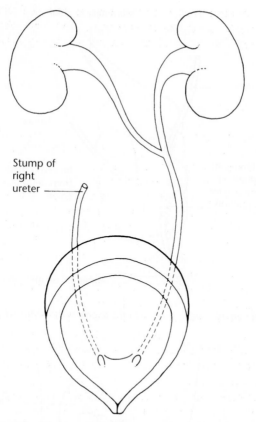

Stump of
right
ureter

Figure 8.9 *Urinary diversion: the Mitrofanoff principle using the right ureter as the continent catheterizable tunnel and the patient's native bladder*

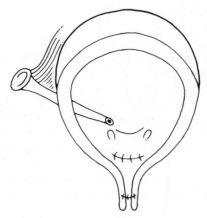

Figure 8.10 *Using the Mitrofanoff principle for a patient with sphincter incompetence. The appendix is used for the tunnel with the patient's native bladder as a reservoir. The bladder neck has been closed*

Many patients have been incontinent for years or have worn stoma bags since childhood. The prospect of being free of these problems sometimes makes them oblivious to anything else they are told about the new diversion. These patients must be prepared for any complication of the surgery and for

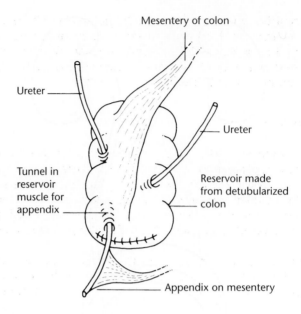

Figure 8.11 Pouch formation using colon with the appendix as the tunnel

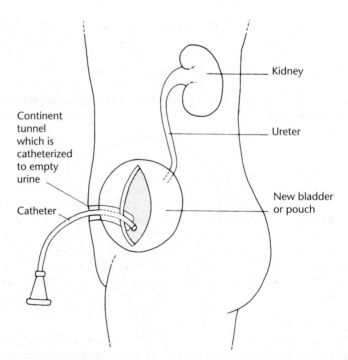

Figure 8.12 Position of neobladder or pouch

subsequent problems, without being made to feel totally negative about the whole procedure. Patients should also have enough manual dexterity to cope with the insertion of the catheter and efficient drainage of the pouch. Preparation for this operation therefore starts in the outpatient department.

Specific preoperative investigations include glomerular filtration rate (GFR) studies and technetium-99m diethylenetriaminepenta-acetic acid (DTPA) scans to ensure the patient's kidneys have adequate function to cope with the change. Urodynamic studies are also carried out to ascertain bladder size, function and pressure, and to test for ureteric reflux.

Admission for surgery

The patient is admitted to the ward 2–3 days before the operation to ensure these tests are complete, and to start bowel preparation. The majority of patients undergo bowel preparation even if preoperative assessment seems to indicate the bladder will be suitable for use as the reservoir. This is a precaution in case, once the operation has commenced, it is felt that some bowel will be needed either to make the bladder larger or to use as part of the channel.

Patients should also be warned about the many drainage tubes they will have inserted during surgery and with which they will return to the ward. Once again they need support and time to ask questions during this period.

Siting the stoma

The stoma is usually sited on the patient's right, low down in the groin (bikini) area. The position varies according to the patient's anatomy, what is being used to form the channel, and if the patient is having any other procedure that will also result in formation of a stoma, such as the Malone antegrade continence enema. The umbilicus is increasingly becoming the site of choice for the exit site of the stoma. This or a site just above it is the best option if the patient is confined to a wheelchair or unable to locate a stoma placed any further down due to any disability.

Postoperative care

Specific postoperative care focuses on maintaining patency of the drainage tubes, to ensure anastomosis of the new pouch and tunnel, and monitoring urine output. The new bladder usually has a catheter inserted into the stoma or channel and a 'suprapubic' catheter. If the patient's ureters had to be reimplanted, the patient may also have one or two ureteric stents in situ. There will also be one or two wound drains and a nasogastric or gastrostomy tube, as well as a peripheral line and sometimes a central venous pressure line (Figure 8.13). This is an impressive amount of tubing to be confronted with if the preparation has not been adequate.

Careful monitoring of the vital signs and urine output is essential to ensure the kidneys are adequately perfused. There is a danger of patients needing extra fluid replacement postoperatively, to replace fluid lost during the procedure, and also because of the 2–3 days of bowel preparation before this. An intravenous infusion is sometimes started preoperatively to start the rehydrating process before surgery. The amount of fluid lost is estimated by monitoring weight loss while bowel preparation is in progress.

The suprapubic and pouch catheters are flushed twice a day with 20 ml of

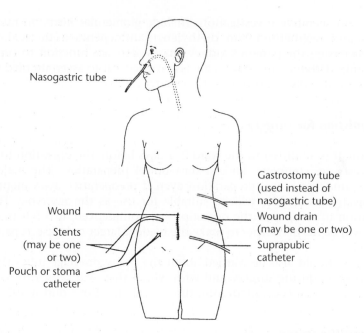

Nasogastric tube

Gastrostomy tube
(used instead of
nasogastric tube)

Wound

Wound drain
(may be one or two)

Stents
(may be one
or two)

Suprapubic
catheter

Pouch or stoma
catheter

Figure 8.13 *Position of drainage catheters and tubes postoperatively*

sterile saline or water for the first 3 days. The ureteric stents may also be
flushed if drainage is not adequate and they are thought to be blocked. As
with the cystoplasty operations, after the fourth postoperative day the pouch
can be washed out gently twice daily to clear the pouch of debris and mucus
produced by the bowel. Once patients are able, they can take over this
procedure, as the skill of washing out the pouch will have to be maintained
once the patient is discharged.

The ureteric stents are gently 'tweaked' on day 7 after the operation, and
generally loosen enough to be totally removed by day 10. After the tenth day
the patient may have a 'pouchogram' or cystogram to check if the new
bladder is intact. If no dye leaks out, the suprapubic catheter may be
removed, leaving the pouch urine to drain out via the pouch catheter in
the stoma. Patients are usually discharged after this, with instructions to
carry on with the bladder washouts at least twice daily, to ensure the pouch
urine drains out and that the pouch is not stretched at any time. Some
patients prefer being discharged home with both the pouch and suprapubic
catheters in situ, though only one is usually on free drainage of urine.

Readmission

The patient is readmitted after 4 weeks (i.e. 6 weeks after the operation). This
gives time for the channel to heal and be ready to be catheterized intermittently. The pouch catheter is clamped and the patient is encouraged to drink
plenty of fluids. This fills the pouch up with urine and helps the patient to
establish what sensation is experienced as this happens. Many patients have
never experienced the feeling of a full bladder before, and some find it
strange, frightening and painful at first. The pouch catheter is released after

2–4 hours, depending on how well the patient can tolerate the discomfort and on the amount of fluid drunk. This process is repeated once or twice more to continue expanding the pouch. The pouches are usually constructed to hold approximately 500 ml. Some patients reach this target easily, while others find that initially they can only tolerate 200 ml or less. It is important to reassure these patients that they will become used to the sensation in time, the pouch will stretch, and they will eventually be able to tell when the pouch needs emptying by the feeling of fullness they experience. Some patients will not have any sensation at all and will have to establish a voiding schedule they can follow. It is vital that the pouch is not allowed to become too full; the patient should be advised to empty it at least every 4–6 hours. If the pouch becomes too full there is a danger of its trauma and rupture, as well as the risk of urine leaking out of the tunnel and the tunnel becoming too compressed to let a catheter into the pouch to drain it. If this happens the urine can be released by insertion of a suprapubic catheter percutaneously into the pouch using ultrasonography. Using a smaller catheter and/or a guidewire down the stoma is sometimes successful. Alternatively, urine can be aspirated out of the pouch via a needle and syringe, until a catheter is able to be pushed into the channel.

After the pouch has been stretched, the catheter is removed and the catheterization procedure is explained and demonstrated (see discharge guidelines). The patient is then supervised catheterizing the pouch until confident about doing this alone, and the supervisor is happy with the patient's technique. Most patients remain in hospital for 1–2 days, and some only require admission as day patients.

Patients are discharged with supplies of catheters and washout equipment, as well as detailed discharge advice to help them through any initial problems. They are encouraged to keep close links with the hospital so that any problems that arise can be dealt with quickly by telephone or by arranging emergency appointments to see the doctor. This is necessary as the procedure is still new and the appropriate care cannot always be obtained from local hospitals or general practitioner surgeries.

Follow-up and complications

Patients are followed up closely after the operation. Follow-up regimens vary, but most include yearly intravenous urograms or kidney, ureter and bladder X-rays, bladder and renal ultrasound scans, GFR tests, pouch pressure studies and blood tests. The latter include measuring the full blood count and urea, electrolytes, creatinine, chloride and bicarbonate levels.

Complications may include:

- incontinence
- stenosis of the stoma
- inability to empty pouch
- metabolic acidosis
- malabsorption
- stone formation
- pouch rupture
- renal damage
- delayed linear growth (in children)

ADVICE FOR PATIENTS ON THE AFTERCARE OF CONTINENT URINARY DIVERSIONS

THIS ADVICE SHEET IS IN ADDITION TO ANY VERBAL ADVICE YOU MAY BE GIVEN BY THE MEDICAL AND NURSING STAFF ON BEING DISCHARGED: PLEASE READ THIS SHEET AND KEEP IT FOR FUTURE REFERENCE

Catheterizing your pouch

Please remember that this is a clean procedure and that it is therefore important to make sure you have everything you need before you begin. Only then should you wash your hands. This avoids unnecessary handling of equipment and potential contamination which could lead to introducing infection into the pouch. Remember that you can catheterize yourself in whatever position is most comfortable or convenient for you (e.g. sitting on the toilet, standing over it, or sitting in your wheelchair or a chair instead).

You may use some lubrication (e.g. K-Y jelly) on the catheter to make it easier to insert, but you may find that this becomes unnecessary in time. The catheter should be inserted gently into the stoma until urine begins to flow out. When the flow has stopped, you should try pushing the catheter in a little further and you may find more urine will flow out. Please do not push it in if you experience any pain. To ensure all the urine has drained out, rotate the catheter gently as you withdraw it. This may dislodge any debris or mucus blocking the tube and allow urine to flow. Once the pouch is empty, withdraw the catheter.

Fluid intake

You must drink at least 3 litres of fluid a day. If your pouch has been made out of bowel or had some bowel added to it, you may find that it can produce a great deal of mucus. This mucus can build up and besides blocking your catheter when you are emptying the pouch, can act as a medium on which bacteria can grow, causing infections. A good fluid intake will keep this mucus diluted, making it easier to flow out of the catheter. Drinks that are high in vitamin C also help keep the urine free of mucus. Cranberry juice, which is available from many large supermarkets or healthfood shops, also helps make the mucus less thick and helps keep the urine infection-free. We recommend you drink two glasses of this daily (approximately 200 ml a glass). If you find the taste too sharp, you may dilute it with other fruit juices.

Diet

If you have had your new pouch made of bowel or if you have had some bowel added to your existing bladder or pouch, you may find it will take some time for your bowels to return to their normal pattern. Try to eat a well-balanced diet with plenty of fruit and vegetables. This will help to prevent constipation. Eventually your bowels will return to normal. If you feel that this has not happened after a few weeks ask your doctor for advice, or ask for advice at your next outpatient appointment.

Work, rest and play

Please allow yourself plenty of time for rest once you are discharged. You should not do anything too strenuous such as gardening, or lift heavy objects (e.g. shopping or children), for the first 4–6 weeks after the operation. It is best to take gentle exercise at first, slowly increasing this as you feel able. You should aim to reach your preoperation level of activity by the time of your first outpatient appointment.

It is very important that before doing any vigorous activity (e.g. sport or sexual activity) you empty the pouch. This will make you feel more comfortable, and ensure any extra pressure on the pouch will not cause a rupture or trauma.

Important

If you find you cannot catheterize your pouch, do not make the stoma sore by repeated attempts. Stop for a few minutes, do not drink any fluids, then try again. If this persists, **contact your general practitioner or the ward. You may have to go into your local hospital to have a catheter inserted into the pouch or you may be directed back to the ward for treatment**.

Finally

Please keep your outpatient appointments. If the one given to you is inconvenient you should contact your consultant's secretary and a new one will be made for you.

> ### Remember
>
> **Contact your general practitioner if:**
>
> ◆   Your urine becomes thick or smelly, you suffer fevers or shivering, feel unwell or your urine contains blood.
>
> ◆   Your operation scar becomes hard, reddened or inflamed, or begins to ooze.
>
> ◆   You have abdominal or back pain that does not get better within 2–3 hours.
>
> **Please contact the ward if you are unable to push the catheter into the stoma to empty the pouch**.

Many of these problems mean further hospitalization and surgery. However, most patients will put up with this, because having a continent diversion, not having to use appliances and being dry enhances their self-image and improves their quality of life. They are in control of their bodies perhaps for the first time in their lives, and the freedom this gives them is immeasurable.

URETEROSIGMOIDOSTOMIES AND RECTAL BLADDERS

Rectal bladders were formed as long ago as the 1800s. The Mauclaire, the Gersuny and the Heitz-Boyer and Hovelaque are all examples of rectal bladders. In these pouches the colon is interrupted and the patient is given an abdominal (Mauclaire) or perineal (Gersuny, etc.) colostomy (Figure 8.14). The ureters were then implanted into the remaining sigmoid-rectal segment and the rectal sphincter was used as the continence mechanism. Urine and faeces were therefore kept separate. These procedures had a high mortality rate and serious complications which included nocturnal incontinence, ureteric obstruction, pyelonephritis and renal function deterioration. Improvements in the technique for the implantation of ureters meant that problems with obstruction and reflux were no longer obstacles and by the 1960s the ureterosigmoidostomy had been developed and was performed clinically. In this procedure the ureters were directly implanted into the sigmoid colon, so that unlike the rectal bladders urine and faeces were now mixed and a colostomy was no longer needed. This procedure also fell out of favour and was perceived to have similar complications to the rectal bladders as well as causing metabolic acidosis. A greater worry was the discovery of the incidence of carcinoma at the ureteric-sigmoid junction in these diversions. Much research has been done in the hope of finding the cause of these changes. It is thought that a high level of nitrosamine compounds (up to 10 times higher than in normal bladders) may be the causative factor and the presence of both urine and faeces may affect the bowel in this way (Woodhouse, 1994). These complications led to ureterosigmoidostomies falling out of favour, and the development of continent urinary pouches as feasible

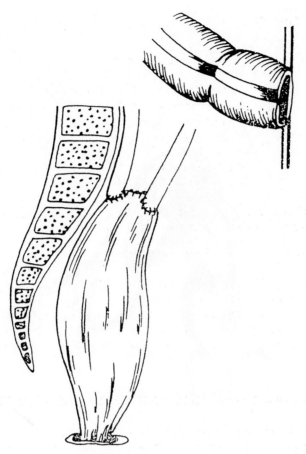

Figure 8.14 *The Mauclaire rectal bladder. The urine and faeces streams are completely separate and the patient has a terminal colostomy. From Wannack R et al., 1995, in* Urinary Diversion: Scientific Foundations and Clinical Practice *(GD Webster and B Goldwasser eds), Isis Medical Media, Oxford. Reproduced with permission*

alternatives. Unfortunately high levels of nitrosamine compounds have been found in ileal and colonic enterocystoplasties (Nurse and Mundy, 1989), and it is feared that history will repeat itself and tumours will also form in these urinary pouches.

In recent years there has been renewed interest in rectal bladders. The problems encountered in the past with ureteric reflux and pyelonephritis are caused by high-pressure peristalsis in the bowel. A rectal bladder has been developed where the uninterrupted colon is detubularized to eliminate these pressures (Figures 8.15 to 8.18). This pouch is called the sigma-rectum pouch or the Mainz sigma II pouch. This procedure results in the elimination of mass contractions and high pressure peaks in the colon and an increase in volume the reservoir can hold.

Preoperative care for these procedures is similar to that for bladder augmentation and reconstruction. However, all rectal bladders require patients to have a competent anal sphincter and be able to hold a 300 ml water enema for 3–4 hours without leaking. This test, together with rectodynamic evaluations which should include an anal sphincter profile, will establish if continence

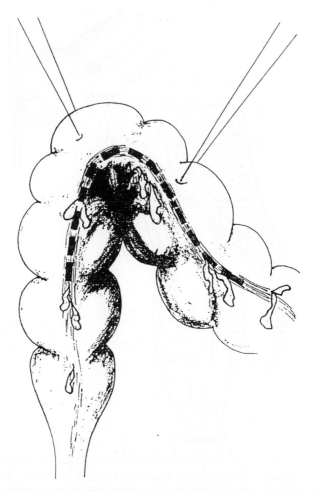

Figure 8.15 *Opening the bowel over a length of 12 cm both distal and proximal of the rectosigmoid junction. From Wannack R* et al., *1995, in* Urinary Diversion: Scientific Foundations and Clinical Practice *(GD Webster and B Goldwasser eds), Isis Medical Media, Oxford. Reproduced with permission*

will be possible after the operation. Patients should also be warned that the mixture of urine and faeces may produce a strong smell which may be offensive and therefore unacceptable to both them and members of their household. Considerations about matters such as separate bathrooms and the problems associated with emptying their bowels in public facilities should also be taken into consideration.

Postoperatively the patient has two rectal catheters, one draining mainly urine while the other drains faeces. Ureteric stents are also inserted. Patients are usually in hospital for 10–14 days; all tubes are removed before discharge home. Some patients may take some weeks learning how to control this bladder.

There are some patients who would find intermittent self-catheterization of their urethra or a continent stoma completely unacceptable or impossible. These patients may not comply with the care such diversions need, which could lead to severe problems. There are those who would also not accept a conventional stoma. For these patients a Mainz sigma II pouch or a ureter-osigmoidostomy may be a suitable option.

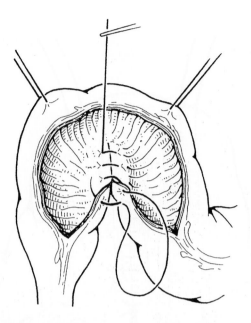

Figure 8.16   *Side-to-side anastomosis of the posterior wall. From Wannack R et al., 1995, in* Urinary Diversion: Scientific Foundations and Clinical Practice *(GD Webster and B Goldwasser eds), Isis Medical Media, Oxford. Reproduced with permission*

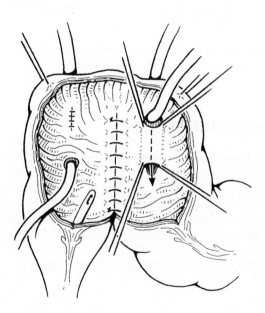

Figure 8.17   *Implantation of the ureters. From Wannack R et al., 1995, in* Urinary Diversion: Scientific Foundations and Clinical Practice *(GD Webster and B Goldwasser eds), Isis Medical Media, Oxford. Reproduced with permission*

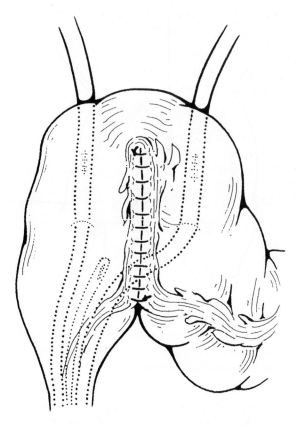

Figure 8.18 *Closure of the anterior pouch wall. Note the position of the ureteric stents and the rectal catheter. From Wannack R et al., 1995, in* Urinary Diversion: Scientific Foundations and Clinical Practice *(GD Webster and B Goldwasser eds), Isis Medical Media, Oxford. Reproduced with permission*

OUTFLOW INCONTINENCE

Outflow incontinence occurs when the intravesical pressure in an overdistended bladder exceeds the urethral closure pressure. The bladder becomes overdistended because of increased resistance to the outflow of urine. This may be because of outflow obstruction such as that caused by an enlarged prostate, or urethral strictures. An unobstructed contractile bladder may also result in the patient suffering from incontinence. Obstruction to the flow of urine from the bladder may occur anywhere along the length of the urethra. This sort of obstruction is more common in men than women.

Bladder outflow obstruction

Causes of bladder outflow obstruction are listed in Table 8.1.

The detrusor muscle responds to the increase in pressure needed to empty the bladder by hypertrophy. The bladder wall becomes thick and coarse, and may show increased irritability while filling with urine. This results in detrusor instability and the involuntary or 'unstable' contractions which cause

1. **Congenital**
   Urethral valves
   Urethral polyps
   Urethral stricture
2. **Acquired**
   Structural causes:
   - benign prostatic hyperplasia
   - carcinoma of the prostate
   - bladder neck stenosis
   - urethral stricture
   - urethral carcinoma
   - urethral calculi

   External compression:
   - faecal impaction
   - pelvic tumour
3. **Functional causes**
   Bladder neck dyssynergia
   Detrusor-sphincter dyssynergia

From Bullock *et al.* (1989).

Table 8.1   *Causes of bladder outflow obstruction*

frequency and urgency of micturition, which may lead to incontinence if the obstruction is not removed. The detrusor will eventually fail, becoming inefficient and giving up its contractions before the bladder is empty. The active, hypertrophied detrusor turns into an inert atonic bag, with a huge volume of residual urine. The patient experiences chronic retention of urine, and only a small quantity of urine is voided at a time. This chronic obstruction can lead to hydroureter and hydronephrosis. The ureters may also be partially obstructed as they pass through the thickened bladder wall, and some patients may suffer from vesicoureteric reflux. If untreated the condition may lead to increasing upper tract dilatation (obstructive uropathy) and a gradual deterioration of renal function.

After the age of 40 years most men suffer from enlargement of the prostate, but only 1 in 10 will have obstruction as a result of it (Blandy, 1992). The degree of obstruction is not always necessarily related to the size of the prostate, and the type and degree of nodular hyperplasia seems to vary from one race to another. Men of Celtic ancestry are thought to have larger glands than Anglo-Saxons, who in turn have larger ones than Mediterranean men (Blandy, 1992). No race is entirely immune, however.

Outflow obstruction may also be a result of a urethral stricture. The patient presents with a poor urinary stream, and may develop the same symptoms caused by detrusor hypertrophy (poor stream, hesitancy, frequency, nocturia and dribbling incontinence). Urine is trapped in the urethra upstream of the stricture and dribbles away after the patient thinks he has finished voiding. Strictures can occur at any time.

1. **Congenital strictures**
   Meatal stenosis
   Bulbar stricture
2. **Acquired strictures**
   Traumatic:
      perineal trauma
      ruptured urethra from pelvic injury
      urethral instrumentation
   Infective:
      gonococcal
      non-specific urethritis
      tuberculosis
   Inflammatory:
      balanitis
      chemical urethritis (e.g. from certain catheter materials)
   Neoplastic:
      squamous carcinoma
      transitional cell carcinoma
      adenocarcinoma

Table 8.2   *Aetiology of urethral strictures*

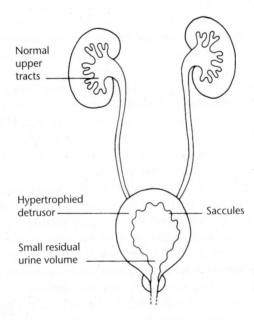

Figure 8.19   *Early pathological changes in urethral stricture*

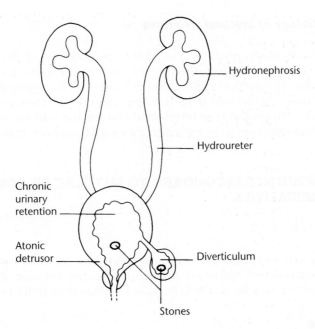

Figure 8.20 *Late pathological changes in urethral stricture*

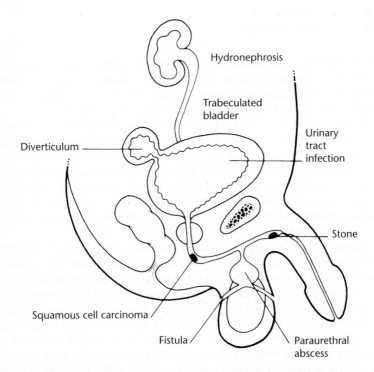

Figure 8.21 *Possible complications of prolonged urethral stricture*

Aetiology of urethral strictures

Urethral strictures may be congenital or acquired (Table 8.2). The late complications of urethral stricture are shown in Figures 8.19 to 8.21.

Whether the outflow obstruction is caused by the prostate or stricture in the urethra, bladder and renal function can only be conserved by removing the cause. The prostate can be resected and strictures dilated or divided (using optical urethrostomy). In extreme cases a urethroplasty may be indicated.

INCONTINENCE SECONDARY TO FISTULAE OR CONGENITAL ABNORMALITIES

Fistulae

Fistulae may be congenital or acquired. A fistula is an abnormal communication between two epithelial surfaces, or to the exterior. Any part of the urinary tract may be affected. Acquired fistulae may result from:

◆ trauma
◆ infection
◆ tumours
◆ surgery
◆ radiotherapy

A vaginal fistula is usually the result of pelvic surgery (e.g. hysterectomy). This is the most common cause in the industrialized countries. Elsewhere, these fistulae often form as a complication of obstructed labour. The prolonged pressure of the baby's head against the symphysis involving much of the back of the bladder, lower ends of the ureters and sometimes the external sphincter, causes tissue necrosis and the resulting sloughing leaves a fistula. The repair is done surgically. If the fistula is small, a vaginal repair may be adequate, but if large, then the repair may have to be via a midline incision in the bladder. The bladder is opened down to the fistula and posteriorly, the fistula is excised, and the vagina and bladder closed. A plug made of greater omentum is mobilized and brought down between bladder and vagina, sealing the vaginal vault.

If the fistula is large it may be seen on speculum examination. A tampon or gauze pack may be placed into the vagina and methylene blue dye instilled into the bladder. If the tampon turns blue this indicates that the fistula is from the bladder. If a ureterovaginal fistula is suspected then an intravenous urogram (IVU) can show the side and level of ureteric injury. Ureters can be damaged during hysterectomy, by being cut, crushed or accidentally caught up in a ligature. Urine escapes through the vault of the vagina, but may not appear for 4–5 days after the procedure. Testing this fluid for its urea content will confirm that it is urine. The ureter may be reimplanted into the bladder, or a flap of tubed bladder used to make up any lost ureteric length (Boari flap); the ureter may also be joined to the unaffected ureter (transureteroureterostomy).

Repair of vaginal fistulae may be done early after the initial procedure, though some units prefer a delay of up to 3 months so that the tissues are not oedematous. Extremely large fistulae may not be successfully closed, and a urinary diversion (continent or otherwise) may be the only option. Such a delay in offering treatment only prolongs the misery suffered by these individuals. The patient is constantly wet and has to wear large pads to cope with this sudden incontinence. The patient's quality of life is poor and she may become isolated and depressed. Such patients should be approached with understanding and sympathy and reassured as to the success of the operation proposed to repair the damage. The possibility of failure and the alternative of having a stoma formed should also be discussed, however, to prepare the patient should the procedure not succeed.

Another type of fistula which is occasionally seen as a complication of prostatectomy is a rectoprostatic fistula. This may be seen especially after an open operation for invasive carcinoma of the prostate, and after severe pelvic fracture injuries with rupture of the membranous urethra and laceration of the rectal wall. Many of these fistulae heal after a period of suprapubic catheterization of the bladder, and diversion of the faecal stream by temporary colostomy. Complex injuries may also involve urethral reconstruction.

Congenital bladder anomalies

Bladder exstrophy is twice as common in males than females and occurs in one in 10,000–40,000 live births. This is only part of a range of defects in which there is failure of fusion of the lower abdomen, genitalia and pelvic bones. The result of this can be defects which range from isolated epispadias to complex anomalies involving the bladder and intestine.

There are other congenital defects which may result in incontinence for the patient. However, many are dealt with immediately after birth with the aim of making the patient continent initially, with reconstructive surgery used as the child grows, to enhance body image and improve quality of life.

REFERENCES

BLANDY J P (1992) *Lecture Notes on Urology*, 4th edn. Oxford: Blackwell Scientific.

BULLOCK N, Sibley G and Whitaker R (1989) *Essential Urology.* Edinburgh: Churchill Livingstone.

ENZELSBERGE H, Kurz C and Mittermayer F (1995) Topical administration of oxybutynin hydrochloride in women with urge incontinence. *Geburtshilfe und Frauenheilkunde* **55**(5): 240–243.

KULBER D A, Davos I and Aronowitz J A (1995) Pseudotumoral granulomatous foreign body reaction to Teflon particles. *Journal of Oral and Maxillofacial Surgery* **53**(6): 719–722.

McKINNEY C D, Gaffey M J and Gillenwater J Y (1995) Bladder outlet obstruction after multiple periurethral polyethyluoroethylene injection. *Journal of Urology* **153**(1): 149–151.

NORTON C (1986) *Nursing for Incontinence.* Beaconsfield: Beaconsfield Publishers.

NURSE D E and Mundy A R (1989) Assessment of the malignant potential of cystoplasty. *British Journal of Urology* **64**: 489–492.

ROSENBAUM T P, Shaw P J R, Rose G A and Lloyd W (1989) *Cranberry Juice and Mucus Production in Enterouroplasty.* Paper presented to the British Association of Urological Surgeons, June 1989.

ROSENBAUM T P, Shaw P J R and Worth P H (1990) Trans-trigonal phenol failed the test of time. *British Journal of Urology* **66**(2): 164–169.

SOKELAND J (1989) *Urology*, 2nd edn. Stuttgart: George Thieme.

WANNACK R, Fisch M and Hohenfellner R (1995) Ureterosigmoidoscopy and the Mainz Pouch II. In: *Urinary Diversions: Scientific Foundations and Clinical Practice*, G D Webster and B Goldwasser (eds). Oxford: Isis Medical Media.

WOODHOUSE C R J (1994) *The infective metabolic and histological consequences of enterocystoplasty.* European Board of Urology - European Urology Update series, vol. 3. Union Europeanne des Medecins Specialistes.

FURTHER READING

BELLINGER M F (1989) The history of urinary diversion and undiversion. *Journal of Enterostomal Therapy* **16** (1): 39–46.

LEAVER R B (1994) The Mitrofanoff pouch: a continent urinary diversion. *Professional Nurse* **9**(11): 748–753.

LEAVER R B (1996) Continent urinary diversions – the Mitrofanoff principle. In *Stoma Care Nursing – a Patient-Centred Approach* Myers C (ed.) pp 166–179. London: Arnold.

LEAVER R B (1996) Cranberry juice. *Professional Nurse* **11**(8): 525–526.

MITROFANOFF P (1980) Cystomies continente trans-appendiculaire dans le traitment des vessies neurologiques. *Chirurgie Pediatrique* **2111**: 297–307.

WAGSTAFF K E, Woodhouse C R J, Rose G A, Duffy P G and Ransley P G (1991) Blood and urine analysis in patients with intestinal bladders. *Journal of Urology* **68**: 311–316.

WOODHOUSE C R J (1991) The Mitrofanoff principle for continent urinary diversion. *World Council of Enterostomal Therapists Journal* **11**(1): 12–15.

WOODHOUSE C R J and Gordon E M (1994) The Mitrofanoff principle for urethral failure. *British Journal of Urology* **73**: 55–60.

PROSTATIC PROBLEMS

9

Contents

The anatomy and physiology of the prostate gland are described in Chapter 1.

PROSTATITIS

Definition

Prostatitis is inflammation of the prostate gland and can be acute or chronic. It can result in the formation of abscesses or urethral strictures.

Causes

Prostatitis may occur if the patient has a history of:

- ◆ sexually transmitted disease
- ◆ tuberculosis
- ◆ urinary tract infection
- ◆ instrumentation (e.g. following cystoscopy)

The affecting organism can reach the prostate gland via the blood stream, rectum or pelvic lymphatic vessels.

Signs and symptoms

The patient usually presents with a history of perineal pain which radiates to the thighs and penis. The patient generally feels unwell and feverish, with dysuria and frequency which may result in retention of urine. Haemospermia (blood in sperm) may occur with pain on ejaculation, which affects sexual function.

Investigations

A digital rectal examination will show a very tender prostate gland which may feel enlarged and hot to the touch. The prostate should not be massaged too long because this can cause septicaemia.

A midstream specimen of urine may identify the causative organism.

Treatment and nursing care

Treatment is based on finding the causative oganism and treating the symptoms.

Pain in perineal area

The patient should be given regular analgesics and their effect should be monitored. A soft cushion to sit on and a warm bath to relieve the pain may be appreciated. The patient is encouraged to rest.

Infection causing general malaise and high temperature

If the causative organism can be found the appropriate antibiotic should be given as prescribed. This may be for several weeks. Temperature should be recorded 4-hourly and antipyretics given as required. Fluid intake is encouraged. If an abscess is present it may be drained.

Difficulty passing urine

To relieve difficulty in urinating, a urethral catheter may be inserted until the inflammation subsides.

Embarrassment about the condition and inability to perform sexually

The patient will need privacy and time to talk and express his concerns. He will require a full explanation of his condition and treatment.

If the prostatitis continues to recur or becomes chronic a transurethral resection of the prostate can be performed, or in extreme cases a total prostatectomy (described later in this chapter).

BENIGN PROSTATIC HYPERTROPHY

Definition

Benign prostatic hypertrophy is the benign enlargement of the prostate gland. This occurs in all men over 40 years of age, and 1 in 10 of these men suffer with urinary outflow obstruction due to the enlargement.

Causes

The cause is unknown, but it is thought to be due to testicular sex hormone changes as the man ages. Some call it the 'male menopause'. An adenoma (benign tumour), which may develop and cause enlargement of the prostate gland, may be implicated.

Signs and symptoms

The patient may present with various signs and symptoms, the severity depending on how long the prostate gland has been enlarged. Common signs and symptoms of prostatic outflow obstruction are:

◆ *Frequency of micturition* – more than 10–12 times daily
◆ *Nocturia* – the patient wakes up in the night because he wants to void
◆ *Hesitancy* – the patient has a delay before he is able to void
◆ *Poor urinary stream* – the patient may need to strain in order to void
◆ *Urinary tract infection* – due to incomplete bladder emptying
◆ *Dysuria* – pain on micturition due to infection
◆ *Dribbling incontinence* – due to incomplete bladder emptying
◆ *Chronic retention of urine with overflow*
◆ *Acute retention of urine*

The patient may present with renal failure or impairment, due to long-term prostatic outflow obstruction. This is caused by the enlarged prostate gland inhibiting the bladder from emptying properly. The bladder compensates by enlarging and thickening. The bladder muscle becomes stretched and ineffective and this results in an atonic bladder. The bladder is therefore unable to contract properly and becomes distended (bladder diverticula may develop). This in time causes pressure on the ureters and possible ureteric reflux occurs which causes back-pressure on the kidneys. This may result in renal failure (Figure 9.1).

Investigations

1. *A history* of voiding problems is taken in detail.
2. *Abdominal examination* may show a distended bladder.

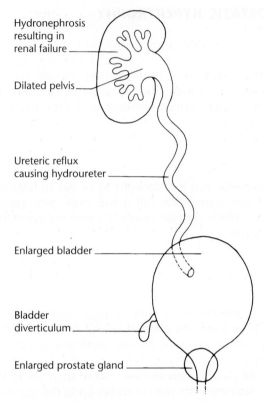

Hydronephrosis
resulting in
renal failure

Dilated pelvis

Ureteric reflux
causing hydroureter

Enlarged bladder

Bladder
diverticulum

Enlarged prostate gland

Figure 9.1   *Effects of prostatic hypertrophy*

3. *A digital rectal examination* will enable the doctor to feel the prostate gland
   and detect if it is enlarged.
4. *A midstream urine specimen* will detect any infection, which can be treated.
5. *Blood samples* are taken to assess renal function, e.g. urea and electrolytes,
   full blood count.
6. *A flow rate* is performed in order to determine the urinary stream.
7. *Urodynamics* may be performed to assess the bladder function.
8. *An intravenous urogram* is performed to show any damage to the urinary
   tract from long-term obstruction (ultrasound may also be used for this).

Treatment

Acute retention of urine

If the patient presents with acute retention of urine it will probably be due to
chronic retention of urine which has not been treated. The patient will be in
acute pain and have a strong desire to void. He should be seen as quickly as
possible and have a catheter inserted. A urethral catheter is tried first. If the
prostatic obstruction prevents this procedure, a suprapubic catheter is
inserted. The patient will require a great deal of support and explanation.
Relief from the symptoms is almost immediate once a catheter has been
inserted.

There is much confusion as to whether the catheter should be clamped after a certain amount has drained from the bladder. This is done in order to prevent a large diuresis which could make the patient go into shock, owing to the pressure being suddenly released from the kidney. In the authors' experience, clamping is of little use and even a small amount of drainage from the kidney will result in a large diuresis if it is going to occur.

One of the important nursing actions here is to ensure the patient has an input which is equal to the output. This is usually achieved by oral intake but intravenous fluids may be necessary. An accurate fluid balance chart is essential.

Haematuria with clots is common after this procedure, and bladder washouts may be needed or bladder irrigation commenced. If blood loss is a problem the patient's pulse and blood pressure should be carefully monitored and symptoms of shock observed for and reported promptly. The bleeding should subside over 2–3 days. Once everything has settled down further treatment can be decided.

The majority of patients present with voiding problems rather than retention of urine and are admitted routinely for treatment.

TRANSURETHRAL RESECTION OF THE PROSTATE GLAND

Transurethral resection of the prostate gland (TURP) involves the passage of a resectoscope via the urethra and the insertion of a loop for cutting and diathermy. This instrument cuts slivers of the gland away, and diathermy is used to control the bleeding. The surgeon has to be very careful not to damage the external sphincter at the base of the prostate gland because this could result in incontinence.

The bladder neck is resected and consequently retrograde ejaculation occurs, i.e. the semen goes into the bladder rather than out through the urethra. When the bladder neck is intact, it closes during ejaculation, enabling the semen to travel down the urethra. If the bladder neck is damaged this does not occur, and semen enters the bladder and is passed out during voiding. It is important to explain this to the patient because fertility will be a problem, but it should not be used as a form of contraception.

It is important that the surgeon does not damage the verumontanum. This is a small projection on the posterior wall of the prostate gland and contains the ejaculatory ducts (Figure 9.2).

The whole of the prostate gland is not removed because of the possibility of damaging the prostatic capsule, causing extravasation of urine, and also the possibility of damaging the external sphincter, causing incontinence.

Specific preoperative care

Explanation of patient care during admission

Full explanations of preoperative and postoperative care should be given to the patient. Many men are not aware that they have a prostate gland until it

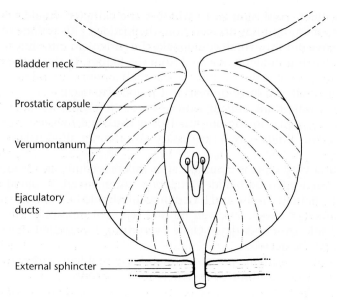

Figure 9.2 *The prostate gland*

causes problems, and then they do not understand why it is causing problems. Time should be spent explaining where the prostate gland is and why it is causing a problem. Draw a diagram of the urinary tract and show where the prostate gland is. It is sometimes easier to compare the prostate to a 'doughnut', the hole in the middle representing the urethra. As the prostate gland enlarges it compresses on the urethra and causes obstruction to the outflow of urine.

Other preoperative care

◆   chest X-ray if the patient has respiratory or cardiac problems
◆   blood specimens for urea and electrolytes and full blood count
◆   cross-match 2 units of blood
◆   electrocardiogram (ECG)
◆   flow rate
◆   antiembolic stockings
◆   midstream specimen of urine

Specific postoperative care

The patient returns to the ward with an intravenous infusion, urethral catheter and bladder irrigation.

Bleeding from the prostate gland following surgery

The prostate gland is highly vascular, and even though diathermy is used during the surgical procedure bleeding and haemorrhage can still be a problem which needs to be carefully monitored.

Blood pressure and pulse are recorded every 15–60 minutes until stable. A sudden drop in blood pressure and rise in pulse with the patient becoming cold and clammy indicates the patient is hypovolaemic, owing to haemorrhage, and the doctor should be contacted immediately. The intravenous infusion may be speeded up or a blood transfusion or plasma expander (e.g. Gelofusine) may be prescribed. The urethral catheter has a bladder irrigation attached and normal saline is used to irrigate the bladder. If the output remains heavily bloodstained then the doctor should be informed. Traction may be applied to the catheter, resulting in the balloon on the catheter being pulled down into the bleeding prostatic area, hopefully stopping the bleeding. The traction should only be applied for 20–30 minutes at a time and then released, even if bleeding continues. If the traction is left longer, necrosis of the area around the catheter balloon will occur. Traction can be applied by tying a piece of gauze around the catheter at the end of the penis and pulling the catheter down or by tying a weight to the end of the catheter and hanging it over the end of the bed. This can be achieved by tying a bandage to the catheter and attaching a 500 ml bag of intravenous fluid to the other end of the bandage (the bag should hang free and not on the floor). If the traction is not effective then the patient may need to go back to theatre for further diathermy.

When bleeding is heavy the irrigation should run fast and this will help to prevent clots forming and blocking the catheter. If the catheter does block the patient usually complains that he wants to void and he will have a distended bladder. If this does occur the bladder irrigation should be turned off to prevent further bladder distension and discomfort. Milking the catheter bag tubing gently may clear any clots. However, a bladder washout may be necessary, but breaking the closed system should be a last resort and performed aseptically to prevent any infection. If a bladder washout is not effective the catheter balloon can be deflated and the catheter gently twisted round. It is important that the catheter is not moved in or out of the urethra because this can cause urethral trauma and introduce infection; also the balloon should be reinflated after this procedure. If after these procedures the catheter is still not draining, it should be changed by the doctor.

Some surgeons also prescribe a drug to help stop the bleeding. An example is tranexamic acid which prevents fibrinolysis (the physiological mechanism that dissolves clots); therefore clotting should occur.

As the urine becomes less bloodstained the bladder irrigation is slowed down and usually after 24 hours the urine is pink in colour and irrigation is discontinued. When the urine is clear or almost clear the urethral catheter is removed. This usually occurs 2–4 days postoperatively.

A full blood count is obtained 24–48 hours postoperatively to detect anaemia.

Maintenance of hydration and monitoring output

The patient comes back to the ward with an intravenous infusion to ensure that he does not become dehydrated and has a good urine output. This is maintained for about 24 hours or until the patient is able to drink without nausea or vomiting. If it is not medically dangerous the patient is encouraged to drink 3 litres of fluid daily to achieve a high urine output and consequently reduce the amount of haematuria. The amount of irrigation has to be carefully monitored and it should be ensured that the total output exceeds the irrigation input. If the irrigation is being absorbed into the blood stream, owing to extravasation, transurethal resection (TUR) syndrome may occur. This is not a common complication but is an emergency if it does occur. Symptoms usually start to become apparent soon after surgery. The irrigation fluid is absorbed into the blood stream and causes dilution of the blood and circulatory overload. The patient becomes confused and disoriented. He may fit, owing to a low plasma sodium, become comatosed and have a cardiac arrest. The doctor should be informed immediately of any significant change in the patient's condition and blood should be taken to check sodium and potassium levels which, in TUR syndrome, will be low. An ECG should be recorded, irrigation stopped and IV fluids reduced. The patient may be transferred to the intensive care unit. Water should never be used as an irrigation fluid because, owing to osmosis, it will be readily absorbed from the bladder and prostate area and cause TUR syndrome. Normal saline as an irrigation fluid reduces this risk, because it is isotonic and therefore not easily absorbed. Absorption principally occurs in theatre, where irrigation solution (devoid of sodium or potassium) is forced under pressure into the prostatic veins.

Infection due to surgery and indwelling catheter

Temperature is recorded 4-hourly and any elevation is reported to the doctor. If the patient is known to have a urinary tract infection, antibiotics are given with the premedication or in theatre and continued postoperatively. However, if symptoms occur postoperatively, a catheter specimen of urine is sent for culture and sensitivity and a broad-spectrum antibiotic is prescribed.

To prevent infection the catheter insertion site is kept clean and dry using soap and water. It is better if the patient is able to clean this area himself.

A closed system should be maintained with the catheter and irrigation, and if it has to be broken an aseptic technique should be used, with sterile gloves being worn.

Pain due to the catheter

Pain due to endoscopic prostatic surgery is unusual. However, patients may complain of either bladder spasm or penile pain, both of which are caused by the large urethral irrigation catheter inserted postoperatively, and are not a result of the surgery.

Bladder spasm (manifesting as acute, spasmodic, lower abdominal pain, which is often positional in nature) is caused by trigonal irritation, from the 30–50 ml balloon, which secures the three-way irrigation catheter in position. Securing the catheter to the leg to prevent 'pulling' will aid comfort and also reduce downward movement of the catheter. This may reduce irritation of the trigone and thus spasm. However, if the spasms are very troublesome, then antispasmodics (e.g. anticholinergic agents such as oxybutynin or propantheline bromide) may need to be prescribed. Usually, this problem is only reduced when the catheter is removed.

Penile pain (usually at the tip of the patient's penis) is also catheter-related and reflects the large diameter of the irrigation catheter. This problem is most effectively treated with lignocaine gel, applied locally to the urethral surface.

Constipation due to restricted mobility and fear of opening bowels

The patient is usually up and mobile the day following his operation. However, constipation can still be a problem because the patient is afraid to strain with a catheter in situ. Therefore a high-fibre diet is encouraged and if the patient expresses difficulty an oral aperient or suppositories are prescribed.

Following removal of catheter

Following catheter removal the patient is at risk from:

- retention of urine
- frequency of micturition
- incontinence

Occasionally when the catheter is removed the patient is unable to void and will develop retention of urine. If the patient is unable to void he is asked to have a warm bath to help him relax. The patient is usually left until he has a strong desire to void and has drunk at least a litre of fluid before another catheter is inserted. Once the catheter has been reinserted it is left in situ for between 2 days and 6 weeks and voiding without the catheter is tried again. If the patient continues to experience retention of urine, further surgery may be necessary.

Most patients suffer with frequency and urgency once the catheter has been removed. This should be explained to the patient. Initially the volumes may be 50–75 ml each void, but this does improve over a few days and the patient is encouraged to try and 'hold on' between voiding.

Dribbling incontinence can be a problem. If this occurs the patient is advised to perform pelvic floor exercises. The situation usually improves over a period of days and this is explained to the patient. While the problem is resolving the patient is given incontinence pads which are changed as required. A supply may need to be given on discharge home.

A fluid chart is maintained and each voided volume is recorded. The patient, if able, is taught how to complete his output chart himself. Fluid intake of 2–3 litres is encouraged but the patient is told to cut down on his intake in the evening to prevent nocturia.

A flow rate is recorded before discharge.

Advice on discharge

An outpatient appointment is made for 6 weeks postoperatively, when a further flow rate test will be performed. The patient is advised to rest during this time and not to perform any heavy lifting. If the patient works this can be resumed after about 4 weeks.

After about 2 weeks an episode of bleeding in the urine is possible due to the 'scabs falling off' in the healing prostate. This is explained to the patient who is advised to increase his oral intake during this period, and if it does not subside to contact his general practitioner.

The patient should also contact his GP if there is any burning on micturition, or fever, which indicates infection.

The patient is advised to refrain from sexual intercourse for 2 weeks; sexual sensation should not be affected.

Complications

Incontinence

One per cent of patients who have had a prostatectomy suffer with long-term incontinence and may require further surgery.

Stricture

Urethral strictures may occur owing to damage to the urethra from instrumentation during surgery.

Impotence

Impotence following TURP has a reported incidence of between 4% and 30% (Tanagho and McAninch, 1992). This wide variation of figures may reflect a reluctance on the part of patients to admit that the problem exists.

Haemorrhage

Postoperative haemorrhage is seen in some 4% of patients. Secondary haemorrhage can occur, which may require the patient to be readmitted to hospital.

Mortality

The overall mortality rate of TURP is less than 1%, and is usually the result of cardiovascular or respiratory complications.

Long-term problems

The long-term follow-up of patients after TURP reveals the resolution of voiding symptoms in some 80–90% at 1 year, though this decreases to 60–75% by 5 years. Some 5% of patients will require a repeat TURP within 5 years of their original operation (Tanagho and McAninch, 1992).

Interestingly, a study by Roos *et al.* (1989), which compared the mortality rates following both TURP and open prostatectomy, found a higher incidence of death from myocardial infarction both at 3 months and later on in patients who had undergone TURP. This information is being investigated, as it would appear to undermine the usual assumptions regarding the safety of TURP when compared with an open procedure.

OTHER FORMS OF PROSTATECTOMY

If the prostate gland weighs over 60 g a TURP is not performed because the operation would take much longer than other methods of prostatectomy. One of the following operations may be performed.

Retropubic prostatectomy

A transverse skin incision is made (Figure 9.3), the prostatic capsule cut and the gland removed using the finger. The prostatic capsule is sutured and the wound closed.

Transvesical prostatectomy

A transverse skin incision is made and the bladder is opened (Figure 9.4). The prostate gland is removed using the finger through the bladder. The bladder is sutured and the wound closed.

Perineal prostatectomy

Perineal prostatectomy is a rare procedure. An incision is made through the perineum to expose the prostate gland. The capsule is opened and the gland removed.

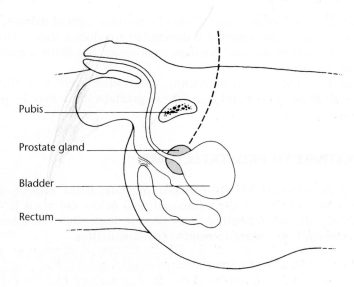

Pubis

Prostate gland

Bladder

Rectum

Figure 9.3 *Retropubic prostatectomy*

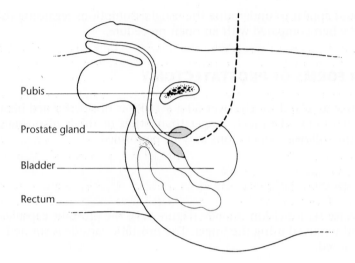

Figure 9.4 *Transvesical prostatectomy*

Nursing care

The nursing care required for these methods of prostatectomy is the same as for a TURP plus the following.

Pain due to abdominal wound reducing mobility

Regular controlled analgesia should be given as required and the patient mobilized with help for the first 2–3 days postoperatively.

Care of abdominal wound and wound drains

The wound is re-dressed as required and observed for signs of redness, oozing and soreness. Sutures are removed as directed by the doctor after 7–10 days. A wound drain is left in situ and drainage monitored. The drain is removed as directed by the doctor.

With all the types of prostatectomy mentioned there is a chance of regrowth of the prostate gland and further prostatectomy may be required in the future.

ALTERNATIVES TO PROSTATECTOMY

Patients may present with an enlarged prostate gland causing outflow obstruction but are not fit for an anaesthesia, or do not want to have a prostatectomy and risk retrograde ejaculation or impotence. Therefore alternative treatment is necessary to combat the obstruction.

Balloon dilatation of the prostate gland

In the balloon dilation procedure (McLoughlin and Williams 1990), a balloon is inserted transurethrally and positioned in the prostatic urethra. The balloon is expanded (usually to 35 mm) for periods of 10–15 minutes.

This procedure can be performed using intravenous sedation and analgesia. Slight bleeding can occur and a urethral catheter may be left in situ for 24 hours. At present results are variable. A study by Gill *et al.* (1989) showed that less than 50% of patients had symptomatic improvement. Perez-Marrero et al (1990) showed 73% had improvement. From the authors' experience the former figure seems more realistic.

At present the improvement in symptoms is short-term; it is therefore usually used for younger patients who are concerned about retrograde ejaculation or loss of potency, and who in later life will go ahead with a prostatectomy.

Prostatic stents

There are two types of prostatic stent – macroporous tubular mesh and prostatic spirals (Chappell *et al.*, 1990; McLoughlin and Williams, 1990).

Macroporous tubular mesh

The stent is made of stainless steel woven into a tubular mesh. It is inserted transurethrally into the prostatic urethra using local anaesthesia. Over a period of 6–8 months epithelium forms around the stent and holds it in place. It can be removed within the first 4–6 weeks if necessary; however, after this time the stent is permanent.

This stent is used for patients who are unfit for anaesthesia and have a limited life expectancy.

Prostatic spirals

A prostatic spiral consists of a tightly coiled metallic spring which lodges in the prostatic urethra. It has a tail which sits outside the external sphincter and can be grasped if it has to be removed (Figure 9.5). Epithelium does not form around the spiral and it is narrower than the macroporous mesh. It is positioned using a cystoscopy and transrectal ultrasound, under a local anaesthesia.

Because it can be removed, this spiral may be suited for temporary relief of obstruction while waiting for a prostatectomy.

With both types of stent the patient is usually able to void following its insertion. If difficulty in micturition occurs a urethral catheter is not inserted owing to the risk of displacing the stent, and a suprapubic catheter is inserted instead. Antibiotic cover is given to minimize the risk of infection. Problems of frequency and urgency following the stent insertion have been reported and these are treated with anticholinergic drugs. The stent can also become

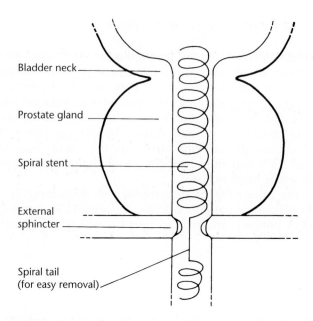

Bladder neck

Prostate gland

Spiral stent

External
sphincter

Spiral tail
(for easy removal)

Figure 9.5 *Prostatic spiral*

displaced and protrude or move into the bladder, necessitating its replacement or removal.

Microwave hyperthermia

Microwave hyperthermia (Strohmaier *et al.*, 1990; Astrahan *et al.*, 1991) involves the prostate gland being heated to a temperature of 42–43 °C. The treatment consists of heating the prostate gland for a period of 1 hour, once or twice weekly for 8–10 sessions. The treatment is given as an outpatient procedure and only requires local anaesthesia for insertion of the urethral equipment.

The equipment consists of a machine comprising a microwave generator, a heat applicator – which can be either a transurethral applicator or a transrectal applicator (this applicator also has a cooling system to protect the rectal wall from heat damage) – and two temperature monitors, one for the urethra and the other for the rectum.

This method of treatment is still being studied and results at present are variable. The treatment appears to be palliative rather than curative and prostatectomy still has to be performed following treatment.

Laser treatment

Laser treatment involves the insertion of a laser fibre via the urethra, and the use of a laser beam at close range in the prostate gland to burn it away.

Medical treatment

It is possible to treat prostatic problems using drugs (Christmas and Kirby, 1991).

Alpha-1 adrenoceptor blockers

The smooth muscle of the prostate gland contains alpha-adrenoceptors, and it has been discovered that by blocking these receptors the tone in the prostatic urethra decreases and hence the urinary flow rate improves. Examples of drugs that block alpha-adrenoceptors are prazosin, indoramin and phenoxybenzamine. Side-effects of these drugs include dizziness, palpitations and retrograde ejaculation.

Research is in progress to find an alpha-adrenoceptor that is specific to the prostate gland.

Hormones

Oestrogen therapy (e.g. stilboestrol) and antiandrogen agents (e.g. cyproterone acetate) are able to reduce the size of the prostate gland but they do have side-effects which are not acceptable. Oestrogens cause sexual dysfunction and gynaecomastia; antiandrogens can cause loss of libido, impotence and hot flushes.

5-Alpha reductase inhibitors

The 5-alpha reductase inhibitors such as finasteride block the enzyme that breaks down testosterone to dihydrotestosterone. Dihydrotestosterone is essential for normal growth of the prostate gland; by stopping the metabolism of testosterone, the growth of the prostate will be reduced, reducing outflow obstruction. The medication needs to be given for 3–6 months before improvement is evident. Impotence can be a side-effect but is easily reversed when the drug is stopped.

Research is in progress on the effect of combining 5-alpha reductase inhibitors with alpha-1 adrenoceptor blockers.

Conclusion

All the treatments stated as alternatives to a prostatectomy are still being researched and are not available as treatment in all urology departments at the time of writing this chapter. An excellent summary is provided by Christmas and Kirby (1991) and Tanagho and McAninch (1992).

CARCINOMA OF THE PROSTATE GLAND

Carcinoma of the prostate gland is the third most common cancer in men, representing 16% of all malignancies in the adult male. The tumour often arises in the posterior prostatic lobe and is hormone-related, depending upon androgens to retain its integrity. The tumour also causes an increase in the secretion of acid phosphatase and prostatic-specific antigen – both of these are reflected in blood serum levels and may indicate a prostatic tumour.

There are no known direct aetiological factors, but carcinoma becomes more common with increasing age, and by the age of 90 years most men have foci of carcinoma in their prostate glands. The incidence steadily increases with age, ranging from 10% in men in their 50s to 80% in men in their 80s, thus every decade of ageing nearly doubles the incidence. Although clinical prostate cancer can and does occur in men in their 40s, approximately 85% of prostate cancer patients are over 65 years old.

Because of its frequency and the fact that early diagnosis can be made in most cases by a digital rectal examination (DRE), all men should be advised to have an annual check-up after the age of 40 years. Nurses are advised to include this advice whenever it is relevant in their health teaching.

Predisposing risk factors for prostate cancer

Genetic factors

There is a higher incidence of cancer among relatives of patients with prostatic cancer. More significantly, when cancer occurs in a patient with an affected father, brother, uncle or grandfather there is an eight-fold increase in risk. In these family clusters disease develops at an earlier age and run a more aggressive course, suggesting that genetic factors influence the biological behaviour of the tumour.

Environmental factors

Mortality rates from prostate cancer appear to be higher in men living in urban areas where exposure to environmental pollution with exhaust fumes, cadmium, chemical fertilizers and other industrial chemical carcinogens is greater. (Cigarette smoke, certain dietary items such as oysters, and soft drinking water are other potential sources of cadmium.) There is little epidemiological evidence that any of these factors substantially influence prostate cancer risk.

Pathology

The majority of prostate cancers are adenocarcinomas. Sarcomas occur rarely in the prostate. The prostatic ducts are lined with transitional epithelium and can, therefore, be involved in urothelial cancer. The most common prostatic cancer is a columnar adenocarcinoma with distortion of normal architecture. Several schemes for assessing differentiation exist, and correlate reasonably well with prognosis.

Staging

The staging of the disease is central to any decision regarding treatment, and to the prediction of outcome. It is based on an evaluation of the extent of the primary tumour and the presence or absence of metastases. Biochemical tumour markers and advances in imaging techniques have improved the accuracy of staging. The system used is the TNM classification (Figure 9.6).

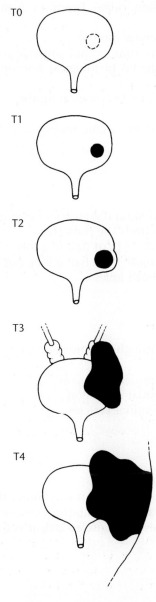

Figure 9.6 *Staging of prostatic carcinoma: T0; one or more foci of impalpable carcinoma, usually a chance finding following TURP; T1, one or more small tumours with no deformity of the capsule; T2, tumour confined to the prostate but deforming the capsule; T3, tumour extending beyond the capsule and/or invading the seminal vesicles; T4, tumour infiltrating other pelvic organs or the pelvic wall*

Carcinoma of the prostate is classified into four stages. These stages are based on the results of digital rectal examination, serum acid phosphatase and prostatic-specific antigen (PSA) levels, and on X-rays of the skeleton and metastases.

Stage 1

Carcinoma in situ is often called latent or focal. Usually there are no symptoms.

T0 – no evidence of primary tumour

T1 – clinically inapparent tumour, not palpable and not visible by imaging

T1a – tumour an incidental histological finding in 5% or less of tissue resected

T1b – tumour an incidental histological finding in more than 5% of tissue resected

T1c – tumour identified by needle biopsy (e.g. because of elevated PSA levels)

Stage II

The nodule may be palpated on digital rectal examination.

T2 – tumour confined within the prostate

T2a – tumour involves more than half of a lobe or less

T2b – tumour involves more than half a lobe but not both lobes

T2c – tumour involves both lobes

Stage III

The growth has spread through the prostatic capsule but no distant metastases are present.

T3a – unilateral extracapsular extension

T3b – bilateral extracapsular extension

T3c – tumour invades seminal vesicles

Stage IV

The tumour is fixed or more invasive.

T4 – tumour fixed or invades adjacent structures other than seminal vesicles

T4a – tumour invades bladder neck and/or external sphincter and/or rectum

T4b – tumour invades levator muscles and/or is fixed to pelvic wall

Presentation

Local disease

Ninety per cent of carcinomas arise in the peripheral zone of the prostate, and therefore small tumours may not interfere with voiding. As they enlarge they obstruct the outflow from the bladder, causing poor stream, frequency and nocturia. Some cancers may grow quite large without causing urinary obstruction, and therefore remain undetected until the prognosis is poor. If the tumour extends upwards it may irritate the trigone and cause bladder irritation. A few extend posteriorly and cause tenesmus (painful straining to empty bowel without effect) or even rectal obstruction. Many men present with bladder outflow obstruction caused by benign prostatic hypertrophy and are incidently found to have carcinoma as well.

Remote disease

Cancer of the prostate metastasizes early to pelvic lymph nodes and bone. About 15% of T1 tumours, 30% of T2 tumours and 60% of T3 tumours have lymph node metastases at presentation (Bullock *et al.*, 1989). Half of those with nodal metastases have bone metastases. Patients may present with bone pain, pathological fractures or even anaemia.

Prognosis

It is very difficult to give a prognosis for an individual patient, as the natural history is so uncertain. Patients with one or two foci of carcinoma, in an otherwise benign gland, and those with small cancers without metastases, have the same life expectancy. The prognosis becomes progressively poorer with increasing stage and grade: the overall survival of T2 cases is about 50% at 5 years. The age of the patient at presentation is irrelevant.

Investigations

The specific investigations into carcinoma of the prostate can not only be physically uncomfortable and generate a high level of anxiety, but also can be extremely embarrassing for the patient, owing to their invasive nature. Therefore, apart from preparing the patient both physically and psychologically for these tests, the nurse should also ensure that the patient's privacy and dignity are maintained as far as possible at all times.

Digital rectal examination

While a digital rectal examination of the prostate gland cannot prove conclusively the presence of a carcinoma, it is certainly an extremely good indicator. This is because a small tumour will feel hard, like a dried pea on the prostate surface, while larger infiltration into the prostatic capsule will make the gland feel generally hard and knobbly. This compares with a healthy prostate gland which should feel smooth and slightly soft, when palpated rectally.

A digital rectal examination is one of the first investigations performed, so if a patient suffering from outflow obstruction seeks help promptly from his general practitioner, the latter will undoubtedly perform a digital rectal examination, and if suspicious, will then order further tests to be done.

Blood tests

The prostate gland, under hormonal control, secretes specific antigens; in a healthy man the level of PSA is 0–4 μg l^{-1}. The level of antigen secretion will be raised, as well-differentiated carcinoma cells have the same enzyme properties as healthy prostatic cells. Therefore if a rise in the PSA level occurs, this may be due to a growth in the prostate size owing to the presence of carcinoma.

Alkaline phosphatase (normal range 80–280 U l^{-1}) and acid phosphatase (normal range below 4Ul^{-1}) are also chemicals detected in the blood and are raised if carcinoma is present in the prostate and metastases have occurred.

All such diagnostic indices are rendered unreliable if the patient has undergone a recent digital rectal examination of the prostate, or has recently had a urethral catheter inserted.

Transrectal ultrasonography

Transrectal ultrasonography should be regarded as complementary to digital rectal examination. This investigation is occasionally carried out during a TURP, but can also be performed independently in the radiology or outpatient department. A small ultrasonic probe is inserted into the patient's rectum, and its head rotated to allow for an optimum assessment. The ulstrasound scan will be able to show prostatic growth and its density, as a malignant growth will appear darker on an ultrasound monitor. Thus the actual staging of the tumour can be diagnosed using transrectal ultrasound as the shape, size and infiltration of the carcinoma will be seen. Antibiotic cover may be given prior to this procedure (e.g. gentamicin 80 mg intramuscularly).

This test can be extremely uncomfortable for the patient, whose dignity must be preserved at all times.

Prostatic biopsy

Obtaining a prostatic biopsy for histological analysis is the most reliable test. If a surgeon suspects the presence of a carcinoma of the prostate during a TURP, a biopsy can be sent to the laboratory for assessment. Otherwise a biopsy can be obtained either transperineally or transrectally, in theatre, on the ward or in the radiology department. Following this procedure the patient should be observed for signs of rectal bleeding.

CT scan

Computed tomographic (CT) scanning can be used in conjunction with the transrectal ultrasound probe to provide accurate staging of the tumour.

MRI scan

A magnetic resonance imaging (MRI) scan of the area can be used to detect node involvement prior to surgery or radiotherapy.

Skeletal survey and bone scan

One of the prime metastatic targets for prostatic tumours is the bones. The symptoms that bony metastases cause range from mild backache to an inability to walk, as a tumour pressing on the spinal cord can weaken the legs. The presence of bony metastases can be detected by two investigations:

- ◆ plain X-ray film of the abdominal area – will illustrate the presence of metastases, shown as osteosclerotic deposits
- ◆ isotopic bone scan

An isotopic bone scan is a much more detailed, accurate and easily identifiable investigation than a plain X-ray. An isotopic agent is injected intravenously and 3–4 hours later films are taken. As a tumour receives a blood supply, if there is metastatic bone involvement, then there will be increased blood flow to these areas. A bone scan should be taken and used as a baseline, but should no longer be repeated as a sequential scan to monitor the course of the disease.

Pelvic lymphadenectomy

The prostate gland has a large lymphatic supply, therefore in the presence of prostatic carcinoma, the possibility of nodal metastases around the pelvic lymph area is high. Nodal staging can be achieved by examination of the nodules after a pelvic lymphadenectomy. The latter is usually performed in conjunction with a radical prostatectomy. It is not performed as a separate procedure, as the patient's future treatment will depend on the extent of the metastases beyond the pelvic lymph area (i.e. the spine, chest, liver), rather than on the pelvic lymph node analysis alone.

Chest X-ray

Radiography of the chest is done if metastases are suspected, as occasionally lung involvement is found and can be detected on a plain chest X-ray.

Liver function tests

Another site for metastatic spread is the liver, so liver function tests can be performed to establish whether tumour infiltration has taken place. This is detected by a blood test.

Treatment

Treatment for carcinoma of the prostate depends largely on the stage of the tumour when it is diagnosed. This particular cancer is usually proved to be present following biopsy analysis taken during a TURP. Usually if the tumour is small enough and a resection has been done, further treatment will not routinely take place unless the patient shows signs in the future of further outflow obstruction, or during a routine follow-up appointment, signs are indicative of further tumour development (i.e. raised PSA levels).

The rationale behind this is that carcinoma of the prostate does have a good prognosis if detected early enough, if the tumours are well differentiated and confined to the prostate, and it would ultimately be unnecessary to submit patients to further surgery or treatment which was not definitely required. Patients who have been diagnosed as having a carcinoma of the prostate will be seen in the outpatient department on a regular basis to ensure that no further problems occur.

However, not all prostatic tumours are detected at an early stage, and for more advanced disease treatment is inevitable. Here the alternatives available are described below.

TURP

If cancer of the prostate has been diagnosed by blood tests and an ultrasound scan and the latter shows that the tumour is within the prostatic capsule, then a straightforward TURP is performed. After discharge the patient will be monitored to ensure that no tumour regrowth occurs.

Radiotherapy

Radiotherapy can be given both to the prostate itself and to areas of metastatic involvement. Radiotherapy to the gland itself can take place prior to surgery such as radical prostatectomy, to limit the chance of tumour spread, and to shrinking it to the smallest possible size preoperatively, or it can be used after radical prostatectomy, depending on the histopathological findings.

This treatment can also be implemented without the patient having to undergo surgery. It may be that radiotherapy will shrink the gland and prevent metastatic involvement. Treatment can be undertaken using the linear accelerator, or by using a more recent technique of actually inserting radioactive iodine implants into the gland to cause tumour regression.

Radiotherapy can also be used as a palliative treatment. Bony metastases are common and cause the patient great pain and discomfort. A course of radiotherapy can relieve the pain and ensures the bones can heal. Usually only a short course is required.

Hormone treatment

Before discussing hormone therapy, let us summarize androgen activity in men.

The anterior pituitary gland secretes two gonadotrophic hormones: follicle stimulating hormone (FSH) and luteinizing hormone (LH). The FSH initiates spermatogenesis, while the LH serves to both develop mature sperm and also bring about the secretion of testosterone. The latter is the main androgen in the male and has a vast effect on the body. It ultimately controls the growth and development of the male sex organs, ensures maturation of sperm and is responsible for the development of the male secondary sexual characteristics.

The prostate gland and any carcinoma present can develop according to androgen secretion. Hypothetically, if testosterone were given to a patient it could stimulate prostatic growth, and if a tumour were present this too would be encouraged to develop. Conversely, if the androgen supply is stopped, any metastic spread from the prostate can usually be prevented or severely reduced (by approximately 70–80%).

Hormone manipulation is usually started in patients when metastases are symptomatic; the aim is to prevent testosterone production, and there are two main ways to achieve this.

First, as oestrogens inhibit the production of gonadotrophin releasing hormone (which in turn initiates the whole cycle of androgen production), if oestrogens are administered the androgen secretion will stop. Commonly used antiandrogen drugs are cyproterone acetate, flutamide, stilboestrol, casodex, leuprorelin acetate (Prostap SR) and goserelin (Zoladex). These drugs do have a number of side-effects, including risk of fluid overload due to sodium retention, cardiovascular involvement, liver disease, gynaecomastia, changes in hair pattern and loss in libido. A small number of androgens are produced in the adrenal glands and an adrenalectomy may be performed (very rarely), or medication given to inhibit adrenal hormone output.

The other hormonal alternative involves surgery: a bilateral subcapsular orchidectomy stops all androgen secretion from the testes. This treatment usually puts an abrupt end to pain caused by metastases. It should be remembered and respected that despite the advantages of a subcapsular orchidectomy, it is a change in body image for the patients, and their psychological feeling towards this surgery should be explored. It is a myth that patients will develop a high-pitched voice, and this should be explained to them. Impotence is not an inevitable consequence of orchidectomy, but is more than likely to ensue. After orchidectomy there is a rise in serum luteinizing hormone releasing hormone (LH-RH) and LH levels, the effects of which are loss of libido and hot flushes.

Chemotherapy

Chemotherapy is not used at present. Certain drugs are on trial for use in cases of prostatic cancer, but their effectiveness has not yet been assessed, and chemotherapy is not considered as a suitable treatment even after other alternatives have been exhausted.

RADICAL PROSTATECTOMY

Radical prostatectomy is the removal of the whole of the prostate gland including the capsule. A retropubic approach is taken and the urethral endings are anastomosed together. This operation is often performed with a pelvic lymphadenectomy and ultimately, if the appropriate preoperative tests have been carried out, the aim is to remove the tumour completely.

Specific preoperative care

Psychological care

The patient should be admitted to hospital at least 1–2 days preoperatively. Psychologically this operation can be extremely daunting for a patient; not only is he about to undergo a procedure which has numerous possible complications (impotence, retrograde ejaculation and incontinence, to name but three), but he will also be aware that he has 'cancer', which is distressing enough anyway. Therefore the patient and his family will need much psychological support. The patient should be given the time and opportunity to discuss any specific fears or anxieties that he may have. The feasibility of the tumour being removed by surgical intervention can be discussed with the patient by the nursing or medical staff, but the patient may wish to discuss the possibility of impotence or infertility with a sexual counsellor if one is available to the hospital.

Physical care

Bowel preparation

This is needed owing to the possibility of bowel mobilization during surgery. Usually the regimen is as follows: 1 day preoperatively the patient is given clear fluids only and two doses of sodium picosulphate with magnesium citrate (Picolax). During bowel preparation ensure the patient takes adequate oral fluids to maintain hydration.

ECG

An ECG is required to exclude any cardiac abnormalities as the patient will be anaesthetized for approximately 3 hours and will probably suffer a significant blood loss.

Blood assay

The patient will most certainly have a blood transfusion either during or after surgery, so blood will need to be cross-matched preoperatively. The patient's full blood count, urea and electrolytes should be analysed to rule out any abnormalities.

Antiembolism stockings

All patients should have a pair of antiembolism stockings as they will be immobile for some time postoperatively. Patients with a history of deep vein thrombosis should be heparinized too.

Shave

Shaving should be performed in theatre from mid-thorax down to the scrotal area.

Specific postoperative care

Postoperatively the patient will return to the ward with both urethral and suprapubic catheters, two wound drains, an intravenous infusion (which may be blood), a central line and an opiate analgesic pump, e.g. epidural or patient-controlled analgesia (Figure 9.7).

The patient should have no difficulty breathing although opiates for pain control may lower the patient's respiratory rate, so this should be carefully monitored. Oxygen will probably be prescribed.

The patient's blood pressure may be lowered in the first 12 hours postoperatively. This may be due either to opiate infusion or to blood loss in theatre (or both). Central venous pressure may be monitored along with the normal blood pressure for the first 24 hours. Blood (or a blood substitute) may have to be given. The catheters and wound drain should be observed to ensure that there is no significant blood loss.

Pain is usually well controlled using opiate infusions; the regimen can be reduced over a few days and if not contraindicated rectal analgesia can be prescribed, e.g. diclofenac.

Urine output must be carefully monitored. Bladder irrigation may be in

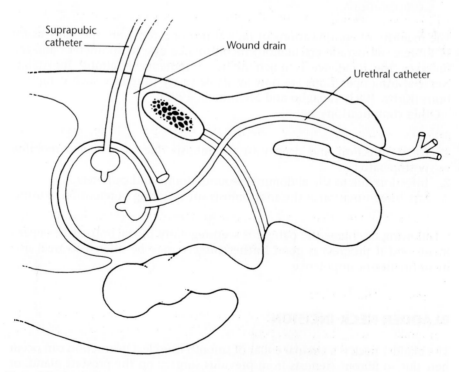

Figure 9.7 *Positioning of drainage apparatus after radical prostatectomy*

progress if the urine is very heavily bloodstained, but usually the catheters are left to drain normally and initially the output is monitored hourly for 24 hours. The urine output should exceed 30 ml per hour; if it is less than this it should be reported to the doctor.

Once bowel sounds have been established the patient is allowed to take fluids as tolerated and commence a light diet. This is usually 2–4 days postoperatively. Wound drains are left in situ until drainage is minimal – again 2–4 days.

Mobility can be a problem postoperatively, especially if epidural pain control is used. Physiotherapy is important, and the patient should be mobilized as soon as possible. Antiembolic stockings are worn until the patient is discharged home.

Intravenous antibiotics are usually administered for the first 3 days following surgery.

The suprapubic catheter is usually removed 2–3 days postoperatively and the urethral catheter is left in situ for 3–4 weeks. The catheter acts as a splint to aid anastomotic healing. The patient is discharged home after 7–10 days with the urethral catheter in place and is readmitted for its removal. A urethogram may be performed prior to removal. Once the urethral catheter has been removed the voiding pattern is recorded on a fluid balance chart. Often the patient suffers with incontinence and has to be supplied with incontinence pads, and will require explanation and reassurance. Referral to a continence advisor would be beneficial.

Complications

The majority of complications of radical prostatectomy are the same as for TURP (e.g. retrograde ejaculation, incontinence due to sphincter damage); however, the incidence is much higher. Impotence is almost inevitable. Nerve-sparing operations are now available to try to reduce such complications (Kirby, 1991; Tanagho and McAninch, 1992).

Other complications are:

1. Chest infection and deep vein thrombosis due to restricted mobility postoperatively.
2. Infection due to the abdominal wound, drains and catheters.
3. Stricture formation at the anastomosis site resulting in retention of urine.

Following discharge the patient is seen regularly in the outpatient department, and if progress is good further surgery may be offered to treat any incontinence or impotence.

BLADDER NECK INCISION

The bladder neck is a circular collar of smooth muscle. Obstruction can occur here due to fibrous stenosis from previous surgery on the prostate gland, or bladder neck dyssynergia, where the bladder neck fails to relax or contracts during voiding. The cause is generally unknown. A video cystometrogram will confirm this diagnosis.

If obstruction occurs a bladder neck incision (BNI) can be performed. A single incision is made from the bladder base down to the verumontanum. A urethral catheter is left in situ for 1–3 days. Haematuria can occur and signs of haemorrhage need to be observed for. Infection is also a complication and any signs should be treated with antibiotics.

It is important that retrograde ejaculation is explained preoperatively to patients undergoing a bladder neck incision.

REFERENCES

ASTRAHAN M A, Ameye F and Dyen R (1991) Interstitial temperature measurements during transurethral microwave hyperthermia. *Journal of Urology* **145**: 304–308.

BULLOCK N, Sibley G and Whitaker R (1989) *Essential Urology.* Edinburgh: Churchill Livingstone.

CHAPPELL C R, Milroy J G and Rickards D (1990) Permanently implanted urethral stent for prostatic obstruction in the unfit patient. *British Journal of Urology* **66**: 58–65.

CHRISTMAS T J and Kirby R S (1991) Conservative treatment for benign prostatic hyperplasia. *Hospital Update* **17**: 635–641.

GILL K P, Machen L S, Allison D J and Williams G (1989) Bladder outflow tract obstruction and urinary retention from prostatic hypertrophy treated by balloon dilatation. *British Journal of Urology* **64**: 618–622.

KIRBY R S (1991) Nerve-sparing radical retro-pubic prostatectomy for localised cancer of the prostate. In: Hendry W F (ed.) *Recent Advances in Urology/Andrology.* Edinburgh: Churchill Livingstone.

MCLOUGHLIN J and Williams G (1990) Prostatic stents and balloon dilatation. *British Journal of Hospital Medicine* **43**: 422–426.

PEREZ-MARRERO R A, Lee L M, Emerson L and Goldberg S L (1990) Endoscopic balloon dilation of the prostate: early experience. *Journal of Urology* **144**(1): 83–87.

ROOS N P, Wennberg J E and Malenka D J (1989) Mortality and reoperation after open transurethral resection of the prostate for benign prostatic hyperplasia. *New England Journal of Medicine* **320**: 1120–1124.

STROHMAIER W L, Bichler K H and Fluchter S H (1990) Local microwave hyperthermia of benign prostatic hyperplasia. *Journal of Urology* **144**: 913–917.

TANAGHO E A and McAninch J W (eds) (1992) *Smith's General Urology,* 12th edn. London: Prentice-Hall.

10 UROLOGICAL CANCERS

Contents

'Cancer' is a generic term, encompassing a variety of different illnesses which individually affect a wide range of organ systems and tissues. Common to all cancers, however, is a deregulation of the normal processes of growth and differentiation, resulting in uncontrolled cellular proliferation. Such proliferation occurs because cancer cells no longer respond to normal mechanisms of growth control, and the unco-ordinated growth pattern that results can then lead to invasion of surrounding tissues and subsequent haematological or lymphatic spread.

It is this characteristic pattern of invasion and spread that accounts for the morbidity and mortality of cancer. In any discussion of cancer-related illness, one needs first to distinguish between the descriptive terms 'malignant' and 'benign', which refer to different types of growth control deregulation. A summary of the differences between these two types of growth is given in Table 10.1.

There are other cancer-related terms in common usage which may result in confusion. To avoid ambiguity, the key terms used in this chapter are listed in Table 10.2 along with their definitions.

Cancer is an increasingly common disease within industrialized populations, and this may reflect the combination of an environmental aetiology and possible genetic predispositions for certain types of cancer. Table 10.3 illustrates the incidence of some specific types of cancer, and includes some of the more common urological cancers for comparison. Clearly, causative agents for cancer are extremely varied and, in many cases, unknown at this time.

MALIGNANT GROWTHS	BENIGN GROWTHS
Do not remain encapsulated	Remain encapsulated
Grow in an invasive manner	Do not grow invasively
Metastasize	Do not metastasize
Are life-threatening	Generally are not life-threatening
Tend to be less well differentiated	Generally well differentiated
Usually grow faster than benign tumours	

Table 10.1   *Malignant and benign growth: characteristics*

TERM	MEANING
Tumour	A distinct region of growth deregulation, resulting in a dividing colony of cells of varying size which may display either malignant or benign characteristics
Differentiation	The process whereby dividing cells maintain a degree of morphological and biochemical similarity to their parental cell type. Loss of differentiation is a characteristic of cancer cells, which may be highly differentiated and thus very different from their cell or tissue of origin. Loosely, the higher the degree of undifferentiated character, the poorer the prognosis.
Malignant	A pattern of tumour growth characterized by uncontrolled cellular division, invasion of surrounding tissues and usually metastatic spread, if untreated
Benign	A pattern of tumour growth characterized by uncontrolled cellular division, but which remains localized, without invasion of surrounding tissues or metastases.
Cancer	A generic term used to describe any malignant tumour
Carcinoma	A malignant tumour of epithelial tissue

Table 10.2   *Some key terms used within the context of cancer*

The typical pattern of urological cancers, in terms of their location and incidence, is shown in Figure 10.1. The problem with cancers of the urothelium is that they have the potential for rapid spread throughout the urinary tract, because of the uniform nature of the transitional cell epithelium. Therefore, a bladder carcinoma may readily spread in a retrograde direction to involve the ureter, or via an antegrade route to involve the urethra and

CANCER SITE	INCIDENCE IN ENGLAND AND WALES (%)
Males	
Lung	**9.15**
Colon	**1.89**
Pancreas	**0.94**
Stomach	**2.23**
Bladder	**1.99**
Prostate	**2.17**
Females	
Breast	**5.96**
Ovary	**1.26**
Colon	**1.65**
Cervix	**1.21**
Lung	**2.42**

Note: Adapted from Muir *et al.* (1987).

Table 10.3 *Incidence of some common forms of cancer*

penis. Likewise, a renal cancer may well spread in an antegrade direction to involve the ureter and perhaps the bladder. This underlines the importance of early diagnosis and treatment.

BLADDER CANCER

Bladder cancer, along with prostatic cancer (see Chapter 9) is by far the most common urological malignancy, accounting for 90% of tumours seen. It is found in approximately 20 per 100,000 of the population and this means that some 8,000 new cases of urothelial cancer present within the UK each year.

Worldwide, a significant geographical variation in incidence is seen, with bladder cancer common within the industrialized world but less common within developing countries (except those where schistosomiasis is common). In the UK and Europe the peak incidence of bladder cancer occurs at around 65 years of age. In other areas the age of presentation is lower, because of the nature of the chronic inflammation and irritation caused to the bladder mucosa by schistosomiasis.

Histology

Histology refers to the study of the type and morphology of cells which make up an organ or tissue. Histologically, certain types of urothelial tumours can be identified. These are:

◆ Benign:
papilloma
fibroepithelial polyp

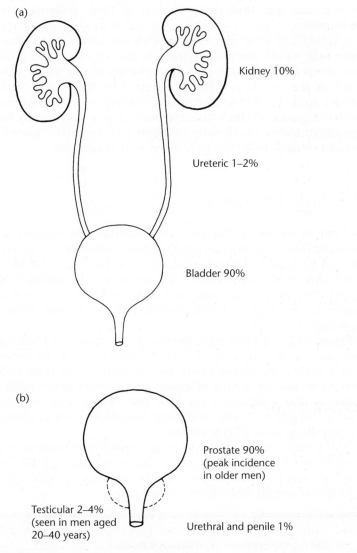

Figure 10.1   *Incidence and location of common urological cancers: (a) upper tract tumours (both sexes); (b) lower tract tumours (men)*

♦   Malignant:
         transitional cell carcinoma (90%)
         squamous cell carcinoma (5–8%)
         adenocarcinoma (1–2%)
         sarcoma (< 1%)
         undifferentiated, highly anaplastic cancer

These categories of malignancy may also present within the upper tracts, such as in the kidney or ureter. However, such upper tract tumours often present later, so that a proportion of them are more advanced at the time of diagnosis and thus the prognosis of these patients may well be less favourable.

A specialized form of cancer, not shown above, but which may present anywhere within the urinary tract, is that of carcinoma in situ. Urothelial carcinoma in situ is analogous to carcinoma in situ within other bodily sites (such as the cervix) and is characterized by malignant change within the surface epithelial lining of either the bladder or upper tract mucosal surface. Such carcinomas in situ within the bladder may occasionally behave in a very aggressive manner with early invasion and metastatic spread, and this can present difficult problems in relation to management.

Staging of bladder cancer

For enhancement of diagnosis and treatment in relation to bladder and prostatic cancer, an internationally agreed system of staging is used, ensuring that all urological units are working from the same uniform diagnostic criteria. This system is the TNM + G stage, where the initials T, N and M stand respectively for *tumour*, *nodes* and *metastases* and the G for *Gleeson*, which relates to the degree of differentiation of the tumour (this is therefore a histological diagnosis).

Figure 10.2 and Table 10.4 illustrate both the use of TNM staging and also how such diagnostic criteria relate to the extent of the presenting disease. The T stage is ascertained both by the histological examination of biopsy specimens and by means of examination under anaesthesia (EUA). Nodal status is also ascertained via EUA and biopsy, and metastatic disease is assessed largely by bodily screening procedures such as ultrasound or computed tomographic (CT) scanning.

It is actually very difficult to stage metastatic disease accurately because, even using CT scanning, magnetic resonance imaging (MRI) or tumour markers, one can never totally rule out the presence of microscopic metastases, which may consist of only one or two cells.

M0	**No evidence of metastatic disease**
M1	**Metastasis present**
MX	**Metastatic state unknown**
N0	**No nodal involvement**
N1	**Single, adjacent node involved, on same side of body as the tumour (i.e. ipsilateral)**
N2	**Bilateral nodal involvement or opposite side nodal involvement (contralateral) or multiple regional nodes involved**
N3	**Fixed, regional nodes involved (i.e. tumour spreading out of nodes into adjacent structures)**
N4	**Regional nodes involved (i.e. wider metastatic disease)**
NX	**Nodal status unknown**

Table 10.4 Staging of metastasis and lymph nodes in bladder cancer

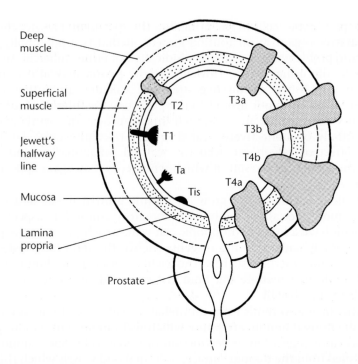

Figure 10.2 Bladder cancer staging: Tis, flat, carcinoma in situ; Ta, papillary, confined to mucosa; T1, invasion of lamina propria; T2 invasion of superficial muscle; T3a, invasion of deep muscle; T3b, invasion of perivesical tissue; T4a, tumour fixed to prostate; T4b, tumour fixed to other pelvic structures (*TNM Atlas*, 3rd edn, 2nd revision, 1992)

Presentation of urothelial cancer

Patients who have developed a urothelial cancer classically present with one or more episodes of painless haematuria. Bullock et al (1994) reported that 20% of such patients are subsequently found to have a urinary tract tumour. Although a common mode of presentation, painless haematuria is thus by no means proof of a urothelial tumour.

Because of the intrinsic sensitivity of the urine testing sticks used for routine health screening, more patients are now being referred for urological investigation, with microscopic haematuria having been discovered on stick testing. Many of these individuals are younger patients and, in the vast majority of cases, the haematuria is idiopathic and no abnormal lesion or disease process is discovered on subsequent investigation. The 'march' haematuria (first seen in soldiers following long route marches) is one such example of idiopathic haematuria. Bullock et al (1994) further reported that approximately 10% of patients with such microscopic haematuria who are over the age of 45 years have a urological malignancy as the cause of the bleeding.

A tumour of the bladder urothelium may also be an incidental finding at cystoscopy for other urological problems (e.g. prostatic resection or recurrent urinary tract infection) and such a method of discovery accounts for about 10% of all urothelial tumours (the vast majority of which are bladder cancers).

Sterile pyuria (pus cells in the urine, but the specimen does not then grow any causative organism on routine growth media) is a potentially sinister presenting problem and is generally indicative of either tuberculosis or cancer within the urinary tract. However, sterile pyuria may also result from recurrent established calculi (e.g. staghorn calculus and other infective stones) because antibiotic agents do not penetrate the interior of such stones and thus viable bacteria are always left intact. Also, sterile pyuria may result from partially or ineffectively treated urinary tract infections. Further, the irritant effect of calculi can lead to localized inflammation and scarring within the kidney, as a result of which white cells may again appear within the urine.

Tuberculous bacilli do not grow on routine growth media and therefore require a more specialized method of laboratory culture, if suspected. Also, such bacilli have a lipid, hydrophobic cell wall, which prevents the penetration of normal acidic staining reagents (hence the term 'acid-fast' bacilli). Thus, a staining method such as the Ziehl–Neelsen procedure is required, which is able to penetrate the lipid cell wall and therefore highlight the presence of such bacilli.

Pus cells may also result from urothelial cancers, because leucocotyes are part of the normal immune response which seeks to prevent tumour growth, and thus cause regression or destruction of cancer cells. Such immune cells may be shed from the tumour surface, or from blood vessels which the cancer has eroded, and thus appear in the urine.

It is useful, therefore, to assume that any patient with sterile pyuria has either tuberculosis or cancer, until it is proved otherwise.

Other problems caused by urothelial cancers, which may cause a patient to present, are shown in Table 10.5. Patients who present with symptoms of urothelial cancer, in association with abdominal or perineal pain, may well have advanced cancer of the bladder or kidney, the pain suggesting that the tumour has begun to infiltrate and invade surrounding tissues, causing both tissue destruction and nerve compression or damage. Generally such pain is

---

Painless haematuria (70–90%), which is *overt* or *microscopic* (i.e. found on routine urinalysis)

Cystitis (some 15% of patients present with symptoms of cystitis and of these 40% have urinary tract infection)

Bladder outflow obstruction (due to tumours which are close to the trigone or bladder neck)

Ureteric obstruction (either at the level of the ureteric orifice or higher up), which can then result in renal failure or loin pain

Non-specific symptoms (e.g. weight loss, anaemia, pyrexia of unknown origin)

Established metastatic disease

Perineal or abdominal pain (this may be a late onset sign which correlates with both soft tissue and nervous invasion by tumour cells)

Table 10.5 Presenting problems which may be caused by malignancy of the urinary tract

characteristic of more advanced urological tumours (e.g. T3–T4 bladder cancers or prostatic tumours).

Investigations

Urothelial cancer is normally investigated by three principal methods. These are:

◆   urinary culture and microscopy
◆   intravenous urography (IVU), ultrasound or CT scanning
◆   cystoscopy and examination under anaesthesia

If IVU or ultrasonography suggests the presence of an upper tract lesion (i.e. within the kidney) then other investigations, such as abdominal CT scanning, are likely to be employed. If IVU or ultrasound scanning suggests a ureteric or bladder lesion, then cystoscopy and EUA are performed, in conjunction with transurethral resection, as this allows effective staging of such tumours.

Tumour staging requires examination under anaesthesia because the abdominal muscles are then completely relaxed, which allows determination of whether the cancer has invaded through the bladder wall into adjacent structures, which could not be discerned by cystoscopy alone.

It must also be stated that a negative urinary cytological examination does not necessary exclude the presence of urothelial cancer, but a positive result is very useful in terms of establishing a diagnosis.

For carcinoma in situ, urinary cytology is a particularly useful investigation because random biopsy of the bladder mucosa, via cystoscopy, in such patients may not actually display a typically malignant histological appearance. However, malignant cells are often shed into the urine in patients with carcinoma in situ, and these may well be detected by urinary cytological investigations, especially in early morning specimens, owing to their increased bladder dwell time.

Management of urothelial cancers

Table 10.6 provides a summary of common approaches for specific types of urothelial cancer, each of which requires specific nursing care measures. The majority of management strategies in Table 10.6 and their nursing implications are covered in other chapters, and therefore are not repeated here. However, tumours of the bladder and also testicular cancers are discussed more fully below.

Management of bladder cancer

As can be seen from Figure 10.2, bladder cancers can either affect very little of the overall mucosal surface, or can be widespread (e.g. carcinoma in situ). Urothelial cancers may either already have invaded deeply into the wall of

LOCATION OF TUMOUR	LIKELY MANAGEMENT
Kidney	**Partial nephrectomy**
	Radical nephrectomy
	Additional therapies:
	radiotherapy
	systemic chemotherapy
	localized chemotherapy via
	nephrostomy
Ureter	**Ureterectomy (partial/total)**
	Ureteral reconstruction once tumour removed
	Additional therapies:
	DXR radiotherapy
	systemic chemotherapy
Bladder	
Superficial tumours	**Systemic chemotherapy (generally poor response)**
	Intravesical chemotherapy (30–50% response rate)
	Cryosurgery, laser surgery
	Immunotherapy
More extensive tumours	**Resection of varying depth according to nature of cancer**
	Additional therapies:
	DXR radiotherapy
	systemic chemotherapy
	intravesical chemotherapy
	Cystectomy and conduit-type diversion
	Cystectomy and continent diversion
	Partial cystectomy (though not advocated by all centres because of the risks of tumour dissemination or further tumour growth in remaining segment)
Prostate	**Resection (TURP)**
	Cryotherapy
	Thermotherapy (microwave)
	Testosterone antagonists or blockers of testosterone synthesis
	Synthetic oestrogens (generally, have significant side-effects)
Penis	**Partial or total amputation, depending on size of lesion at diagnosis**
	Additional therapies:
	DXR radiotherapy
	systemic chemotherapy
	Lymph node dissection if required

Testes (*e.g. seminoma, teratoma*)	DXR radiotherapy (especially for seminoma, which is very radiosensitive) Orchidectomy Systemic chemotherapy (sperm save prior to treatment) Monthly tumour markers (e.g. AFP or HCG) to follow response to treatment, for up to 2 years, then 6-monthly for 5 years and annually until 10 years

Note: AFP, alpha-fetoprotein; DXR, deep X-ray; HCG, human chorionic gonadotrophin.

Table 10.6 *Summary of management strategies for specific urothelial cancers*

the bladder by the time of presentation (e.g. T3–T4) or be far more superficial in nature (e.g. Ta or T1).

Bladder cancer usually presents with one of three appearances. These are:

◆   *Papillary* – a 'fronded' appearance, projecting outward from the mucosal surface into the bladder lumen

◆   *Solid* – usually more invasive tumours, remaining within the bladder wall

◆   *Ulcerated or erythema type* – often mistaken for regions of cystitis or cystitis affecting the whole mucosal surface (biopsy at the time of cystoscopy is therefore very important)

Certain histological types of cancer are also common. Within Europe, by far the most common (approximately 95%) are transitional cell carcinomas, which reflect malignancy of the normal transitional cell lining of the urinary tract. The problem with such tumours is that they may rapidly spread to involve other parts of the urinary tract, and thus cancers originating within the bladder or kidney may undergo either retrograde or antegrade spread, sometimes with alarming rapidity. It is therefore normal, if removing a kidney for cancer, to remove the associated ureter (to minimize the risk of recurrence), or, if removing the bladder, also to remove the lower part of the ureter and the urethra.

Outside Europe, other histological types of bladder cancer are more common, and transitional cell carcinoma in such regions is rarely seen. Thus, in parts of Africa where schistosomiasis is endemic, squamous cell carcinoma of the bladder is far more common, as a result of the chronic irritation and inflammation caused to the mucosal lining of the bladder by the schistosome parasite. Squamous cell bladder cancers are seen in Europe, but far less commonly than transitional cell tumours, and are not usually associated with parasitic infestation. Squamous cell bladder carcinoma may also present within a poorly draining diverticulum, where the constant irritant effects of urine and infection (caused by urinary stasis within the diverticulum) can induce squamous metaplasia and then cancer. Thus, bladder diverticula, which do not empty upon voiding, are potentially serious and require treatment. Squamous cell bladder carcinoma is commonly associated with longstanding irritation to or inflammation of the bladder mucosa.

Adenocarcinoma is also seen within the bladder, as one might expect of a secretory (glandular) epithelium, such as that lining the bladder (which is mucus-secreting). Most commonly, adenocarcinoma is a result of chronic infection over a prolonged period, but can occur de novo anywhere within the bladder lumen, most commonly in the region of the vault from possible urachal remnants (embryological remnants of the bladder). Generally, adenocarcinomas and squamous cell carcinomas of the bladder carry a poorer prognosis because they are more dedifferentiated (i.e. less like their tissue of origin) than many transitional cell tumours.

Overall, the most common sites for metastatic spread from malignant bladder tumours (and also prostatic cancer, because the lymphatic and venous drainage of the two organs are very similar) are the bony pelvis, upper femurs, rib cage and liver.

Staging and treatment

An overview of staging and possible management is shown below.

Tumour in situ or tumour stage I

1. Intravesical chemotherapy.
2. Cryotherapy.
3. Laser therapy.
4. Bacille Calmette–Guérin (BCG) treatment.

Recurrent, invasive tumour in situ may require cystectomy and urinary diversion to prevent advancement of the disease.

Tumour stage II

1. Transurethral resection, with or without radiotherapy and systemic chemotherapy.
2. Cystectomy may be performed if viable tumour remains within the bladder 6 months after radiotherapy or if invasive cancer recurs after initially successful treatment.
3. Cystodiathermy is usually employed for superficial recurrences following radiotherapy.

Tumour stage III

1. Radiotherapy is the mainstream treatment, especially in younger patients. This can then be followed by salvage cystectomy if recurrence occurs or if severe side-effects result (e.g. bladder contracture or fistula formation, as a result of radiotherapy).
2. Conduit-type diversion.
3. Continent diversion with the formation of a neo-bladder.
4. Possibly systemic chemotherapy.

Tumour stage IV

Stage IV treatment falls within the realm of palliative care. Radiotherapy may be used to help control pain caused by both local tumour spread and also bony metastases. Radiotherapy may also be useful in helping to reduce haematuria, should this be a problem. Temporary urinary diversion (e.g. ureterostomy) may also be employed.

The methods of treatment of bladder tumours and their associated nursing care are described below.

SUPERFICIAL BLADDER TUMOURS

Intravesical chemotherapy

Intravesical chemotherapy is generally used for superficial bladder cancers (Ta or T1) or for regions of Tis (see Figure 10.2). Usually such patients will be treated as day cases. The principle behind this treatment is to expose the bladder mucosa to uniform treatment with a chemotherapeutic agent, thus killing as many of the malignant cells as possible, but preventing or minimizing damage to the normal mucosa. Such chemotherapeutic agents directly disrupt the normal cell cycle, either by blocking synthesis of key components required for cellular division (e.g. ribonucleotides) or by disrupting the process of division itself (e.g. by inhibiting microtubule formation). They are instilled via a urinary catheter, which remains in situ for the duration of the treatment.

The patient is asked to lie first supine, then prone, then on either side (laterally), typically for approximately 15 minutes each time, giving a total dwell time of 60 minutes. A key problem with such an approach is that the agents used are often very irritant (as one might expect) and therefore not all patients may be able to retain them for the full treatment period. Thus, patients require both support and encouragement during treatment, and perhaps simple diversional measures such as music, reading or conversation with the nurse. Normally, patients are asked to void prior to the instillation of the drug, to reduce the likelihood of dilution or voiding during treatment. At the end of the specified time period (usually 1–2 hours in total) the drug is allowed to drain out, and the catheter removed. Because of the irritant effect of the drugs used in treatment, some centres prefer to use a catheter without a balloon, such as a 10 FG Nelaton catheter. This is passed into the bladder, and care is taken to ensure the bladder is completely empty before the drugs are instilled. The catheter is removed immediately following instillation and the patient is required to 'hold' the chemotherapeutic agent in the bladder for the specified time. Voiding of the drug takes place after the patient has left the clinic. The patient should be warned prior to voiding that the urine is likely to be coloured, especially as some of the drugs used are red and give the impression of haematuria for the first or second void. After urine has been successfully passed, the patient is encouraged to drink normally, while the voiding pattern is monitored to ensure that a normal pattern for that individual has been restored (cystitis and frequency are common for the first 24–48 hours after the procedure).

Usually a series of treatments is given for 6–8 weeks (approximately one per week) and the patient is examined endoscopically after 3 months, to assess the response to treatment. Instillation of such anticancer drugs (because of their inherent toxicity) requires precautions such as eye protection and the wearing of gloves on the part of all staff.

Patient responses to such intravesical chemotherapy may vary, but only 50% of patients show any response at all. Thus, intravesical chemotherapy is not a particularly successful treatment for superficial bladder tumours.

Laser therapy

The acronym 'LASER' stands for 'light amplificatiion by stimulated emission of radiation'. In essence, particles within a laser medium are raised to a high energy state by the application of energy from a suitable external power source. These unstable, excited particles then return to their normal resting state via a photon release of light energy (stimulated emission of radiation). In a laser, such photon release itself is caused by the impact of a separate photon, and thus the process can rapidly generate a chain reaction which effectively amplifies the light to very high energy levels. For a detailed consideration of laser therapy within urology, see Etchells (1988).

Simply, lasers with a frequency range within the infrared region of the visible spectrum are used for incision, vaporization of tissue and coagulation (i.e. thermal mechanisms). In contrast, lasers of lower frequency interact with naturally pigmented tissues or with compounds added to cells (i.e. photo-sensitizers), inducing cellular disruption and cell death.

Not all lasers are suitable for endoscopic use, however. The carbon dioxide laser, for example, does not function well urologically, because its wavelength is absorbed by fluid within the bladder.

The most versatile laser for urological use is the neodymium–yttrium aluminium garnet (Nd-YAG) laser, which can be used either as an alternative to conventional treatment or as an additional treatment following the electro-excision of tumour, via cautery. The Nd-YAG laser can induce bulk tissue necrosis, which allows it to be used for the destruction of bladder cancers. Because of its infrared wavelength (1,064 nm) the Nd-YAG beam is invisible to the naked eye; thus it is used with a 'pilot' laser (helium–neon) which provides a red light beam, which can be aimed on to the target area. Activation of the Nd-YAG beam increases the temperature of tissues within the target area to approximately 60°C, which is more than sufficient to denature most of the intracellular proteins. Thus, even though the gross architecture of the treated area remains intact, the cells composing it die. The wavelength of the Nd-YAG laser means that such thermal damage to tissues is possible up to a depth of 1 cm, and the laser also has the advantage that it can be directed down a fine, flexible quartz fibre, fed down the channel of a suitable endoscope. Fowler (1991) reported that such laser energy can be transmitted either by specialized 'contact tips' which allow the fibre to penetrate below the tissue surface, or the beam can simply be applied to the surface alone. For such 'non-contact' application, the laser is usually held 0.25–0.75 cm away from the tumour surface, and pulses of less than 5 seconds are applied to the tumour.

Laser treatment requires strict precautions to protect the eyes of both operator and patient, and thus safety goggles or glasses of appropriate colour (this will vary according to the type and frequency of the laser) are mandatory for both staff and patient. An anaesthetized patient's eyes may be taped closed. Black instrumentation is also needed, to prevent reflection. A comprehensive consideration of such safety methods is given by Etchells (1988).

Patients generally report only minor discomfort following laser treatment of superficial bladder cancers, such as suprapubic burning pain or 'prickling' type pains. Fowler (1991) reported that this type of postoperative pain can be avoided or lessened by moving the laser beam during treatment so that local heating of adjacent healthy tissues is reduced. Also, instillation of 20 ml lignocaine solution (1% or 2%) into the bladder, 20 minutes prior to the procedure, has been used to reduce the sensitivity of the urothelium.

Laser treatment produces very little bleeding, so that postoperative urethral catheterization is usually unnecessary (unlike endoscopic resection, where postoperative loss may be significant), and thus patients can be treated on a day-case basis. Follow-up of such patients seems to indicate that the rate of tumour recurrence is no more than for other treatments, and the procedure has the advantage of being suitable for day-case use.

However, although lasers reduce the time the patient stays in hospital, they remain extremely expensive. Safety precautions must be used and rigidly enforced to protect both the users and patient from retinal damage. All surfaces that could reflect must be dulled, and doors alarmed and locked to prevent unshielded people entering during treatment. According to Fowler (1991), the main danger from the use of Nd-YAG laser in treating bladder cancer is late perforation of the bowel, caused by heating of bowel loops adjacent to the bladder wall. As the wall of the heated bowel begins to necrose (because the cells die), intestinal enzymes begin to digest the necrotic tissue, resulting in the possibility of perforation up to 72 hours after laser treatment. Using limited power settings on the laser seems to reduce the incidence of this complication to very low rates.

The nursing care of patients undergoing laser treatment is minimal, especially if they are receiving their treatment under local anaesthesia. Adequate preparation and explanation are vital, as is support during the procedure. It should be ascertained that the patient has voided postoperatively, and that urinary bleeding is not significant. Monitoring the patient for pain is an important aspect of postoperative care.

Photodynamic therapy

Photodynamic therapy (PDT) is a major application of laser therapy, relevant to urology. Photodynamic therapy is a method whereby superficial solid cancers, containing a previously injected photosensitizer, are destroyed with a laser beam of suitable frequency. Red (633 nm) is common but green and other colours are also used.

The patient receives an intravenous injection of photosensitizing agent (e.g. a haematoporphyrin derivative or its purified form, dihaematoporphyrin) which is then taken up by both normal and cancerous tissue. Cancer cells, because of their altered metabolism, retain such drugs, whereas they are gradually removed from normal cells and excreted via the kidneys in urine.

Normal cells when exposed to laser energy suffer a reaction similar to sunburn (just as people with porphyria suffer if they go out in bright sunlight) which normally subsides after a few days, and thus cell death is avoided because of the lower concentration of drug within such cells. Cancer cells, however, retain far more of the pigment and therefore are much more susceptible to damage and death. Thus, if a laser is applied to a localized area of bladder tumour, effective cellular destruction should occur with minimal damage to other normal tissues.

Patients are prepared for surgery, having received the photosensitizing drug beforehand. In theatre, the patient's eyes are protected and the tumour then treated with the laser under direct visual control. After the procedure the patient is observed for pain, urinary output and voiding pattern.

Commonly patients experience frequency and suprapubic pain, and usually require analgesia. They may also be given prophylactic antibiotic treatment. When discharged the patient is warned to stay away from bright sunlight for 2–3 weeks until all the photosensitizing compound has been metabolized.

Irritation can be experienced for up to 3 months, and tissue fragments (e.g. sloughed urothelium) or blood can appear in the urine. Patients may also suffer bladder contracture, though significant contracture appears to be uncommon. Patients require comprehensive information, in a form that they can easily understand, especially as this type of treatment is still new within the UK.

Patients receiving PDT are followed up at 3 months with a check endoscopy and urinary cytological examination, to assess response to treatment.

Bladder thermotherapy

Thermotherapy of the bladder remains a new development in the treatment of superficial bladder cancers, and really falls within the realm of an experimental technique offered at present in only a few centres in the UK.

Thermotherapy of the bladder is based upon the principle of application of microwave energy to localized areas of tissue via a modified flexible endoscope (a metal endoscope cannot be used because of heating effects). Such localized thermotherapy is designed to cause extensive damage to intracellular proteins and thus cell death within the specified treatment area. The treatment is usually performed under local anaesthesia, as a day-case procedure, but its efficacy remains debatable.

Patients are discharged once they have voided, and should be advised that some haematuria and loss of tissue fragments may occur after the procedure.

Thermotherapy of the bladder mucosa (i.e. to areas of superficial tumour growth) poses the same risk as that of laser therapy: the potential heating of adjacent bowel loops, which could then necrose and subsequently perforate.

Cryosurgery

Cryosurgery is another 'experimental' procedure, which still awaits comprehensive evaluation and, like thermotherapy, is offered only in a very few centres within the UK.

Cryosurgery uses a specialized probe, inserted into the bladder under direct vision (via an endoscope), which has the ability to become extremely cold, very quickly. The probe is applied to areas of localized tumour growth, and the intense cold generated by the probe is sufficient to kill cells within the immediate vicinity, by destroying the integrity of cellular membranes.

Patients are usually treated as day cases, and should be advised that some urinary blood loss and loss of tissue fragments may occur during the immediate period following the procedure.

Biological response modifiers

Biological response modifiers (BRM) are naturally occurring proteins which form the basis of the genetic treatment known as cancer immunotherapy. Such immunotherapy is based upon the assumption that if the host immune system is able to recognize invading tumour cells as foreign, they will be targeted and destroyed by immunoactive cells and proteins. Thus, biological response modifiers can either augment or both augment and direct overall immune function. At present, such treatments remain experimental and regimens are changing constantly.

Three major subdivisions of BRM are recognized. These are:

1. Proteins that restore, enhance or modify mechanisms of immunity (e.g. interferon and interleukin-2).
2. Cells that have direct anticancer activity (e.g. monoclonal antibodies).
3. Proteins that have other biological effects, such as interfering with the ability of cancer cells to survive or metastasize, or undergo malignant transformation (e.g. bacterial agents such as bacillus Calmette–Guérin).

Two of the above categories have particular relevance to the treatment of superficial bladder cancer, and these are discussed below.

Interferon

It was discovered in 1957 that cells produce a specific substance that helps them defend effectively against invading pathogens such as viruses. The substance was named interferon because it seems to 'interfere' with viral replication and also to protect bodily cells from infection. Interferon was also found, in the early 1960s, to possess antitumour potential. However, it was not possible, until the advances of molecular biology in the early 1980s (e.g. the cloning of genes and their insertion into a suitable vector) to produce enough of the substance for clinical testing. It was then discovered that interferon was not a single protein but in fact an aggregate of proteins, and could be divided into three major subtypes, alfa, beta and gamma.

Interferons belong to the same group of biological response modifiers as do the group of compounds known as interleukins, and this collective grouping is called the lymphokines. The lymphokines (and thus interferon and interleukin) are produced by specific white blood cells, namely the activated T lymphocytes.

Interferon appears to have three major functions. These are:

1. *Inhibition of DNA replication in viruses*, once these have invaded cells, and also protection of the infected cell from invasion by other viruses.
2. *Interaction with T lymphocytes*, stimulating the production of other cellular products. Such T-cell products then signal monocytes, natural killer cells and other T lymphocytes to recognize and destroy cancer cells.
3. *Inhibition of the growth and division of cancer cells*. It also stimulates the expression of HLA and tumour-associated antigens onto the surface of cancer cells, making such cells more recognizable to the immune system.

It is not understood exactly how interferon causes specific types of cancer to regress, although in some types of tumour (e.g. renal cell carcinoma) its effect seems to be dose-related, suggesting direct cytotoxic activity.

Interferon alfa has been more fully studied than interferon beta or gamma. The maximum tolerated dose is dependent on the route, the administration schedule and its frequency, but generally not more than 30 megaunits per m^2 are given daily and not more than three such doses are given per week. Intermittent dose schedules seem more effective than daily doses, because the build-up of serum interferon levels can suppress some aspects of immune response. Once interferon has been given (usually subcutaneously or via slow intravenous infusion), key nursing responsibilities centre upon support of the patient and observing for side-effects. Acute side-effects include fever (up to 40°C), rigors, headache, muscle pain, fatigue, malaise and confusion. Tolerance to side-effects generally occurs with increasing treatment frequency.

Interferon-induced toxicity is common with doses of greater than 1 $MU\ m^{-2}$, becoming more severe as the dosage is increased. Such toxicity can also be seen with moderate to high doses of interferon if given for longer than 1 month and can manifest as unacceptable fatigue, anorexia, weight loss, confusion, leucopenia and possible problems with liver enzymes (e.g. transaminase). Less severe toxic side-effects, which are usually reversible once treatment has stopped, include nausea, vomiting, diarrhoea, hypotension, central nervous system depression, paraesthesia and proteinuria.

Interferon should be used with caution in patients with a history of cardiovascular disease, because acute cardiac failure with arrhythmia and/or ischaemia can occur.

Interleukin-2

Interleukin-2 is more commonly used in the USA but has been used in trials in the UK for renal cell carcinoma. It can be administered by intravenous bolus injection, continuous IV infusion, subcutaneous injection, intrahepatic infusion or by peritoneal infusion. The pattern of dose frequency can vary; the drug can be given three times a week, or as a weekly 24-hour infusion, a weekly IV bolus or by continuous infusion over 5–6 days (the dose is usually calculated in micrograms per kilogram of body weight).

Interleukin-2 affects every major bodily system and patients must therefore be relatively well before receiving treatment. As with interferon, side-effects are varied and can include malaise, flu-like symptoms, nausea, skin desquamation, anorexia, peripheral oedema, vasodilation and hypotension (this reverses rapidly when treatment is stopped). Most symptoms resolve within 96 hours of stopping interleukin-2 treatment.

Both interferon and interleukin-2 may result in the patient becoming drowsy or confused, and memory loss may be seen. Thus, the nursing care of patients centres upon observation for and assisting in the alleviation of such side-effects. To date, both interferon and interleukin-2 have been used on a trial basis only, and remain essentially experimental treatments.

Bacillus Calmette–Guérin therapy

The use of BCG to treat cancer in humans was first reported in 1935. Modern usage began in 1969 when Mathe *et al.* (1969) demonstrated the successful use of BCG in the treatment of acute childhood leukaemia. Morales *et al.* (1976) then reported the application of BCG in the management of bladder cancer.

Bacillus Calmette–Guérin is now recognized as an effective biological agent for the treatment and prevention of recurrence of superficial bladder cancers. The therapy is currently used more in North America than in the UK and some reservations have been expressed within the UK regarding the long-term effectiveness and potential complications of intravesical BCG therapy.

Several vaccine strains are available, and these differ in the number of colony-forming units (CFU) per ml of solution (e.g. Pasteur 6×10^8 CFU ml^{-1}, Evans $1\text{–}5 \times 10^9$ CFU ml^{-1}).

Mechanism of action

Numerous mechanisms have been proposed for the effects of BCG upon urothelial tumours. These include sensitization of lymphoid cells against tumour cell antigens (lymphoid cells are then more likely to attack the cancer), activation of macrophages (which then cause lysis or inhibition of cancer cells) and increased natural killer cell activity.

The production of interleukin-2 has also been reported as a response to BCG treatment in the urine of patients, and this may constitute a further mechanism of action. Other mechanisms centre upon enhanced immunological recognition of cancer cells, similar to the process seen in autoimmune disease. However, the exact mode of action is as yet not understood.

Patients receiving BCG are those with Ta and T1 tumours. It is also increasingly being used for Tis tumours (carcinoma in situ), especially in patients who have not responded to intravesical chemotherapy. Prior to treatment, all visible papillary-like lesions are removed by transurethral resection or laser, and multiple biopsies are also taken. Urinary cytology also forms an important assessment for gauging response to treatment.

Administration

Therapy with BCG is started within weeks of endoscopy. Mukherjee *et al.* (1992) suggested a 10-day limit for treatment initiation, because the disrupted urothelium may facilitate localization of bacterial antigens (i.e. cellular components) to areas of previous tumour growth.

Freshly prepared BCG vaccine is mixed with 50–200 ml normal saline, and administered intravesically via an indwelling urethral catheter. The BCG suspension is then kept within the bladder for 1–2 hours, with the patient lying alternatively supine, prone and laterally to coat the urothelium evenly with suspension. The bladder is then emptied and the catheter removed. Intravesical BCG can also be administered using a non-indwelling catheter. The catheter must be inserted and removed with care, to minimize urethral trauma. Should bleeding ensue, BCG therapy should not be used for at least 48 hours, to avoid bacterial inoculation into blood and the induction of a possible bacteraemia. Initially, patients were also given BCG intradermally, to try to create plasma antibodies to BCG, so that its effect would only be exerted within the bladder (i.e. any organisms absorbed intravenously would therefore be destroyed). However, this practice has been abandoned because no value has been demonstrated from such 'additional' dosage.

Usually, six to eight BCG instillations are given, at weekly intervals. Patients then undergo further endoscopic examination at 12 weeks, with associated biopsy and urinary cytology, to assess response to BCG therapy. If complete remission has occurred (i.e. no recurrence on biopsy and negative urinary cytology), a monthly maintenance dose can be given, with regular endoscopic checks at 3–6 month intervals. However, no standard protocol has yet been developed, and the need for maintenance therapy is not firmly established.

One protocol which has been suggested includes weekly administration for 6 weeks, biweekly twice, 3-monthly for 2 years, 6-monthly for 2 years and then yearly after that. A further protocol simply suggests weekly instillations for 6 weeks, then no further treatment. Others suggest weekly instillations for 6 weeks, followed by weekly instillations for another 6 weeks if tumour recurrence occurs.

Nursing care

Nursing requirements include support of patients during instillation of the BCG suspension, effective safe catheterization and catheter management, and ensuring the patient is able to void after the procedure. Adequate explanation is also vital.

Side-effects and complications

Patients may experience haematuria and dysuria lasting 2–7 days on average. In addition, BCG treatment requires a high frequency of urethral catheterization; therefore skilled aseptic practice is essential.

Mukherjee *et al.* (1992) reported that the effects of BCG seem to be localized to the urothelium, because some patients found to be free of tumour on endoscopic follow-up had coexisting metastatic disease (though the number of such patients was very small). Further, Lamm *et al.* (cited in Mukherjee *et al.*, 1992) has reported serious side-effects from BCG therapy, in a study consisting of 2,589 patients. These include fever (over 39°C), haematuria, granulomatous prostatitis, joint pain, epididymitis, sepsis, skin rashes, ureteric obstruction and bladder contraction.

Much remains to be discovered about the exact mechanism of action of BCG and its optimum administration regimen, and nursing staff may need to support patients particularly because of this.

Renal use

Therapy with BCG has now been used in the treatment of some renal cancers, especially those in the pelvicalyceal region, where the BCG suspension is administered via a nephrostomy tube directly into the renal pelvis.

Overall, BCG appears to be a useful alternative to intravesical chemotherapy for the treatment of superifical bladder cancer, although it has still to be fully evaluated.

Systemic chemotherapy

Systemic chemotherapeutic agents are sometimes used in the treatment of superficial bladder cancer, but generally they are reserved for patients with more advanced tumours. Commonly administered drugs include cyclophosphamide and methotrexate. However, such drugs have a limited role because both bladder and prostatic cancers are usually poorly responsive to systemic agents. Also, such drugs can cause serious side-effects, which require skilled and co-ordinated nursing and medical management. Systemic chemotherapy may also induce problems with wound healing, should subsequent surgery be required.

STAGE II BLADDER CANCERS

Stage II tumours, by definition, are more invasive than superficial bladder cancers, and around 15% of bladder cancers fall into this category. The management of such patients involves methods that penetrate beyond the superficial layers of the bladder mucosa.

The main method of treatment employed is that of endoscopic resection (which also has the advantage of allowing staging to be performed) in association with radiotherapy or chemotherapy. Resection is performed under general or spinal anaesthesia, using diathermy and cautery (high-frequency electric current, in a suitable liquid medium such as glycine), which is exactly the same method employed for transurethral prostatic resection.

Patients normally return from theatre with a three-way urethral irrigation catheter in situ, which remains for the initial 24–48 hour period, along with isotonic normal saline bladder irrigation if required (i.e. if significant haematuria is present postoperatively, which could cause obstruction from clot formation). The urinary catheter is removed when the urine is a suitable colour (approximately 24 hours postoperatively) and the patient can be discharged once voiding is adequate. Thus, care of such patients, apart from routine postoperative measures, centres upon catheter and irrigation management, and ensuring a normal voiding pattern is restored once the catheter is removed.

Most units will obtain a midstream urine specimen once the catheter is removed, to screen for possible urinary infection. However, the use of testing sticks containing leucocyte esterase and nitrite assay pads is sufficiently accurate to render this practice unnecessary.

Patients may also receive radiotherapy and intravesical chemotherapy, depending on the nature of the tumour and the degree of differentiation (gained from histological examination). If a residual mass is palpable in the bladder wall following resection (i.e. on EUA) or if the cancer is poorly differentiated, then radiotherapy and/or cystectomy are usually advised.

Patients with both superficial and T2 tumours will be given regular endoscopic checks for at least 10 years, to ensure no recurrence occurs and also to monitor the effectiveness of treatment given. (Most units advocate that if an individual patient remains free of recurrence for 10 consecutive years, then no further checks are required.) Thus, if a superficial or T2 tumour is diagnosed and treated, the patient is likely to undergo endoscopy 3-monthly for 12 months, 6-monthly for 2 years and then yearly for 10 years, assuming no recurrence is seen. Bullock *et al.* (1994) stated that if viable cancer is present in the bladder 6 months after radiotherapy, or if an invasive tumour recurs, then cystectomy is the treatment of choice. However, if the recurrence is superficial following radiotherapy, then treatment by cystodiathermy is indicated.

STAGE III BLADDER CANCERS

Stage III cancers of the bladder are potentially far more serious threats to the patient's survival and may involve profound management measures which require intensive nursing care. By definition, such tumours have already invaded deeply into the muscular wall of the bladder and will spread outside the bladder if left untreated. As for all stages of bladder cancer, metastatic disease may already be present at the time of presentation, and this is more likely as the staging of the tumour advances. Stage III bladder cancers are usually treated initially with radiotherapy, though they will often bring the patient into the realm of cystectomy and either conduit-type diversion (traditional) or neobladder reconstruction (more recent) with removal of the urethra in both cases.

Some centres advocate the use of aggressive radiotherapy prior to surgery, as some tumours may respond with a reduction in size and vascularity, which makes their subsequent removal easier (radiotherapy and salvage cystectomy). Overall, however, this policy may not be a good one because if the tumour fails to respond to radiotherapy, it will be more advanced by the time of surgery, and metastatic disease is correspondingly more likely.

Wound healing problems are more likely following radiotherapy, and therefore earlier surgical intervention is common, with follow-up radiotherapy later on. The combination of surgery and radiotherapy appears to offer a better prognosis than either in isolation. In addition, pelvic node dissection may be added to cystectomy if CT scanning reveals regional nodal disease (present in some 30% of patients with T3 disease). If there is recurrence following treatment with radiotherapy alone, or side-effects such as bleeding or bladder contracture, fistulae or incontinence, then cystectomy and some form of urinary diversion are advocated. Generally, systemic chemotherapy for advanced bladder cancer is a poor treatment option, as such bladder tumours are often unresponsive to systemic agents.

Patients may experience profound problems with body image change, especially because operative procedures such as cystectomy (owing to the disruption to pelvic nerves) result in a virtually 100% impotence rate for men, and problems with orgasm and pelvic sensation in both sexes. Such problems may be combined with adjustment to a new urinary stoma. Helping such patients begin the process of coming to terms with such changes is a key nursing responsibility.

The exact nature and nursing management of the types of surgery undertaken for T3 tumours (e.g. conduit diversions or continent reservoir formation) are described in Chapter 11.

Prior to surgery it is essential that the nodal and metastatic status (if any) of the patient is ascertained accurately, because such surgery is not undertaken in patients with metastases. Thus, included in the preoperative work-up will be ultrasound, CT and bone scans to try to ensure that no metastatic disease is present. This should ensure that only patients with tumours localized to the bladder are exposed to the significant stress associated with cystectomy and diversion or neobladder formation.

STAGE IV BLADDER CANCERS

As shown in Figure 10.2, T4 tumours have invaded through the bladder wall into adjacent structures (e.g. prostate in males, uterus in females) and are thus 'fixed' and therefore cannot be surgically removed. It is usual to find significant metastatic disease in such patients and, for these reasons, the treatment and nursing management of patients with T4 tumours falls within the realm of palliative care. Common methods for managing such patients include the following.

1. *Temporary urinary diversion.* If the cancer is blocking urinary outflow at the level of the bladder neck, or is blocking the ureteric orifices, then ureterostomy or nephrostomy is likely to be undertaken. Renal failure is often the terminal event in advanced bladder cancer owing to this process of ureteric obstruction. Temporary urinary diversion may also be undertaken if extensive haematuria is resulting from a bladder cancer, and causing anaemia (embolization of the internal iliac artery has also been used to try to control this).
2. *Nephrostomy* if the renal pelvis is obstructed.
3. *Effective, potent analgesia* (e.g. continuous opioid infusion), as pain from both invasion of soft tissues and bony metastases is common.
4. *Radiotherapy* for palliation of bony pain (e.g. directed to pelvis or femurs) or to reduce tumour size and thus relieve compression on soft tissues or nerves, or nervous invasion by cancer cells. Radiotherapy may also be used for relief of haematuria, but the benefits of X-ray treatment need balancing against the likely side-effects; because the bladder is low down within the pelvic cavity, the intestinal tract is likely to receive radiation.
5. *Psychological care*, as for all terminally ill patients, taking account of the grieving process, etc.
6. *Other care measures*, as for any patient with a terminal illness.

Thus, the effective treatment of bladder cancer at each stage of tumour development requires skilled and insightful nursing management.

Table 10.7 shows the approximate 5-year survival rates for various types of bladder carcinoma. Bullock *et al.* (1994) suggested that lower-risk bladder

TUMOUR STAGE	PROGNOSIS* (%)
Tis	30–40
Ta	90–95
T1	40–75
T2	55
T3	25
T4	5–10

Notes: *Percentage of patients likely to survive for 5 years.
From Bullock *et al.* (1994).

Table 10.7 *Bladder tumour stage and likely prognosis*

tumours include small, well-defined cancers (e.g. Ta, G1), single tumours (i.e. affecting only a small part of the urothelium) and malignant disease where the rest of the bladder is essentially normal on biopsy. Conversely, high-risk cancers in terms of survival include large, poorly differentiated tumours (e.g. T2–T3, G2–G3), large areas of mucosal dysplasia (i.e. multiple areas of pre-malignancy), multiple tumours and also carcinoma in situ (owing to the often aggressive pattern of infiltration that characterizes this type of malignant change).

RENAL CANCER

Cancers of the kidney can result from malignant transformation of the urothelium (lining the collecting duct system) or of the renal parenchyma itself. Urothelial tumours of the kidney account for approximately 9% of total urothelial cancers. In terms of malignancies of the renal substance (parenchyma), the two most important histological types of cancer are adenocarcinoma (accounting for some 80% of renal tumours) and nephroblastoma (Wilms' tumour – usually seen in children). There are, however, a range of other types of renal tumour, both malignant and benign (Table 10.8). Of these tumours, adenocarcinoma of the kidney is by far the most common. The peak incidence of adenocarcinoma occurs at 65–75 years of age, and thus it is generally a cancer of older age groups. The incidence is twice as high in men and some 3% of patients develop bilateral adenocarcinoma, either synchronously (at the same time) or asynchronously.

Adenocarcinoma of the kidney can present as a discrete nodule or as a nodule with satellite nodules spreading outward around the original tumour. With higher G stage tumours (i.e. less differentiated cells), far more infiltration into normal tissue may be seen (i.e. a more diffuse pattern of spread is evident). Spread of renal adenocarcinoma is either by invasion, into adjacent organs via the perinephric fat, or by vascular spread. Vascular spread may be either lymphatic, to the para-aortic nodes; local venous spread via invasion of the renal vein and thus the inferior vena cava; or more distant venous spread to sites such as the lungs, liver, bones and brain.

Renal carcinoma has a similar TNM staging pattern as for that of bladder cancer, summarized in Table 10.9.

Patients can present with a wide range of problems, not all of which may be

Tumours of renal parenchyma
Benign:
  adenoma
  haemangioma
  angiomyolipoma

Malignant:
  adenocarcinoma (formerly called hypernephroma)
  Wilms' tumour (nephroblastoma)
  sarcoma
  secondary tumour deposits from other primary cancers are seen, but
  remain rare

Tumours of the renal pelvis
Benign:
  papilloma

Malignant:
  transitional cell carcinoma
  squamous cell carcinoma
  adenocarcinoma

Note: From Bullock *et al.* (1994).

Table 10.8   *Types of renal tumour*

Tumour stage	
T1	**Small tumour with no distortion of overall kidney structure**
T2	**Large tumour distorting the kidney, but confined within the renal capsule**
T3	**Spread through the renal capsule to perinephric tissues**
T4	**Invasion into the abdominal wall or adjacent organs**
Nodal status	
N0	**No regional nodes involved**
N1	**Tumour present in single regional node**
N2	**Multiple regional nodal involvement**
N3	**Regional nodes fixed owing to tumour invasion from nodes to adjacent structures**
N4	**Lymphatic involvement beyond regional nodes**
Metastases	
M0	**No distant metastatic illness**
M1	**Distant metastatic disease present**

Note: From *TNM Atlas Illustrated Guide to the TNM/pTNM Classification of Malignant Tumours*, 3rd edition, 2nd revision, 1992.

Table 10.9   *Staging for renal cancers*

directly suggestive of a renal malignancy. Haematuria, loin pain and a palpable mass in the area of the kidney are typical signs (the 'classical triad'), but other problems may be weight loss, fatigue, anaemia or fever, and many of these non-specific symptoms may be the result of 'toxohormones' produced by the cancer cells. Varicocele may be seen, caused by invasion of the renal vein, which decreases venous drainage from the scrotal sac. Inhibition of venous drainage may also cause oedema of the leg. Hormone-related problems may result from ectopic hormone secretion by renal tumours; thus, hypertension (due to renin secretion) and hypercalcaemia (due to ectopic parathyroid hormone secretion) are both possible.

Investigations

Intravenous urography or (more commonly) ultrasonography can be used to diagnose renal tumours; ultrasonography has the advantage of being able to distinguish a cyst from a solid mass. Computed tomographic scanning can be used to stage a renal tumour (i.e. assess the degree of spread, if any) and also will allow detection of metastases within the mediastinum and lungs, if of sufficient size.

Venography and bone scanning may also be used (see Chapter 2) to help assess the degree of tumour infiltration into the vena cava or metastatic spread to bone. Needle biopsy of possible malignant lesions is not advocated, because this may disseminate cancer cells along the needle track.

Management

If no metastatic disease is present, treatment of renal cancer centres upon radical nephrectomy (i.e. removal of the kidney, adrenal gland and surrounding fat, together with the upper ureter and any enlarged para-aortic nodes). The kidney is commonly removed via a thoracoabdominal approach (the peritoneum is opened via an abdominal incision and the kidney removed anteriorly), as this allows ligation of the renal blood vessels prior to mobilization of the kidney, preventing tumour cells from becoming dislodged and possibly spreading to other sites.

Postoperative nursing management may involve caring for a patient who has undergone a modified thoracotomy, which is clearly different from the more traditional nephrectomy approach, a loin incision without direct penetration of the thoracic cavity. Radiotherapy may be given postoperatively if invasion into fat or para-aortic nodes is present. The care of patients undergoing nephrectomy is described in Chapter 7.

If a patient has only one kidney, then partial nephrectomy may be undertaken, via extracorporeal cooling. Bullock *et al.* (1994) described the procedure of 'bench surgery', whereby the kidney is cooled, removed, the tumour enucleated and the remnant of the kidney then autotransplanted back into the patient's iliac fossa (the normal site chosen for renal transplantation). If it is not possible to remove a malignant tumour from a solitary kidney, then dialysis will be required postoperatively, with possible transplantation later (either live donor or cadaveric) if the patient remains well.

Nephrectomy may also be undertaken in patients with metastases, but only if intractable bleeding or pain is causing particular problems. Radiotherapy may be equally effective.

Metastatic disease following renal adenocarcinoma is generally poorly responsive to treatment, particularly to chemotherapy. Currently medroxy-progesterone and interferon are under trial for treatment of renal carcinoma. Overall, renal adenocarcinoma results in a 5-year survival of some 30–50% of patients. If penetration of the capsule or lymphatic invasion is present, then the prognosis becomes much worse. A summary of likely prognosis in terms of 5-year survival is shown in Table 10.10.

Nephroblastoma (Wilms' tumour)

First described in 1899 by Wilms, this tumour accounts for approximately 10% of childhood malignancies. Some 80% of nephroblastomas are seen prior to the age of 5 years, with a peak at 3 years (about 5% of patients have bilateral disease). However, a small number of cases are also seen in adults.

Nephroblastoma is usually a soft, pale tumour and may be either cystic or contain haemorrhagic areas. The degree of differentiation ranges from well-differentiated tumours to anaplastic or spindle cell lesions with an unfavourable prognosis. As for adenocarcinoma, nephroblastoma may present with a variety of symptoms, not all of which are urological. A palpable mass is common (approximately 80% of cases), as are abdominal pain and haematuria. However, anorexia, weight loss, anaemia, hypertension, fever and metastatic illness, affecting the lungs, bone and liver, can also be seen.

Nephroblastoma is investigated by IVU, ultrasonography, CT scanning for staging and also bone scanning and chest X-ray (to ascertain the extent of any metastases). The patient's urine may also be sampled for catecholamines to help differentiate nephroblastoma from neuroblastoma (another retroperitoneal tumour).

The treatment of nephroblastoma centres upon surgery, radiotherapy and chemotherapy; all three have implications for nursing care. Initially nephrectomy is undertaken, using an abdominal approach (i.e. laparotomy) which also allows visual examination of the opposite kidney.

The most significant recent advance in the treatment of nephroblastoma

EXTENT OF TUMOUR GROWTH	FIVE-YEAR SURVIVAL (%)
Tumour confined to kidney	75
Invasion of perirenal fat	50
Invasion of regional lymph nodes and/or tumour in renal vein or vena cava	35
Metastatic illness	<5

Note: From Bullock et al. (1994).

Table 10.10 *Renal adenocarcinoma: prognosis*

has been that of chemotherapy, and agents such as doxorubicin (Adriamycin), vincristine and cyclophosphamide, in combination or as single agents, can achieve good response rates, even in advanced disease. Bullock *et al.* (1994) reported an overall 5-year survival of 80% and cure in most patients who present early on in the disease. Thus, patients are likely to require both nursing management following initial surgery and also supportive care measures while they undergo chemotherapy or radiotherapy.

Other renal tumours

Other forms of renal tumour (both benign and malignant) may be hard to distinguish from adenocarcinoma, until operative removal or histological analysis is available.

Renal sarcoma

Renal sarcoma is fortunately rare (less than 3% of renal malignancies) as it is a highly invasive tumour (both locally and via vascular spread) and thus carries a very poor prognosis.

Secondary tumours

Tumours can also arise in the kidney which are actually metastases from other primary cancers. This may reflect the high vascularity of the kidney, although generally it is rare to see such secondary tumour deposits within the kidney. The most common primary tumours which may then involve the kidney by metastatic spread are carcinomas of the bronchus and breast, malignant melanoma and also lymphoreticular cancers (e.g. lymphoma). Secondary renal tumours usually cause loin pain and haematuria, in addition to the symptoms caused by the primary tumour. The prognosis for such patients is very poor and symptoms are treated via radiotherapy or by nephrectomy.

Oncocytoma

Oncocytomas are malignant tumours of proximal tubular cells, composed of oncocytes (well-differentiated granular eosinophilic cells). This tumour carries a good prognosis, compared with, say, adenocarcinoma, because it generally has a low rate of metastatic spread.

Benign renal tumours

Benign renal tumours include adenomas, which tend to vary in size (typically up to approximately 3 cm) but rarely cause symptoms. However, as in the case of the ileum, such adenomas can undergo malignant change.

Angiomyolipoma

Angiomyolipoma, as the name suggests, is a tumour composed of three tissues, namely blood vessels, smooth muscle and fat cells. A CT scan may be helpful in diagnosis because fat has a characteristic tissue density. Generally, haematuria is the most common presenting symptom and angiomyolipomas can usually be removed via partial nephrectomy.

Mesoblastic nephroma

Mesoblastic nephroma is a very rare benign tumour and is usually only seen in very young children and infants. It is composed of mesenchymal tissues, and nephrectomy is usually the treatment of choice.

CANCERS OF THE URETER AND RENAL PELVIS

Cancers of the ureter and renal pelvis are rare, accounting for 2–4% of urothelial cancers. Again, these types of cancers are seen in older people, with a peak age of 65 years, and a male to female ratio of approximately 2: 1.

Patients with a single upper tract tumour are at risk of subsequent bladder carcinoma (about 30–50%) and also upper tract tumours in the adjacent (contralateral) kidney (about 2–4%). Conversely, patients with primary tumours of the bladder appear to be at low risk of developing subsequent upper tract tumours (Oldbring *et al.*, 1989).

Aetiology

As with bladder cancer, smoking and exposure to certain industrial dyes or solvents are associated with an increased risk of upper urinary tract transitional cell carcinomas (Shinka et al, 1988).

The majority of ureteric and renal pelvic tumours are transitional cell tumours (ureteric approximately 95%, renal pelvic approximately 90%). Squamous cell cancers account for approximately 10% of renal pelvic tumours and are extremely rare within the ureter. The majority of squamous cell tumours are identified in patients with a history of chronic inflammation, from infection or calculi, and are often already invasive at the time of presentation.

Staging

The TNM staging of ureteric and renal pelvic cancers is shown in Table 10.11. Patients generally present with gross haematuria, which may also be associated with colicky pain in the loin, due to ureteral obstruction (caused by blood clots or tumour fragments). The renal pelvis and ureter may also be obstructed, or the tumour may already have spread to involve local tissues. Cancers of the ureter or renal pelvis have traditionally been diagnosed using IVU and retrograde ureterography. However, a ureteroscope (ureteropyeloscope) can now be used to visualize directly upper tract abnormalities, at

STAGE	PATTERN OF SPREAD
Ta, Tis	**Confined to the mucosa**
T1	**Invasion of the lamina propria**
T2	**Invasion of the muscularis mucosae**
T3	**Spread through the muscularis mucosae, into fat or the renal parenchyma**
T4	**Spread into adjacent organs**
N+	**Lymph node metastases present**
M+	**Systemic metastases present**

Note: From the American Joint Committee on Cancer (1988).

Table 10.11 *Staging of uretic and renal pelvic cancers*

which time biopsy of any lesions can also be undertaken. Laser vaporization of such tumours may also be possible at the time of ureteroscopy.

Treatment

Treatment is based upon the size and staging of the tumour. Normally, nephroureterectomy is the standard treatment, owing to the possibility of spread into the collecting system on the same side as the tumour mass. When the tumour is within the proximal ureter or in the renal pelvis, the entire ureter is removed, along with a small cuff (patch) of bladder. Tumours of the lower ureter may be treated by partial ureterectomy followed by ureteral reimplantation. Small-volume upper tract tumours may also be treated by the instillation of BCG alone (Studer *et al.*, 1989).

Radiotherapy appears to have a limited role in the treatment of upper tract tumours, and metastatic disease is usually treated with a similar chemotherapeutic regimen as for metastatic cancer of the bladder.

Nursing care

The nursing care in these conditions involves caring for patients undergoing nephroureterectomy or reconstruction of the ureter following partial ureterectomy. Both of these procedures, and their nursing implications, are described in Chapter 7.

PENILE CANCER

In Europe, penile cancer accounts for approximately 2% of all male tumours. Interestingly, circumcision at birth confers complete immunity against this form of neoplasm. The risk of occurrence is increased where there is a high degree of penile irritation from conditions such as balanitis. The risk of malignant change is also present in some skin diseases of the penis. Histologically, penile cancer is typically a squamous cell carcinoma, and evidence of keratinization is usually present. Some 75% of such tumours are usually well differentiated. Two types of growth are normally apparent. These are:

◆　　　a shallow, ulcer-like tumour, typically with 'rolled' edges
◆　　　a fungating, papillary-like tumour

Tumour spread

Early spread of such cancers is usually lymphatic, either from the glans and prepuce to the superficial inguinal nodes, or from deeper channels in the corpora, which may then carry the tumour to the deep inguinal, obturator and iliac nodes. Blood-borne spread is rare, and usually arises at a later stage in the disease, involving sites such as the lung, liver and bones. Direct spread to the urethra is usually a late feature.

Treatment

Treatment of penile cancer centres around two principal options: radiotherapy and surgery. Penile tumours are usually radiosensitive, and the penis is readily accessible for radiotherapy. However, tumours that are poorly responsive or very advanced at the time of presentation may require surgery also.

Surgery for penile cancer involves one of two procedures:

1. Circumcision, where the lesion is contained within the prepuce only (this is rare).
2. Penectomy, which may either be partial or total.

For these procedures and their nursing implications, see Chapter 12.

TESTICULAR CANCER

The incidence of testicular cancer has increased throughout the twentieth century. It is the most common solid tumour in men aged 15–35 years and accounts for 19% of total male cancer deaths within this age group (Stanford, 1988). The cause of testicular cancer is not known, but there are a number of factors that appear to be related to the aetiology of such tumours.

Men with undescended or late-descending testes (either naturally or surgically assisted) have an approximately 11–15% chance of developing a testicular malignancy. Trauma and infection (especially viral infection) have also been implicated in some patients, but neither of these appears to be a generalized factor. Thus it is likely that some unrecognized factors are involved which could be either environmental or genetic. Four main types of testicular malignancy are recognized. These are:

◆　　　*Teratoma* – 5–10% of all testicular tumours and prevalent in young children and infants, though also seen in adults.
◆　　　*Seminoma* – the most common testicular tumour, and carries

the best prognosis (i.e. is usually most responsive to treatment). Accounts for approximately a third of all cancers.

◆ *Embryonal cancer* – characterized by rapid growth and spread. Accounts for approximately a quarter of all cancers.

◆ *Choriocarcinoma* – 1–3% of testicular tumours. Carries a poor prognosis at this time.

Patients may also present with a histologically mixed tumour, possessing a combination of the above characteristics.

Treatment

Treatment of testicular cancer is dictated by the staging of the tumour. This is achieved by CT scanning to allow assessment of the tumour and also any metastatic disease. Besides scanning, blood samples are also taken and assayed for levels of alpha-fetoprotein (AFP), human chorionic gonadotrophin (HCG) and placental alkaline phosphatase (PAP). The plasma levels of these specific tumour markers not only help with staging but also allow monitoring of treatment response, as well as providing an indication of any subsequent tumour recurrence.

Tumour staging

Testicular tumours are usually staged using the Royal Marsden staging system (Table 10.12).

Nursing care

The care of patients undergoing orchidectomy is considered in Chapter 13. Chemotherapy plays a crucial role in the treatment of testicular tumours, particularly when the tumour has spread outside the testicle. The regimen

Stage 1	**Disease confined to testes**
Stage 2	**Infradiaphragmatic nodal involvement (i.e. nodes below the diaphragm level)**
	(a) < 2 cm in size
	(b) 2–5 cm in size
	(c) 7 cm in size
Stage 3	**Supradiaphragmatic nodal involvement**
Stage 4	**Extralymphatic disease**
	L_1 Lung metastasis > 3 in number
	L_2 Lung metastasis > 3 in number but < 2 cm in size
	L_3 Lung metastasis > 3 in number but > 2 cm in size

Table 10.12   *Royal Marsden staging system for testicular cancer (cited in Stanford, 1988)*

commonly employed is a triple therapy of three drugs, bleomycin, etoposide and platinum (normally cisplatin), usually abbreviated to BEP.

The side-effects of BEP therapy can be very significant, and include pulmonary fibrosis, alopecia, nausea, vomiting, nephrotoxicity, ototoxicity, peripheral neuropathy, low plasma magnesium levels and also hypersensitivity reactions. The monitoring for and prompt treatment of such side-effects are key aspects of nursing management and can do much to minimize the harmful effects of the drugs upon the patient. In cases of recognized renal impairment, carboplatin may sometimes be substituted for cisplatin. Newer antiemetic drugs such as granisetron and ondansetron have helped to reduce some of the more distressing side-effects of drug treatment.

The nursing management of these patients may include supportive measures during the administration of chemotherapy, and postoperative nursing measures following orchidectomy or laparotomy (for staging and removal of para-aortic metastases) or even thoracotomy (for removal of pulmonary metastases). A partnership between nursing and medical staff with a team approach to overall care is essential.

Testicular cancer can profoundly harm the patient's concept of body image, particularly because the testes are closely identified with 'masculinity', sexual potency and the ability to father children. Further, the combination of surgery and drug therapy can have a dramatic effect not only on the patient but also upon the family and significant others, particularly as some of the side-effects of treatment become apparent. The patient's status and role within both family and society may be threatened by the required treatment and hospitalization periods, and sexual performance may be temporarily impaired. Such patients should be offered 'sperm banking' facilities prior to treatment so that any lasting infertility (occurring as a result of treatment) will not prevent them fathering children.

Blakemore (1989) stated that the nursing management of patients with testicular tumours is primary concerned with two key areas, namely patient education and psychological support. By educating patients about their

1.	**Examination should be performed at least once a month**
2.	**The skin around the scrotum must be relaxed. A good time for examination is therefore after a warm bath or shower**
3.	**Support the testicles and scrotum within the palm of the hand. Note the size and weight. A testicle that appears larger or heavier than usual requires a medical opinion**
4.	**Examine each testicle in turn using both hands. The testicle should be gently rolled between the thumb and fingers. The epididymis is found at the back of the testicle and should be soft, spongy and often is slightly tender to touch**
5.	**Check each testicle for any small lumps or irregularities, slight enlargement or a change in firmness. All of these require a medical opinion, especially if there is a lump or irregular area of swelling**

Table 10.13 Guidelines for testicular self-examination

cancer, the required surgery and treatment, possible complications and side-effects, and by providing continuing support and encouragement, nurses can assist patients to work through their sense of self-loss and come to a more optimistic and positive outlook for their future. Early detection and treatment means that most testicular cancers now carry an excellent prognosis. Testicular self-examination should therefore be taught and encouraged, just as breast self-examination is taught to women. Nurses have a pivotal role to play as health educators, and testicular self-examination should thus be an integral part of nurse education. Guidelines for testicular self-examination are shown in Table 10.13.

REFERENCES

AMERICAN JOINT COMMITTEE ON CANCER (1988) *Manual for the Staging of Cancer. Philadelphia: Lippincott.*

BLAKEMORE C (1989) Altered images. *Nursing Times* **85**(12): 36–39.

BULLOCK N, Sibley G and Whitaker R (1994) *Essential Urology*, 2nd edn. Edinburgh: Churchill Livingstone.

ETCHELLS J (1988) Photodynamic laser therapy: a bladder cancer protocol. *AORN Journal* **48**(2): 221–234.

FOWLER C G (1991) Flexible cystoscopy and laser surgery. In: *Recent Advances in Urology/Andrology*, Hendry W F (ed.). Edinburgh: Churchill Livingstone.

LAMM D L, Steg A, Boccon-Gibod L et al (1989) Complications of bacillus Calmette–Guérin immunotherapy: review of 2602 patients and comparison of chemotherapy complications. In: EORTC Genitourinary Group Monograph 6: *BCG in Superficial Bladder Cancer*, Debruyne F M J, Denis L, Van der Meijden A P M and Alan R (eds). New York: Liss.

MATHE G, Ameil J and Schwartzenberg L (1969) Active immunotherapy for acute lymphoblastic leukaemia. *Lancet* **i**: 697–699.

MORALES A, Eidinger D and Bruce A W (1976) Intracavitary BCG in the treatment of superficial bladder tumours. *Journal of Urology* **116**: 180–183.

MORALES A and Nickel J C (1986) Immunotherapy of superficial bladder carcinoma with BCG. *World Journal of Urology* **3**: 209–214.

MUIR C, Waterhouse J and Mack T (1987) Cancer incidence in 5 continents. *IARC Scientific Publication* **5**: 88.

MUKHERJEE A, Persad R and Smith P (1992) Intravesical BCG treatment for superficial bladder cancer. *British Journal of Urology* **69**: 147–150.

OLDBRING J, Glifburg I, Mukulowski P and Hellsten S (1989) Carcinoma of the renal pelvis and ureter following bladder carcinoma; frequency, risk factors and clinicopathological findings. *Journal of Urology* **141**: 1311.

SHINKA T, Uekado Y, Aoshi H et al (1988) Occurrence of uroepithelial tumours of the upper urinary tract after the initial diagnosis of bladder cancer. *Journal of Urology* **140**: 745–746.

STANFORD J R (1988) Testicular cancer. *Nursing* **26**: 157–160.

STUDER U E, Casanova G, Kraft R and Zingg E J (1989) Percutaneous bacillus Calmette-Guérin perfusion of the upper urinary tract for carcinoma in situ. *Journal of Urology* **142**: 975.

UROLOGICAL STOMAS

Contents

'Urostomy' is the general term given to all urinary stomas. Even with the rapid and sophisticated advances in reconstructive surgery, urinary stomas are still commonly formed, with an approximate annual incidence of 2,000 (ConvaTec helpline, 1996). All the stomas included in this chapter are considered 'incontinent' and necessitate the use of an external urinary appliance.

Primary reasons for urinary diversion are as follows:

- *Tumour* – radical pelvic clearance
- *Tumour* – obstructive (usually palliative)
- *Trauma* – resulting in fistula formation
- *Congenital abnormalities* – bladder exstrophy, spina bifida
- *Bladder failure* – neuropathic, severe incontinence, interstitial cystitis

Types of urostomy include:

- cutaneous vesicostomy
- cutaneous pyelostomy
- jejunal conduit
- cutaneous ureterostomy
- colonic conduit
- ileal conduit

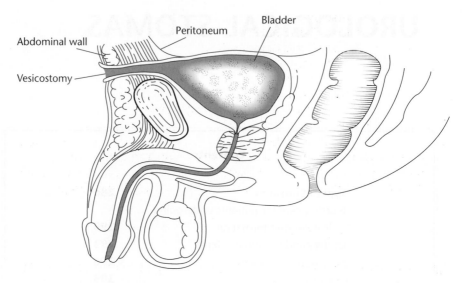

Figure 11.1 *Cutaneous vesicostomy*

TYPES OF UROSTOMY

Cutaneous vesicostomy

Although now a rather outdated procedure, cutaneous vesicostomy was generally performed in children with congenital abnormalities. The bladder is brought out onto the abdominal wall and an opening is made into the bladder to form a cutaneous vesicostomy (Figure 11.1). Surgically this is a simple procedure which preserves the upper tracts.

Stenosis is a common problem. Appliance fitting can be difficult because of the flush stoma, although babies and young children usually wear nappies.

Cutaneous pyelostomy

Cutaneous pyelostomy is a rarely formed stoma, usually in children where the pelvis of the kidney is brought to the abdominal surface creating a cutaneous stoma. Problems include stenosis and a high, flush stoma.

Jejunal conduit

A jejunal conduit is usually only indicated in cases of extensive previous surgery, irradiation, active disease or congenital abnormalities which prevent the use of ileum or colon.

An electrolyte imbalance known as jejunal conduit syndrome may be caused when using the jejunum. This is characterized by salt loss, potassium absorption, azotaemia (increase of urea in urine), acidosis and hypochloraemia.

◆ Salt loss leads to:
metabolic acidosis

uraemia
hyperkalaemia
◆ Retained potassium leads to:
hydrogen loss
alkalosis in cells
alkalization of urine
increased urinary bicarbonate levels

The clinical symptoms include anorexia, nausea, vomiting, cramps, pain, personality changes, weakness and eventually coma. Patients with jejunal conduit may require continuous salt replacement. Serum electolytes should be monitored on a regular basis and medication adjusted accordingly.

Cutaneous ureterostomy

Cutaneous ureterostomy may be a temporary or permanent measure. The ureters are brought to the abdominal surface either singly, bilaterally or as a double-barrelled procedure. This form of stoma is often the choice in ill, debilitated patients with poor renal function, in those with thickened, dilated ureters, and when less extensive intra-abdominal surgery is indicated.
    The benefits of this procedure are:

◆   relative ease of surgery
◆   reversible
◆   ureters easily catheterized
◆   preferred choice in cases of poor renal function and dilated ureters
◆   avoids extensive intestinal surgery
◆   no excessive mucus production
◆   no electrolyte reabsorption

The disadvantages are:

◆   the stoma is very small
◆   stoma is flush to skin
◆   stoma is prone to stenosis
◆   urinary reflux
◆   urinary tract infections lead to pyelonephritis
◆   difficulties maintaining leak-proof appliance

Colonic conduits

Colonic conduits are generally fashioned from the sigmoid colon, occasionally from the transverse colon. Colonic conduits are indicated for patients with neurogenic bladder and normal upper tracts (Broadwell and Jackson, 1982). This procedure can also be regarded as a temporary measure after reversible bladder damage occurs. One of the major benefits is the natural formation of antireflux valves at the ureterocolonic anastomosis, preventing the backflow of urine from conduit to ureter.

Complications include:

◆ high degree of mucus formation
◆ large stomas (often difficult to manage)
◆ sigmoid conduit have a poorer blood supply than transverse ones, and the stoma is usually darker in colour

A transverse conduit has a richer blood supply, and a lower incidence of residual urine, pyelonephritis and ureteric stenosis.

Ileal conduit

Described by Bricker (1950), the ileal conduit has become the most popular form of urinary diversion (Figure 11.2).

1. A section of ileum approximately 15–25 cm long (P. Worth, 1996 personal communication) is resected from close to the ileal caecal valve with the mesentery intact. Nowadays the ileal loop is considerably shorter than when first described by Bricker, to avoid the development of a large, floppy loop that would act as a static reservoir. A maximum amount of the terminal ileum is preserved in order to maintain its function in reabsorption of vitamin B_{12} and bile salts.
2. A segmented piece of ileum is well mobilized and the distal end securely fixed to the peritoneum.
3. The remaining ends of the ileum are anastomosed to restore continuity (Figure 11.3).
4. The proximal end of the isolated segment is closed and the ureters are implanted following resection from the bladder. Methods of ureteric anastomosis vary: some urologists prefer to implant the ureters separately, while others favour the methods described by Wallace (1970) and Clarke (1979) (Figure 11.4).
5. The distal end of the stoma is brought through a previously marked

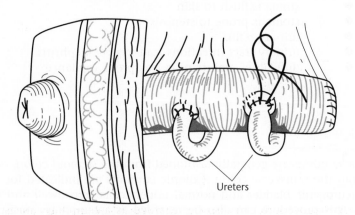

Ureters

Figure 11.2   *Ileal conduit (Bricker, 1950)*

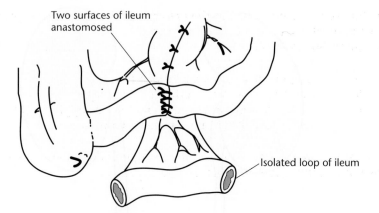

Two surfaces of ileum
anastomosed

Isolated loop of ileum

Figure 11.3   *Section of ileum isolated*

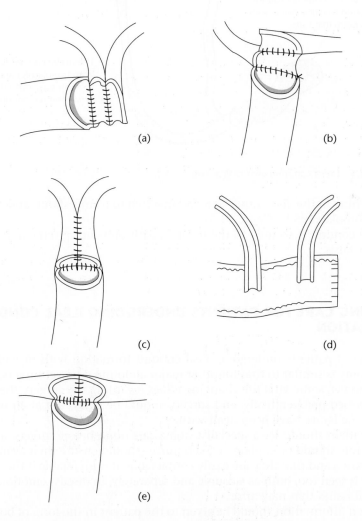

(a)

(b)

(c)

(d)

(e)

Figure 11.4   *Types of ureteroileal anastomoses: (a) Wallace I; (b) Wallace II; (c) Y anastomosis (Clark 1979); (d) nipple anastomosis; (e) modified Wallace (1970)*

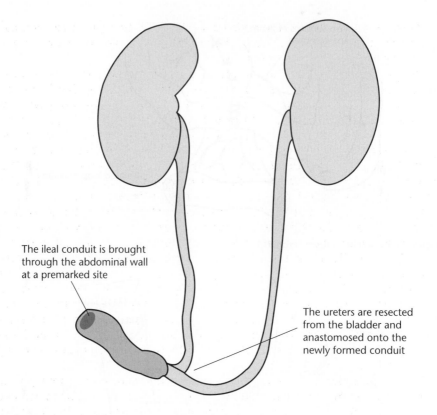

The ileal conduit is brought through the abdominal wall at a premarked site

The ureters are resected from the bladder and anastomosed onto the newly formed conduit

Figure 11.5   *Ureters anastomosed to ileal loop*

opening in the abdominal skin and inverted to form a spout, as described by Brooke (1952) (Figure 11.5).

6. The conduit is secured to the rectus sheath preventing retraction due to peristalsis.

NURSING CARE FOR PATIENTS UNDERGOING ILEAL CONDUIT FORMATION

The care of patients undergoing ileal conduit formation with or without a cystectomy is similar to that for other major abdominal bowel surgery. There are, however, some vital life changing issues regarding the surgery that must be addressed preoperatively, and surgery should be delayed if at all possible until these issues have been dealt with.

The patient should see a specialist stoma care nurse before surgery, and the nurse's role should be explained. Such nurses should ensure their availability is advertised and that they are easily contactable. It is preferable if the client's partner is seen too, both as a couple and separately, to discuss emotional and personal issues that may arise.

Written information should be given to the patient in the form of booklets, fact sheets, pamphlets, etc., so patients have something to refer to for information. If this is not an appropriate medium, then there are plenty of audiotapes, videos, slides and models available from the appliance manufacturing companies and nursing organizations that will give the client a greater appreciation of life with a stoma.

The patient should be aware of the risks and benefits of the operation as stated in the Ostomy Patients' Charter (designed for the Campaign for Impartial Stoma Care in association with the British Colostomy Urostomy Associations and the Royal College of Nursing Stoma Care Forum) and will need to give informed consent to the surgery. The site for the stoma should be chosen preoperatively and clearly marked in accordance with the standards of care formulated at either national or local level (RCN, 1992). An ileal conduit is normally sited on the right-hand side of the abdomen below the umbilicus, a third of the way from the umbilicus towards the iliac crest (Figure 11.6).

The stoma should be brought to the surface within the rectus abdominis muscle to supply the stoma with a good foundation, and there should be at least 5 cm^2 of smooth, evenly contoured abdomen to ensure a good appliance seal. However, when siting the stoma other considerations must also be taken into account. A left-handed person may want the stoma on the left side of the abdomen, which although more technically difficult is perfectly feasible. Avid golfers may prefer the stoma to be on the opposite side to their golf swing. Anatomical features such as the costal margin, iliac crest and symphysis pubis bone should all be avoided. Old scar sites should be avoided and enough distance allowed between the umbilicus and the stoma to allow the flange to lie flat.

It is essential that the site is chosen when the patient is conscious, so the patient can bend and stretch, sit down, lie down and be as mobile as possible without the appliance affecting the movement or its adhesion being undermined. Natural body contours that crease when the patient sit must be noted and avoided as stoma sites, as should areas concealed by pendulous breasts.

The client should have the opportunity to look at a range of appliances before surgery and to wear the product for a trial period (maybe with a little

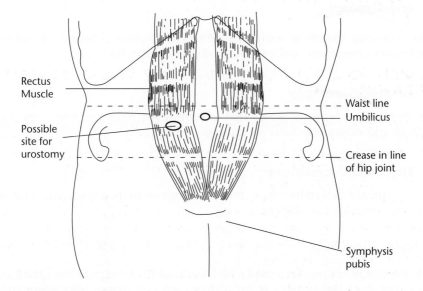

Figure 11.6 *Urostomy site*

water in the bag to represent urine). It is important to wear the product under normal day clothes and night attire in order to determine if the position interferes with waistbands, bras or other garments.

Patch testing for allergies to stoma products must be done preoperatively to ensure that there is no sensitivity to the materials. The test sites should be away from the operation site, ideally on the patient's back or shoulder, so that if a reaction does occur it will not affect the surgical area. Samples of the products should be left on for 12–24 hours to determine any sensitivity.

The patient's social and cultural situation must also be addressed, and an opportunity provided to discuss religious or spiritual problems that may arise from stoma surgery; for example, Jewish patients may need to consult the views of their Rabbi before feeling able to commit themselves to surgery (Susser, 1993). It is essential that we respect other cultural considerations and respond appropriately (Elcoat, 1986).

The client should be introduced to voluntary organizations that provide support and information to ostomists. These organizations may be able to put the patient in touch with other people with stomas of similar age, sex and social status, who can provide encouragement and help.

Psychologically and emotionally, the effect of a stoma can be devastating (Jones *et al.*, 1979). The impact of surgery must be assessed preoperatively to ensure that the quality of life is increased and not decreased. The client must be aware preoperatively of the probable changes in sexual function and difficulties that may occur. Following radical cystectomy a high incidence of male erectile dysfunction has been recorded (Devlin and Plant, 1979). For further details, see Chapter 12. In women, the destruction of nerves may lead to vaginal dryness and dyspareunia.

Preoperative care

Investigations

The following specific investigations must be completed before the patient undergoes cystectomy and formation of an ileal conduit.

Intravenous urography

An intravenous urogram is required to outline the renal and lower drainage system and detect structural or drainage problems.

Computerized tomography

A CT scan will determine the extent and severity of any malignant disease, within or outside the bladder.

Renal function tests

Glomerular filtration rate should be measured to determine the creatinine clearance from the kidneys. If the kidneys are not able to filter adequately, surgery may not be appropriate.

Bowel preparation

Bowel preparation is required to clear the bowel of faeces and is undertaken according to local procedure. For example, 2 days preoperatively intake is restricted to fluids only, and on the day prior to surgery clear fluids only are given and two 10 mg sachets of sodium picosulphate (Picolax) one in the morning and one in the early afternoon. Overnight, intravenous fluids may be given to maintain hydration.

Postoperative care

Postoperative care of the patient must be individualized. There are a number of problems that may occur with regard to the stoma. It is therefore essential that regular observation is carried out and any changes reported and acted upon. Table 11.1 lists possible complications that may occur following formation of a urinary diversion.

UNDERSTANDING URINARY STENTS

Following ureteroileal anastomosis, fine-bore catheters – most commonly paediatric feeding tubes (approximately 4 FG) – are inserted into the newly formed stoma and beyond the point of anastomosis where they are sutured. This maintains patency and protects the suturing until primary healing is completed. Stents remain in situ for 7–10 days, depending on the surgeon's preferences. If the patient has had radiotherapy then stents are left in longer, e.g. 14 days.

Care of stents

Patency of stents should be checked hourly in the first instance. Rarely, stents become blocked with mucus plugs. Very gentle flushing with saline will remove any debris and allow free flow of urine.

Drainage from urinary stents should be observed closely, and it is essential that a two-piece appliance with a floating flange is used after surgery for ease of removal from the pouch. Stents should be inserted through the non-return section of the pouch so that the urine collected is prevented from coming into continual contact with the newly formed stoma and the base-plate hydrocolloid section. Potential trauma of the stoma will also be avoided if lengths of catheter are not left on the stoma.

Removal of stents

It is important to reassure the patient that removal is not a painful procedure. The stents are removed by simply pulling them out, although a certain degree of traction may be required. If resistance is felt the stents should be left in,

OBSERVATIONS	VIABLE STOMA	PROBLEM STOMA	POSSIBLE CAUSES AND ACTIONS TO BE TAKEN
STOMA			
Colour	Pink	Dark, dusky or black	Bruising is very common initially and may cause discolouration
			A constricted or absent blood supply to stoma may cause
Texture	Soft	Hard	darkening, but this should pink up within 48 hours. May be
			caused by difficult surgery, the flange constricting the stoma or
Temperature	Warm	Cool	oedema constricting the blood supply. If the stoma does not pink
			up and the discoloured portion necroses the end of the stoma will
Moisture	Moist	Dry to touch	slough off and the client will be left with a shorter loop
			Oedema from surgery should resolve within the first 3 days
Shape	Regular	Irregular, oedematous	The shape may be irregular owing to difficulty during surgery
			to maintain a regular shape
URINE OUTPUT			
Quantity	Urine must be produced immediately from the stoma	Urine output not congruent with input	Unequal fluid balance may be an indication of:
			1. Dehydration
			2. Obstructive problem with ureteric stents
			3. Breakdown of anastomosis, leading to urinary leak. This could later lead to pain and peritonitis (see urinary stents)
Colour	Light haematuria or clear urine	Heavy and/or persistent haematuria. Obvious bleeding from the stoma	Probably caused by an unligated blood vessel at the end of the surgical procedure. If the bleeding persists the client will have to return to theatre to have the bleeding point ligated

Urinary stents	Will have a patent stent for each ureter, extending from the mid-ureter, through ureteric/stoma junction, out of stoma and into drainage bag. The stent protects anastomosis of ureteric loop junction from breakdown.	May have a poor urine output via the stents, or the stents may fall out and be found at the bottom of the drainage bag	Decreased urine output from the stents may indicate that they are blocked with mucus, formed from the ileal loop. May be necessary to flush the stents with 0.5–1 ml of saline to release blockage
			Stents may not drain as urine is extravasating from the ureteric anastomosis. The urine is leaking into the abdominal cavity and will produce pain and peritonitis. If the leak persists then septicaemia may occur and IV antibiotics must be administered. If small, the leak may resolve spontaneously or it may necessitate further surgery.
			Ureteric stents may fall out if they have been inadequately sutured to the ureter. Stents are normally removed after 10 days when the suture has dissolved and allows for release
			If the stents expel spontaneously then do not try to reinsert them. The client should be observed carefully for pain, tenderness and urine quantity.

Table 11.1 Postoperative observations

and the procedure repeated daily. Stents often fall out spontaneously by 8–10 days.

UROSTOMY APPLIANCES

Manufacturing companies are constantly working towards providing the client with a wider choice. Urostomy appliances continue to provide them with their most difficult challenge in comparison with other drainable or closed pouches. The majority of patients in the UK use lightweight disposable pouches with hydrocolloid base-plates in a one-piece or two-piece system. Reusable appliances made from more durable materials such as rubber are still manufactured. Intended for long-term use, these are most commonly found where there may be financial constraints, although occasionally remain the product choice for some well-established ostomists.

Modern urostomy appliances incorporate a non-return valve to prevent urine pooling on the flange and stomal area. All patients put security and freedom from leakage as their top priority. Specific products are chosen with regard to:

- ◆ patient choice (Ostomy Patients' Charter)
- ◆ manual dexterity
- ◆ skin contours
- ◆ patch testing results
- ◆ visual ability

Assessment of the individual's ability to open the drainage tap and empty urine must be taken into consideration. If night drainage bags are to be used the patient must be able to connect and disconnect without difficulty.

Appliance choice

Certain considerations should be borne in mind when helping a client choose a suitable appliance.

- ◆ Despite recent improvements to patient choice, it still remains possible to show the complete range of products available to the client.
- ◆ One-piece or two-piece appliances: there is no superiority of one system over the other, and the choice is the client's own.
- ◆ It must be remembered that a urostomy is constantly active. The ideal time for changing an appliance is first thing in the morning before any oral fluid is taken.
- ◆ Manual dexterity. Companies offer a choice of mechanisms such as drainage taps and pouch and flange fixation, so a suitable one can always be found.
- ◆ Eyesight. Impaired sight requires a straightforward appliance. If the stoma is poorly sited, i.e. on the other side of a rotund

abdomen, the use of a small adjustable or full-length mirror may be required. Another person may need to help.

♦ Physique is relevant, as a smaller pouch is available for the shorter person, who cannot accommodate a regular pouch under their clothes.

♦ Mobility may necessitate the need for the stoma bag to be connected to extra drainage, i.e. a leg bag or night drainage bag if the person is unable to empty the pouch regularly. Chairbound patients may benefit from a drainage tap extension tube to allow easier emptying into toilets that they cannot get close to. The needs of paraplegic and tetraplegic patients may also differ. Body braces may have to be worn for spinal support and these interfere with wearing stoma appliances. Hemiplegic patients may prefer a one-piece appliance.

The client ultimately wants a product that is comfortable, manageable, secure and aesthetically pleasing. Because of the nature of the effluent and its continual flow, the reliability of the appliance is of utmost importance and a great deal of product development has gone on, especially into durable adhesives that can withstand the constant attack of urine.

Teaching the new urostomist

Urostomists cannot be discharged from hospital until they or their carers are practised at caring for the stoma. It is important to help create an individual teaching programme for each client.

♦ Tailor the learning experience to the patient's capabilities and needs.

♦ Do not push the patient to learn more than can be easily taken in, in one lesson.

♦ Some patients will find it very distasteful to touch their stomas with bare hands. They may feel more comfortable with gloves on.

♦ Sometimes it may take several appliance changes before the client will even look at the stoma.

♦ Cleaning the stoma. Mucus is formed in the ileum and this will always be present; it is not harmful or an indication that something is wrong. It should be washed away with water, a wet flannel or gauze. The adhesive residue should be cleaned away with water and gauze until the skin is clean. Cotton wool should not be used as it leaves a fibrous residue. All lanolin-based soaps and oil-based cleansers should be avoided as they prevent the flanges sticking to the skin. Perfumed cleansers may irritate the skin under the flange and are best avoided.

♦ If the skin does become sore from urine a barrier application specific to urostomy care may be used. Patch-test these prior to use in an inconspicuous area. Check also that the flange size is accurate. The stoma may shrink during the first month following surgery and the flange size will need frequent revision.

◆ The ureteric stents will be removed on or after day 10 following surgery.

◆ It will be much easier for the client to manage the stoma with the stents out.

◆ As with any new skill, the client gains confidence and dexterity with practice. It is helpful to write down a step-by-step plan to take them through an appliance change. This can be written on a small card which can be kept with the stoma products as an *aide-mémoire*.

◆ The teaching of partners and significant others is also an important stage in patient teaching. The patient will feel less isolated after discharge if their partner is familiar with the new procedure, and may be the major provider of care in times of sickness or disability.

◆ Prior to discharge it is important to explain the need and use of urostomy accessories. It is preferable to keep the amount of equipment required to a minimum. This reduces cost and makes the change quicker and simpler. Pastes, adhesives and protective lotions should only be used when indicated and not on a routine basis. They can be explained to the patient as and when they are needed.

◆ Night drainage bags allow the urine to be collected overnight without the need to disturb sleep for constant pouch emptying. The maximum urine capacity of a pouch is only about 400 ml.

◆ Pouch covers are available to keep the plastic pouch off the skin. There are now pouches which have a 'comfort backing' that feels like cloth.

◆ Belts may give the patient added security.

Guidelines for changing a urostomy appliance

The following equipment is needed:
new appliance of correct size and type
stomal measuring and cutting guide (template) if peristomal wafer/flange is not pre-cut
pen
clean gauze swabs, wipes or tissues
scissors
disposal bag
bowl of warm water
additional requirements such as skin barrier cream, protective film sachet and applicator, gel or spray
disposable gloves (latex) and disposable apron (if procedure is to be carried out by nursing staff)
jug
The procedure is set out in Table 11.2.

NURSING ACTION	RATIONALE
1. Give appropriate explanation to patient	To reduce anxiety and obtain patient's co-operation
2. Screen the bed, ensure patient is in a comfortable position and stoma is easily accessible	To ensure patient's privacy and comfort
3. Put on plastic disposable apron. Wash and dry hands	To reduce risk of cross-infection
4. Arrange equipment at patient's bedside	Stoma can act at any time
5. Prepare new stoma equipment. Prepare wafer/flange, if used, as follows:	
Remove flange from packaging. Follow arrows. Place template on the paper-covered side of the wafer and draw around the hole with pen	To transfer shape of stoma onto peristomal wafer/flange
Cut out marked hole in wafer. Keep template for subsequent changes	To ensure wafer fits snugly around stoma and protects skin
Smooth around roughened edges	To prevent laceration of stoma by wafer/flange
6. Preparing different drainage systems *Two-piece pouch and flange – alternative methods*	
(a) Attach pouch to flange ring (a click should be heard)	To avoid pressing pouch and flange together on patient's abdomen
Remove backing paper from flange and place this adhesive side upwards where it will be readily available for use	To prevent direct handling of adhesive surface and to ensure pouch is ready for immediate use when skin is dry
Ensure drainage tap is off	To prevent leakage of urine
(b) If floating flange is used, remove backing paper and place adhesive side upwards	Pouch can be applied to flange without direct pressure on abdomen. Can therefore be applied as a second stage
One-piece pouch The pouch is ready for use when backing paper is removed from adhesive area. Place ready for use adhesive side upwards	Rationale as for two-piece system
7. Place incontinence sheet or paper towel beneath patient	To protect patient's clothing and bedding

Table 11.2 Changing a urostomy appliance

8. Put on disposable gloves and give explanation to patient of why *staff* must wear gloves but unnecessary for patients to do the same	It may be psychologically damaging to the patient to feel that procedures are 'dirty'; therefore careful explanation of local policy on handling body fluids can overcome this
9. Disconnect night drainage system or empty stoma bag contents into jug and record drainage on intake and output chart	To make disposal of old appliance easier To maintain accurate intake and output chart
10. Peel the old appliance gently from the skin, working from highest point downwards	To reduce trauma to skin
Place index finger on skin	To reduce trauma and pulling
If ureteric splints in situ, leave old appliance close to patient so that splints may drain into this. If no ureteric splints in situ then remove appliance completely and place in disposal bag	To reduce likelihood of urine spillage and to maintain an accurate intake and output chart
11. Place clean gauze swab over stoma. Clean peristomal skin with warm water and swabs	To absorb leakage of urine from stoma
12. Check stoma size with template. Make a new template for next bag change if stoma has shrunk	New stoma may alter in size and shape, particularly during the first postoperative month
13. Observe stoma for colour, temperature, moistness, oedema, texture, prolapse, retraction, necrosis. Observe peristomal skin for erythema, excoriation	Report adverse changes to nurse in charge or stoma care nurse so that prompt remedial action can be taken
Observe splints for patency so that any change can be reported	To ensure free flow of urine
14. Dry skin with swab carefully	To prevent urine dripping onto skin, thereby promoting adherence of bag to clean dry skin
15. Barrier cream protective film gel or spray may be applied to peristomal skin at this time	To protect skin and provide additional adherence

Table 11.2 Continued

16. Guide ureteric splints into new pouch. Ensure stents enter lower section of pouch. Apply this centrally over stoma and smooth wafer/flange down onto skin	**To prevent urine pooling over stomal area**
17. Apply belt, if worn. This should be attached to the pouch and be positioned level with the stoma	**To avoid upward drag on appliance and subsequent damage to stoma. To increase patient's feeling of security**
18. Apply cotton pouch cover if worn	**To prevent plastic of appliance causing discomfort due to sweating and increase patient's feeling of safety and comfort**
19. Measure urine in used stoma pouch (if used to collect urine drainage from ureteric splints). Record on intake and output chart	**To maintain accurate input and output chart**
20. Dispose of all items in yellow disposal bag	**To ensure clinical waste is incinerated**
21. Wash and dry hands	**To reduce risk of cross-infection and comply with local policy**
22. Record observations and care on nursing computer information system	**To comply with local regulations and maintain continuity of care**

Table 11.2 *Continued*

Guidelines for obtaining a urine specimen

It may be necessary to collect a catheter specimen of urine from a patient with an ileal conduit for microscopy and culture
  The following equipment is needed:
  sterile dressing pack containing gloves and gauze
  sterile, disposable single-use catheter, 8–14 FG
  sterile specimen pot
  disposable plastic apron
  skin cleansing lotion (water or normal saline)
  clean stoma appliance
  disposal bag
  sterile gauze swabs
  incontinence pad, paper towel
The procedure is set out in Table 11.3.

NURSING ACTION	RATIONALE
1. Explain procedure to the patient and ask patient to drain urostomy appliance and record output if indicated	To gain patient's consent and co-operation. To maintain an accurate fluid balance chart
2. Ensure that the patient is in a comfortable position, e.g. sitting up, supported by pillows, and that the stoma is easily accessible	To maintain patient's comfort
3. Screen the bed	To ensure patient's privacy
4. Put on disposable plastic apron	To comply with local infection control policy
5. Wash and dry hands	To prevent cross-infection
6. Prepare new stoma equipment	So that equipment is ready for use immediately. To minimize urine spillage by reducing the time when there is no appliance over the stoma
7. Position an incontinence pad/paper towel under patient	To protect patient's clothing and bed linen
8. Prepare the sterile dressing pack in accordance with local aseptic technique policy	To reduce risk of contaminating sterile area
9. Remove the appliance from stoma, place in disposal bag. Cover stoma with sterile guaze swabs	To absorb spillage from the stoma
10. Wash and dry hands. Open sterile field. Put on sterile gloves	To reduce the risk of contaminating sterile field during the procedure
11. Clean around the stoma with skin cleansing lotion (e.g. saline) and gauze swabs from the centre outwards. Dry the area	Good cleansing of the skin reduces the risk of introducing infection into the stoma during the procedure
12. Insert the catheter tip gently into the stoma to a depth of 2.5–5 cm only; wait for urine to drain through. Collect 2–5 ml in sterile container	Gentle handling reduces the risk of trauma to the mucosa. Sterile container to prevent contamination of urine and to supply adequate volume of urine for microbiology department

Table 11.3 Collecting a catheter specimen of urine

13.	Remove the catheter and seal the specimen container	To prevent contamination of specimen
14.	Check peristomal skin is clean and dry – wash and dry again if necessary	To clean and dry skin and promote adherence of appliance
15.	Apply new stoma bag in accordance with local protocol	To ensure collection of urine and maintain patient comfort
16.	Remove gloves. Dispose of equipment in soiled dressings bag	To ensure that rubbish is incinerated and comply with local infection control policy
17.	Wash and dry hands	To comply with local infection control policy
18.	Check that the specimen is labelled correctly and send to laboratory with the appropriate request form as soon as possible	To ensure correct specimen is processed promptly

Table 11.3 Continued

COMPLICATIONS

Peristomal hernia

A peristomal hernia may occur months or years after the original surgery. The appearance is usually of a bulge around the stomal area. The patient may be asymptomatic but if the segment of loop becomes strangulated in any way severe pain and cessation of urinary output may require emergency surgery.
Possible causes include:

◆ initial placement of stoma outside the rectus muscle
◆ multiple surgical procedures
◆ loss of muscle tone – weight increase, ageing process

Nursing care

Encourage a gentle return to exercise after surgery, and advise the patient against excessive weight gain. The patient should be referred for support belts and corsets, and given advice on appropriate appliance change to accommodate raised areas.

Prolapse

Prolapse may be caused by:

- inadequate fixation of the stoma to the abdominal wall
- increased abdominal pressure

In severe cases the only option may be surgery.

Conservative treatment includes reducing stoma with cold compresses, iced water and gentle pressure to the distal portion of the stoma. Appliances may need to be changed to a larger size. Two-piece pouches are generally more convenient.

Patients with a prolapsed stoma require a great deal of psychological support. The stoma is often regarded as unsightly and difficult to manage.

Retraction

Possible causes of retraction of the stoma include:

- insufficient mobilization of the mesentery
- tension on the suture line at the fascial layer
- weight gain

Nursing care

Retraction can cause numerous management problems including flush stomas and concaved 'dipped' areas. Development of products with built-in convexity, detachable inserts, belts and malleable seals and pastes have helped the situation greatly, but occasionally the only resolution to the problem is surgical revision to mobilize the stoma and release tension.

Stenosis

Stomal stenosis and strictures have been found in up to 25% of patients with ileal conduit. A variety of causes have been identified, including:

- severe infection – both acute and chronic
- scar tissue – trauma, infection
- inappropriate technique when stoma is fashioned (Corman, 1989)
- inflammation and fibrosis of mucosa due to constant contact with alkaline urine (Jeter and Lattimer, 1974)
- prior irradiation of the bowel segment (Johnson and Smith, 1986)

Symptoms

Symptoms are often slow in presentation. The patient gives a history of:

◆ constant or recurring urinary tract infection
◆ visible shrinkage of stoma
◆ appliance changes becoming more difficult because of urine shooting from stoma in a projectile fashion
◆ urine output reduced and not congruent with intake
◆ eventually flank pain

Diagnosis

Diagnosis is based on the following investigations:

◆ digital examination
◆ high residual volumes of urine from ileal loop on catheterization
◆ intravenous urogram
◆ 'loopogram'
◆ ultrasound scan

Nursing care

In the early stages patients should be advised to increase their oral intake of fluids. Treatments include:

◆ acidification of urine (see below)
◆ long-term catheterization (eventual scarring may result and occasionally trauma)
◆ dilation of the stoma (may only be of short-term benefit)
◆ surgical removal of area of stenosis
◆ stomal reconstruction if an extensive area is involved

Urinary pH

Both dip-stick (Multistix) and litmus paper tests should be carried out on freshly produced urine. Urine that has been left to stand is usually alkaline; this is caused by bacterial breakdown, resulting in ammonia formation.

The ideal range of urinary pH is 6–7.5. Many postoperative complications concerning the stoma and peristomal skin are associated with alkaline urine, i.e. a urinary pH of 7–8. Alkaline urine has been known to cause stomal bleeding, ulceration, urinary tract infection, strong odour and urinary calculi. Stoma stenosis and pseudoepithelial hyperplasia and hyperkeratosis may eventually occur (Walsh, 1992). Various bacterial and fungal organisms find the alkalinity of surrounding skin (skin pH is normally 5) and urine a perfect medium for growth. Oxalate crystals which form mainly from alkaline urine can cause both irritation to the stoma and mucosal bleeding. Untreated these may lead to ulceration (Abrams, 1984).

There are various methods for restoring acidity to urine and surrounding skin.

Vinegar

Equal parts of white distilled vinegar and warm water are applied to the stomal area. This can be achieved using a small appliance with no antireflux valve. The vinegar solution is added to the pouch and allowed to wash over the stomal area for at least 30 minutes. Alternatively, the solution can be put into a small container and the area douched a number of times.

Ascorbic acid

Research has shown not only that high doses of ascorbic acid are necessary to produce acidification of urine (Young, 1984) but also that the amount should be given in regularly divided doses to ensure maximum urine levels. Studies argue that the recommended dosage should be anywhere between 4 g and 12 g daily. In the authors' experience general practitioners are reluctant to prescribe doses higher than 4–6 g daily due to potential toxic effects, which can include:

◆ nausea
◆ vomiting
◆ heartburn
◆ diarrhoea
◆ crystalluria

(Young, 1984)

Ascorbic acid may also affect other medications; it reduces the effects of amphetamines, tricyclic antidepressants, drugs used in alcohol dependence (e.g. disulfiram) and antipsychotics (e.g. prochlorperazine). In combination with digoxin it may cause arrhythmias; and it increases the effects of sulpho-namides to produce crystalluria.

Acetic acid preparations

Application of Aci-Jel – acetic acid 0.92% in a buffered base jelly (pH 4) – topically to stomal mucosa is more effective if done regularly (at least twice daily), and is therefore most useful if the patient uses a two-piece appliance.

Ash diet

The Ash diet is a now rarely used method of attempting to produce acid urine. It may be contraindicated for patients who are overweight, or who have cardiac or circulatory problems. Included in the diet are an increased intake of:

meat protein and fats
cheese
butter
and a decreased intake of:
green vegetables
citrus fruits

Many patients find it difficult to accept the fact that citrus fruits although a rich source of vitamin C, may result in alkaline urine; but the effect on urinary pH after ingestion has been well researched (Abrams, 1984; Fischbach, 1988; Walsh, 1992).

Cranberry juice

The cranberry, in both juice and capsule format, has become widely used in urology for the control of:

◆   urinary tract infection (Soloway and Smith, 1988)
◆   mucus formation (Rosenbaum *et al.*, 1989)
◆   formation of urinary stones (Woodhouse, 1994)

A native North American wetland fruit, cranberry (unlike most citrus fruits) does actually acidify the urine (Walsh, 1992). Early studies (Fellers et al, 1933) identified the production of hippuric acid which had a bacteriostatic effect on the urinary pH (i.e. pH 5.5), although the concentrations required to achieve this was argued. Later studies advocated the use of cranberry juice in combination with oral medication, e.g. ascorbic acid and methenamine hippurate (Papas *et al.*, 1966).

Escherichia coli is a natural inhabitant of the gut and is therefore present in small amounts in the stomal urine. If large amounts of mucus are produced in the urostomy loop and remain static, *E. coli* has an ideal medium in which to colonize and the patient may become symptomatic with fever, malaise and offensive urine. Under these circumstances the patient would be given antibiotics. The effect of hippuric acid is to reduce mucus formation, thus inhibiting the adherence of *E. coli* (Busuttil-Leaver, 1996).

Propolis

Stoma care nurses are frequently given recommendations by patients about herbal and alternative therapies that they have found to be beneficial. Propolis is such a substance. Ghisalberti (1979), in the Department of Organic Chemistry at the University of Western Australia, reviewed various studies carried out on the chemistry and pharmacology of bee propolis. Propolis is a resinous substance collected by bees from various plant sources, particularly the black poplar tree; it is used in a thin layer as a natural defence lining for hives. Chemical analysis has shown numerous properties (Grange and Davey, 1990) but has failed to identify any one of particular benefit. Propolis has proved to be effective in:

- ◆ inhibiting the growth of gram-positive rods
- ◆ inhibiting the growth of *Staphylococcus aureus*
- ◆ mouth ulcers
- ◆ streptococcal throat
- ◆ bladder antiseptis

Available in capsule form, it is a chewable substance with a slightly antiseptic taste and has a mild anaesthetic effect. The minimum effective dose required is stated to be 1.5 g (Grange and Davey, 1990).

PREGNANCY AND THE UROSTOMIST

Urostomies are formed in people of all ages. They are becoming the less common choice in the young owing to continued improvements in continent pouch surgery, eliminating the need for an external appliance to be worn. However, for some people this surgery may be too complicated and a urostomy may be the chosen option.

It is always the aim of surgery to return the patient to a full and active life, with participation in the activities normally associated with their peer group. In younger women this will include the chance to become a mother. However possible pregnancy may be, it is not without its problems. While the subject of pregnancy has been well reviewed in various studies, no single urologist or obstetrician has amassed a large personal experience of the problems that arise after stomal surgery.

Conception may be difficult for various reasons. Major abdominal surgery requires a period of recovery before a pregnancy is considered. Sexual intercourse may be difficult or painful as a previous cystectomy may have reduced or heightened sensation in the vaginal vault. The absent bladder may also allow the uterus to fall forward, which may lead to difficulty in conceiving.

Diagnosis of pregnancy may be difficult because of the nature of the test. Urine samples taken from the ileal loop will have been subject to reabsorption of electrolytes and hormones in the ileal canal, therefore the concentration of human chorionic gonadotrophin may be altered. This can lead to false positive or negative results when carrying out conventional pregnancy testing. Blood samples need to be taken for accurate diagnosis. This may also be the case for testing of diabetic urine.

Once diagnosis is confirmed, subsequent developmental testing may also prove difficult. The absence of a functioning bladder makes ultrasound scanning more difficult. Later on in development the baby's head may well be lying directly behind the conduit, so it can be difficult to measure parietal diameters that determine the baby's growth and development. Ultrasound scanning jelly also contains liberal quantities of alcohol, which will erode stoma appliances and quickly cause leakages. It is therefore advisable to change the complete appliance after scanning to ensure no mishaps occur.

Urostomists experience all the expected difficulties with their stoma during pregnancy. As the abdomen swells the stoma can no longer be seen. Difficulty in changing appliances is experienced. Careful positioning with pillows may be needed in order to sleep, prevent damage to the stoma and to enable drainage into a night bag.

Infection in the urostomate is potentially very serious during pregnancy. Any urinary tract infection must be treated as serious. Pyelonephritis may induce premature labour and can potentially lead to renal failure. If possible the status of renal function should be known prior to conception. During pregnancy the expanding uterus may constrict the ureters which are abnormally situated across the vertebrae to reach the conduit. This can cause the uterus to go into sympathetic contractions. If renal function becomes compromised nephrostomy tubes will need to be inserted to ensure renal failure does not develop.

Other problems include stomal bleeding, which may increase as the urostomy becomes more vascular. Urinary tract infection and hormonal changes may increase leakage problems. Renal calculi may develop if the flow from the kidney is restricted or impaired. Urostomists are advised to drink 2.5 litres daily to increase urine output, reduce urine stasis and potential urinary tract infections.

Erectile dysfunction

Radical pelvic surgery, cystourethrectomy and formation of stoma will invariably lead to erectile dysfunction (Jones et al, 1980). The effect of the ability to achieve erection on the patient's overall psychological wellbeing has been well documented (Sidi et al, 1990). Zolar (1982) proposed that the nurse is an ideal member of the health team to counsel patients in an area as sensitive and highly charged as human sexuality. Nurses must ensure that they have the necessary knowledge, skills and expertise to fulfil this role (Topping, 1990). See Chapter 12 for management of erectile dysfunction.

Urine colour and odour changes

Having an abdominal collecting device for urine increases the patient's awareness of both colour and odour changes. It is important to warn patients that certain medication and food products may change the appearance and smell of urine (Table 11.4).

CONCLUSION

Evidence produced by Jeffries et al. (1995) showed that when patients are assured of knowledgeable management they will feel supported. It is rare for a urostomy to be created as an emergency as it is generally undertaken as an elective procedure, therefore early referral to the stoma care department in either the hospital or the community is usually possible. Although this chapter has been restricted to urology, it has been necessary to include some general aspects of stoma care. Patients with urological stomas consistently present with specific, complicated needs and problems. Therefore the nurse working in specialist areas must have, in addition to expert knowledge, an ability to encompass other issues such as advocacy, counselling and education (Allison, 1996).

MEDICATION OR FOOD	COLOUR OR ODOUR
Amitriptyline	Blue-green
Anthraquinones	Red-brown (in alkaline urine)
Chloroquine	Rusty brown, yellow
Danthron	Orange
Ferrous salts	Black
Ibuprofen	Red
Indomethacin	Green
Levodopa	Darkens
Methyldopa	Darkens (red-black on standing)
Metronidazole	Red to brown
Nitrofurantoin	Brown or rust yellow
Phenolphthalein	Pink (alkaline)
Phenothiazines	Pink to red-brown
Rifampicin	Red to brown
Senna	Yellow-brown (acid urine; yellow-pink (alkaline urine); darkens on standing
Sulphonamides	Greenish blue
Triamterene	Blue
Warfarin	Orange
Certain antibiotics	Offensive smell
Alcohol	Lightens colour
Beetroot	Pink to dark red
Red fruit drinks	Pink to dark red
Oily fish	Fishy
Total parenteral nutrition	Offensive
Certain food smells appear to pass through into the urine, e.g. onions, garlic, some spices	

Note: Data from Watson (1987).

Table 11.4 *Effects of drugs or foods on the urine*

THE UROSTOMY ASSOCIATION

The Urostomy Association is a self-help organization in the UK which can provide support and advice for its members.
Urostomy Association
Central Office
Buckland
Beaumont Park
Danbury
Essex CM3 4DE

REFERENCES

ABRAMS J S (1984) *Abdominal Stomas: Indications, Operative Techniques and Patient Care*. Boston: John Wright.

ALLISON M (1996) Discharge planning for the person with a stoma. In Myers C (ed.), *Stoma Care Nursing: A Patient-centred Approach*, pp. 267–82. London: Arnold Publishing.

BRICKER E M (1950) Bladder substitution after pelvic evisceration. *Surgical Clinics of North America* **30**: 1151.

BROADWELL D and Jackson B (1982) *Principles of Ostomy Care*. St. Louis: Mosby.

BROOKE B N (1952) The management of an ileostomy including its complications. *Lancet* **ii**: 102–104.

BUSUTTIL-LEAVER R (1996) Cranberry juice. *Professional Nurse* **11**: 525–526.

CLARKE P B (1979) End to end uretero-ileal anastomosis for ileal conduits. *British Journal of Urology* **51**: 105–109.

CORMAN M L (1989) Colon and rectal surgery, 2nd edn. Philadelphia: Lippincott.

DEVLIN B and Plant J A (1979) Sexual function – an aspect of stoma care. *British Journal of Sexual Medicine* **6**: 33–37.

ELCOAT C (1986) *Stoma Care Nursing*. Eastbourne: Baillière Tindall.

FELLERS C R, Redmon B C and Parrott E M (1933) Effect of cranberries on urinary acidity and blood alkali reserve. *Journal of Nutrition* **6**: 455–463.

FISCHBACH F T (1988) *A Manual of Laboratory Diagnostic Tests*, 3rd edn. Philadelphia: Lippincott.

GHISALBERTI E L (1979) Propolis: a review. Department of Organic Chemistry. University of Western Australia. *Bee World* **60**(2): 59–84.

GRANGE J M and Davey R W (1990) Antibacterial properties of propolis (bee glue). *Journal of the Royal Society of Medicine* **83**: 159–160.

HAMPTON B and Bryant R (1992) *Ostomies and Continent Diversions. Nursing Management*. St Louis: Mosby Yearbook.

JEFFRIES E, Butler M, Cullum R et al (1995) A service evaluation of stoma care nurses practice. *Journal of Clinical Nursing* **4**(4): 235–242.

JETER K F and Lattimer J K (1974) Common stoma problems following ileal conduit urinary diversion. *Urology* **3**: 399–403.

JOHNSON D G and Smith D B (1986) Urinary diversions. In: *Ostomy Care and the Cancer Patient*. Orlando: Grune & Stratton.

JONES M A, Breckman B and Hendry W (1980) Life with an ileal conduit. Result of questionnaire surveys of patients and urological surgeons. *British Journal of Urology* **52**: 21–25.

PAPAS N P, Brusch C A and Ceresia G C (1966) Cranberry juice in the treatment of urinary tract infections. *Southwestern Medicine* **47**(1): 17–20.

RCN (1992) *Standard of Care. Stoma Care Nursing*. Harrow: Royal College of Nursing Scutari.

ROSENBAUM T P, Shah P J R, Rose G A and Lloyd-Davis R W (1989) Cranberry juice and the mucus production in entero-uroplasties. *Neurourology and Urodynamics* **8**(4): 55; 344–345.

SIDI A, Becher E F, Zhang G and Lewis J H (1990) Patient acceptance of and satisfaction with an external negative pressure device for impotence. *Journal of Urology* **144**: 1154–1156.

SOLOWAY M and Smith R (1988) Does cranberry juice help in urinary infections? *Journal of the American Medical Association* **260**: 1465.

SUSSER J (1993) *Stoma Surgery and the Orthodox Jewish Patient*. ENB 980, unpublished paper.

TOPPING A (1990) Sexual Activity and the Stoma Patient. *Nursing Standard* **4**(41), 4 July, pp. 24–26.

TURNBULL R B and Weakley F L (1967) *Atlas of Intestinal Stomas*. St. Louis: Mosby.

WALLACE D M (1970) Uretero-ileostomy. *British Journal of Urology* **42**: 529–534.

WALSH B A (1992) Urostomy and urinary pH. *Journal of Enterostomal Nursing* **19**; 119–123.

WATSON D (1987) Drug therapy – colour changes to faeces and urine. *Pharmaceutical Journal* **236**: 68.

WOODHOUSE C R J (1994) The infective, metabolic and histological consequences of enterocystoplasty. *European Urology Update Series* **3**(2): 10–15.

YOUNG C (1984) Ascorbic acid. *Journal of Enterostomal Nursing* **11**: 157–158.

ZOLAR M K (1982) Role preparation for nurses. In: *Human Sexual Functioning. Nursing Clinics of North America* **17**(3): 351–363.

12 PENILE DISORDERS

The general anatomy and physiology of the penis are described in Chapter 1. This chapter describes pathological conditions of the penis and their nursing care. These conditions include:

- ◆ phimosis
- ◆ paraphimosis
- ◆ circumcision
- ◆ balanitis
- ◆ cancer of the penis
- ◆ priapism
- ◆ Peyronie's disease
- ◆ venous leaks

The erectile process is described, together with the causes, investigation and management of erectile dysfunction.

Certain congenital conditions of the penis such as chordee, hypospadias and epispadias are described in Chapter 15.

THE MALE PELVIS

Blood supply

The blood supply to the male perineum is shown in Figure 12.1.

Arterial

The right and left internal pudendal arteries divide into superficial and deep arteries of the penis which arise from the internal iliac artery. The deep artery supplies separate branches to the spongiosum, urethra and corpora cavernosa. Arterioles connect the spongiosum and dorsal vessels.

Venous

The veins form two main channels – superficial and deep. The superficial dorsal vein passes beneath the skin to the pubis and there divides into branches which empty into the saphenous system or directly into the femoral veins. The deep dorsal vein follows a similar course but additionally drains via the prostatic plexus. The network of dorsal veins drains the peripheral blood from the penis during detumescence.

Lymphatic drainage

The skin of the penis is drained into the medial group of superficial inguinal nodes. The deep structures of the penis are drained into the internal iliac nodes.

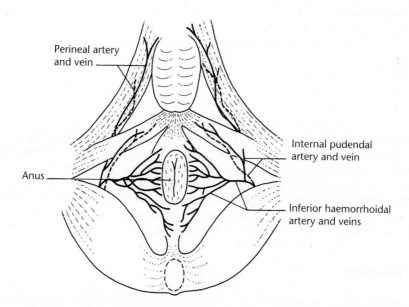

Figure 12.1 *Blood supply of male perineum*

Nerve supply

The penis is supplied by autonomic and somatic (voluntary) nerves:

- internal pudendal nerve – cerebrospinal system
- hypogastric plexus to the erectile tissue – autonomic system

The sensory nerve supply to the penis is via the pudendal nerve. The erectile mechanism is controlled by the nervi-erigentes, the nerves of erection originating from the pelvic plexus which is situated on the pelvic side wall. The word pudendal originates from the Latin *pudeo* (I am ashamed). In polite society the genitalia were once called the pudenda.

The pudendal nerve arises from S2 to S4 of the sacral region of the spinal cord, supplying the musculature of the levator ani, pubococcygeus and the muscles of the penis, the ischiocavernosus and the bulbospongiosus. The nerves supplying the blood vessels to the genitalia and involved in the neural control of vasocongestion derive from the sympathetic and parasympathetic systems.

PENILE CONDITIONS AND THEIR TREATMENT

Phimosis

Phimosis is the inability to retract foreskin back over the glans. This can result in a 'pinhole' meatus, thus impeding flow of urine, and can cause urinary retention, meatal infection and symptoms of lower urinary tract obstruction.

Treatment

If symptoms do not subside within 6–8 weeks, an elective circumcision may be performed.

Paraphimosis

Paraphimosis is the swelling of a retracted foreskin and the inability to pull the foreskin forwards over the glans penis (Figure 12.2). This condition may arise after sexual intercourse, masturbation or surgical instrumentation of the penis, e.g. cystoscopy or transurethral resection of the prostate. It is therefore important to check that the patient's foreskin has been pulled forward following instrumentation. If unresolved the compression of the glans may become so severe that gangrene of the glans may ensue.

Treatment

Paraphimosis can be treated conservatively in the early stages. Application of an anaesthetic gel, e.g. lignocaine, and gentle, firm compression may be

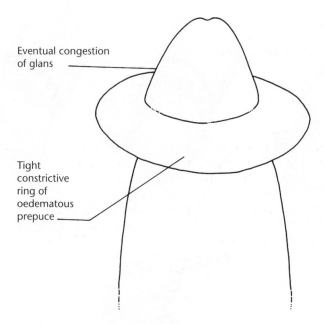

Eventual congestion
of glans

Tight
constrictive
ring of
oedematous
prepuce

Figure 12.2 *Paraphimosis*

sufficient to reduce the oedema and restore the foreskin over the glans. If this is unsuccessful it may be necessary for the patient to undergo emergency circumcision. For individuals who have had paraphimosis initially treated successfully without surgery, an elective circumcision should be performed within 6–8 weeks (Bullock *et al.*, 1994).

Circumcision

Circumcision is the surgical removal of the foreskin and is indicated as treatment for balanitis, phimosis and paraphimosis. This procedure is also commonly performed within certain religious communities (Fuller and Toon, 1988). The incidence of carcinoma of the penis is rare in Jewish men and in other religious groups where they practise circumcision at birth (Bullock *et al.*, 1994).

Procedure

A dorsal slit is performed and the foreskin excised to the base of the glans. The individual bleeding vessels are ligated and interrupted catgut sutures circumscribe the base of the glans (Figure 12.3).

Nursing care

The complications of circumcision and their nursing care are listed in Table 12.1.

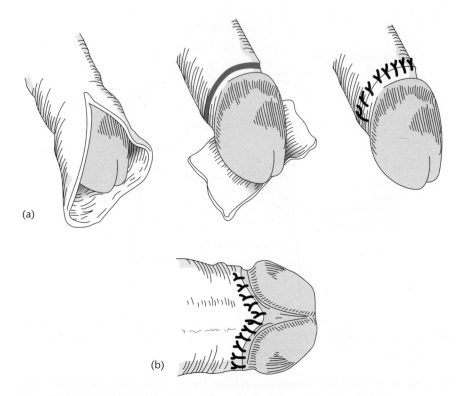

Figure 12.3 *Circumcision: (a) dorsal view; (b) ventral view*

PROBLEM	ACTION
Bleeding – close proximity of dorsal vein and frenular arteries	**Regular observation**
	Light paraffin dressing
	Inform medical staff immediately of any excessive bleeding and possible return to theatre as an emergency
Pain – particularly postoperatively if patient has erections	**Regular analgesia**
	Surgeons may prescribe diazepam to reduce erections
	Applications of anaesthetic gel
Oedema	**Supportive pants and pad with penis in upright position**

Table 12.1 *Complications of circumcision and specific nursing care*

Balanitis

Inflammation of the foreskin and penis is often a result of poor hygiene. A resulting infection can produce itching and burning. The foreskin and glans penis can be exposed to a number of potential infections (Figure 12.4). In the

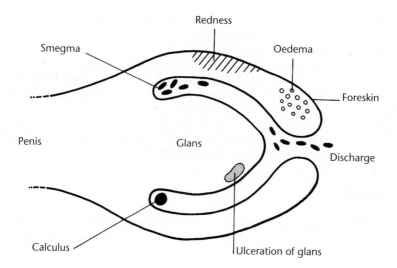

Figure 12.4 *Sources of infection*

presence of any additional problems of maintaining hygiene, e.g. phimosis, the underlying infection may produce oedema, exudate, erythema and scarring. Sources of infection include:

- poor hygiene
- urethral discharge of bacterial origin
- certain skin diseases, e.g. psoriasis, lichen planus, leucoplakia
- vulvovaginitis – cross-infection from an infected partner
- underlying illness, e.g. diabetes, resulting in secondary infection

Treatment

The main aim of any treatment will be to eradicate any infection and to maintain hygiene. Local washing and careful drying are extremely important. The use of systemic antibiotics may be necessary, accompanied by the use of localized antibiotic cream or lotion. Circumcision may be considered if there is no improvement owing to tightness of the foreskin.

Priapism

Priapism is painful, persistent penile erection. This is accompanied by venous congestion of the penile cavernous structures. While the corpora cavernosa become rigid, the corpus spongiosum and the glans penis usually remain flaccid. The prolonged erection is not accompanied by sexual desire or excitement. Possible causes include:

- Venous thrombosis in the vessels that drain the penis in certain blood disorders, e.g. sickle cell, anaemia, leukaemia

- Obstructive tumours around the base of the penis, bladder, prostate or rectum
- Spinal cord injuries
- Idiopathic – often no definite cause can be found, but there may be a history of prolonged vigorous sexual intercourse
- Drugs (often in overdose) – anticoagulants, phenothiazine, marijuana, antihistamines
- Intracorporal injection of drugs used to produce erection when injected into the base of penis; erections should subside naturally but occasionally do not

Treatment

This condition should be recognized as a urological emergency. Initially the erection may be resolved by sedation, e.g. with diazepam. Other methods used include:

- Intravenous procyclidine hydrochloride (Kemadrin). The patient may complain of a dry mouth, dizziness and blurred vision after administration and should be reassured that this will resolve.
- Aspiration of the corpora with a butterfly needle and syringe and flushing with heparinized saline. This may thin and relieve the pressure of the thick, viscous blood.
- Metaraminol (Aramine) or phenylephrine hydrochloride – drugs used in the treatment of acute hypotension – can be injected intracorporally into the penis.

If medical management is unsuccessful, or the patient only receives temporary relief, it will be necessary for the surgeon to bypass the blocked channel by means of a shunt. This can be created by one of three routes:

- glans – cavernosus
- spongiosus – cavernosus
- corporosaphenous

By providing this escape route for the blood, the erection will then subside. The effect of performing shunts is often a damaged erectile system and permanent impotence.

Specific nursing care is described in Table 12.2.

Peyronie's disease

Peyronie's disease is characterized by the formation of plaques of fibrous tissue (Figure 12.5) in the sheath of the corpora cavernosa, which are adherent to the overlying Buck's fascia (Blandy, 1991). These plaques prevent the penis from distending fully on erection, producing varying degrees of curvature. Although the aetiology is unknown, the tissue is similar in its histological appearance to that found in Dupuytren's contracture and retroperitoneal fibrosis. This is a benign condition.

PROBLEM	ACTION
Potential sudden severe hypertension	Frequent monitoring of the patient's blood pressure for the first hour is essential
Psychological effects of: embarrassment, worry about impotence	Provide privacy. Keep patient informed before each treatment is commenced
Pain and discomfort	Provide reassurance. Analgesia as required. Studies have shown that giving information reduces anxiety and pain (Hayward, 1975)
Potential bruising and bleeding around injected site	Provide scrotal support/pants and a soft sterile pad. The penis should be supported upwards to prevent further oedema

Table 12.2 Specific nursing care for priapism

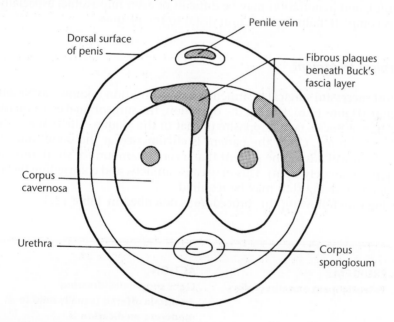

Figure 12.5 Peyronie's disease: position of plaque

Clinical examination

Diagnosis is generally confirmed by injection of an intracorporal vasodilator into the corpus cavernosum which will produce an erection. The degree of curvature can then be assessed. During erection the area of fibrous tissue fails to distend. Varying degrees of bend are produced according to the site and overall area of scarring which can be confirmed using cavernosography. On

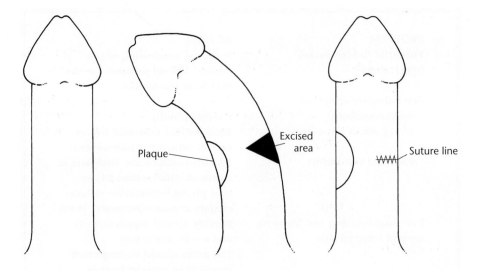

Figure 12.6   *Peyronie's disease: Nesbitt's procedure*

questioning the patient may report that there is a tendency for his erection to be painful, and penetration may be difficult or even impossible, especially if there is complete failure of erection distal to the plaques.

Surgical treatment

The most successful surgical treatment for this condition is known as Nesbitt's procedure (Figure 12.6). During the operation, the surgeon makes an incision in the area of Buck's fascia opposite to that of the plaque. The tissue is then reefed and sutured. Often the patient is circumcised at the same time. The medical staff will advise the patient that a certain amount of shortening will occur (approximately 1 cm). This may cause anxiety, and counselling by both medical and nursing staff may be required.

Nursing care following this procedure is described in Table 12.3.

PROBLEM	ACTION
Potential pain and discomfort	Light supportive dressing Analgesia offered (usually mild to moderate medication is sufficient)
Potential haemorrhage	Frequent checking of sutured areas Inform medical staff promptly as patient may require further suturing if bleeding is excessive

Table 12.3   *Nursing care following correction of Peyronie's disease*

Venous leaks

In the event of a venous leak there will be failure of the erectile bodies to fill with blood and therefore inability to form an erection. Causes may be:

◆   Congenital: the patient may always have been unable to achieve erection caused by congenital leakage within the venous system of the spongiosus or glans. Abnormal veins may also be present.
◆   Acquired:
     after surgery, e.g priapism or urethral surgery
     atheroma
     after fracture of the pelvis

Diagnosis

A detailed history will establish the onset of erectile dysfunction. An intra-cavernosal injection of a vasoactive drug will produce an erection providing the blood supply is not obstructed or leakage present. Impairment of the arterial blood supply may be shown by Doppler studies of the penile blood flow. The site and extent of the leakage can be more specifically identified under X-ray conditions using pelvic angiography or a cavernosogram

The position of the major blood vessels is shown in Figure 12.7.

Venous leak repair

The operation will vary in severity depending on the site and extent of the leak. The aim of the surgery is to restore penile vascularization. This is neither

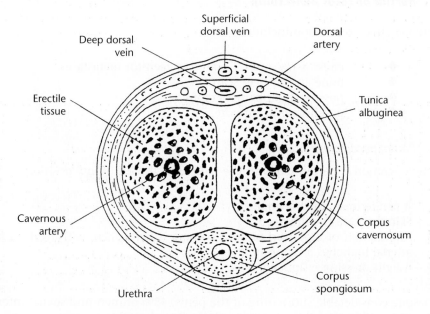

Figure 12.7   *Major veins and arteries of the penis*

PROBLEM	ACTION
Embarrassment and anxiety about success of operation	**Obtain information from surgeon for patient as to nature of operation and success rate. This is essential, as the operation may be fairly minor, or the patient may return to the ward with intravenous infusion, wound drains and large wound incision**
	Reduce embarrassment by providing privacy for patient as far as possible

Table 12.4   Specific nursing care for venous leak repair

an easy nor always a successful task. The surgeon's aim is to either reroute blood flow or ligate veins to improve venous leaks.

Nursing care is described in Table 12.4.

Carcinoma of the penis

For incidence, tumour spread and alternative treatments please see Chapter 10. Tumours of the penis that are poorly responsive to radiotherapy or are very advanced at time of presentation may require surgery.

Partial or total penectomy

Preoperative preparation includes:

◆   chest X-ray and CT scan to screen for metastases
◆   bone and/or liver scan
◆   possible lymphangiography
◆   psychological support

Partial penectomy

The operation is performed with the patient in the lithotomy position.

1. A penile tourniquet is applied.
2. Skin flaps are then marked.
3. Amputation of a portion of both corpora is performed, with ligation of arterial branches as appropriate.
4. A light dressing is applied.

Despite considerable shortening of the penis, 45% of men find sexual intercourse possible after this procedure (Bullock *et al.*, 1994).

Total penectomy

The patient is placed in the lithotomy position.

1. A circular incision is made around the penis and extending into the perineum.
2. The roots of both corpora are exposed and excised.
3. The penis is amputated and the blood vessels ligated.
4. A perineal urethrostomy is fashioned by anastomosing the bulbar urethra to the skin of the perineum.
5. An indwelling catheter is then passed and wound drainage inserted.
6. After closure of the incision a perineal dressing is applied firmly to help reduce postoperative oedema.

Nursing care

Nursing procedures after partial or total penectomy are described in Table 12.5.

ERECTION AND EJACULATION

The penis consists of three cylindrical bodies of erectile tissue. These are the two corpora cavernosa and the corpus spongiosum. The corpora cavernosa consist of a network of fibrous tissue which becomes filled with blood during erection of the penis. The two corpora cavernosa lie next to each other and have a deep central artery – a branch of the internal pudendal artery. The corpora separate posteriorly to form the two crura which are attached to the ischiopubic rami of the pelvis. The crura are covered by the ischiocavernous muscle, which provides the penis with a secure attachment to the pelvis. The corpus spongiosum is expanded to form the glans penis anteriorly and the

PROBLEM	ACTION
Potential excessive blood loss due to arterial involvement	Frequent observation of wound pad and drains
	Regular monitoring of pulse and blood pressure
Risk of oedema	Maintain supportive dressing for first 24 hours with mild compression
Risk of infection	Observe wound exudate
	Monitor temperature and pulse
Pain	Administer regular analgesia
Inability to pass urine	Indwelling catheter for first 48 hours
Profound change in body image and sexual function	Referral to psychosexual or cancer counsellor

Table 12.5 Postoperative care for partial or total penectomy

bulb of the penis posteriorly. The bulb is covered by the bulbospongiosus muscle which has many fibres closely associated with the corpus spongiosum which surrounds the urethra. The muscle has an important role in propelling semen along the urethra during ejaculation. The bulbospongiosus reflex is elicited by stimulation of the glans penis and this results in reflex contraction of the bulbospongiosus muscle. The reflex requires the integrity of the sensory and motor branches of the pudendal nerves and of the segments S2 to S4 of the spinal cord.

Sexual response cycle

Erection in the male is gradually built up as a consequence of various sexual stimuli. Four phases have been identified which rather than being distinct tend to overlap each other.

The excitement phase is initiated by whatever the individual finds sexually stimulating, thus resulting in the bombardment of the central nervous system by afferent stimuli (Figure 12.8). Efferent nervous impulses pass down the spinal cord to the parasympathetic outflow in the second, third and

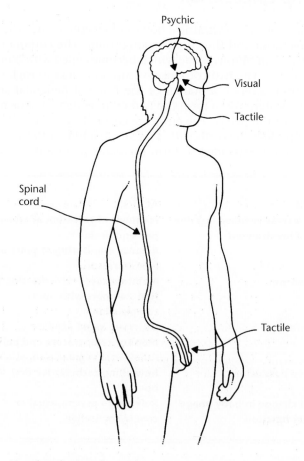

Figure 12.8 *Neural mechanisms for erection*

fourth sacral segments. If the stimuli are interrupted for any reason the cycle may stop here or become extended.

If stimulation continues sexual tension increases, entering the plateau phase. During this phase the efferent nerve impulses pass into the tissue at the root of the penis. Vasodilation of the arteries now occurs producing a great increase in the blood flow through the blood spaces of the erectile tissue.

The third phase – the climatic or orgasmic phase – involves a completely involuntary response. The corpora cavernosa and corpus spongiosum become engorged with blood and expand while compressing the vessels of venous drainage against the surrounding tissue, thus retaining the blood, causing rigidity and an increase in both length and diameter of the penis. Secretions from the bulbourethral glands moisten the glans penis and continued friction results in increased nervous impulses along the sympathetic nerve fibres to the smooth muscle of the duct of the epididymis, vas deferens, the seminal vesicles and the prostate. On contraction of the smooth muscle the spermatozoa are discharged into the prostatic urethra along with seminal fluid. Ejaculation from the penile urethra occurs as result of rhythmic contractions of the bulbospongiosus muscles which compress the urethra. During this phase the sphincter of the bladder contract to prevent reflux of sperm into the bladder.

The fourth or final phase, resolution, is characterized by decreased sexual tension as the individual returns to an unstimulated state. The arteries supplying the erectile tissue undergo vasoconstriction and the penis returns to its flaccid state.

Erection is a neurovascular phenomenon dependent on the flow of blood in and out of the penis.

◆ Arteries dilate owing to relaxation of smooth muscles.
◆ Veins partially constrict resulting in corpus cavernosa and corpus spongiosum becoming engorged.

Erectile dysfunction and impotence

Erectile dysfunction is defined as the inability to sustain an erection sufficiently rigid to allow sexual intercourse to take place. Causes of erectile dysfunction are:

◆ vascular (e.g. diabetes, atherosclerosis)
◆ neurological (e.g. cerebrovascular accident, head injury, diabetes, pelvic fracture, surgery)
◆ endocrine (e.g. pituitary dysfunction, hypothyroidism)
◆ congenital (e.g. exstrophy, epispadias, hypospadias)
◆ acquired (e.g. Peyronie's disease, carcinoma of penis)
◆ drugs (e.g. antihypertensives, anticonvulsants, alcohol)
◆ radiotherapy damage
◆ psychogenic

Clinical diagnosis

The medical staff will take a detailed history of onset of impotence. Questions will be asked about the following:

- ◆ early morning erections – presence suggests psychogenic origin
- ◆ gradual or sudden onset:
     gradual onset is usually organic in origin
     sudden onset is usually psychogenic in the absence of known injury
- ◆ lifestyle:
     smoking can cause atheroma in the arteries of the penis
     drinking habits
- ◆ history of any pelvic injury
- ◆ drug history – problems can be caused by hypotensive therapy, narcotics, oestrogenic agents, cimetidine, digoxin, antidepressants and antipsychotics

Examination of the patient will include observation of facial hair, development and pitch of voice, and neurological and vascular examination of sacral sensation and peripheral pulses.

Investigations include the following:

- ◆ blood tests to establish hormonal levels, e.g. testosterone, prolactin, pituitary follicle-stimulating hormone and luteinizing hormone, oestrogen, thyroxine
- ◆ urine test for glucose
- ◆ Doppler ultrasound flowmeter – assesses blood flow in penis
- ◆ intracorporal injection
- ◆ cavernosogram – X-ray to establish venous drainage
- ◆ nocturnal penile tumescence study – this test requires an overnight stay in hospital
- ◆ rigiscan – a clinical computerized ambulatory device for the evaluation of erectile dysfunction. Measures penile rigidity and tumescence.
- ◆ bulbospongiosus reflex test (Bullock *et al.*, 1994)

Nocturnal penile tumescence study

Gauges are attached to the penis to record changes in penile length and circumference. Erections occur naturally several times during the night, especially in deep sleep during periods of rapid eye movement. The results are computerized; graphs showing no movement suggest erectile dysfunction of neurogenic origin, while graph activity shows erectile dysfunction of a psychogenic nature.

Snap gauge

A snap gauge consists of a non-stretchable fabric band which joins together by hook and loop closure. Three plastic elements are attached to the device requiring three specific levels of force. The device is worn around the penis at night. If all three remain intact, insufficient erectile activity has occurred. This test can be carried out at home; however, for patients complaining of an inability to maintain erections nocturnal penile tumescence studies are recommended.

TREATMENT OF IMPOTENCE

Once investigations establish the cause of impotence, the possibility of treatment can be discussed with the patient. If noctural tumescence studies show night-time erections, the patient can be referred to a psychosexual counsellor. If surgery is not advisable or desired, alternative therapies can be discussed. These include injection into the corpora cavernosa and vacuum therapy.

Drug therapy with agents such as yohimbine has been proved to be effective in certain cases. This should be taken 2 hours before intended sexual activity (Alexander, 1994). Glyceryl trinitrate in patch form is effective in some cases: 5 mg patches stuck onto the skin of the penis increase the amount of blood flow to produce an erection.

Surgical treatment

Prosthetic implants

Prosthetic implantation involves the insertion of materials into the corpus cavernosum. This treatment tends to be reserved for men who have not responded to non-surgical treatments and whose erectile dysfunction has a physical cause.

Malleable prostheses

Malleable prostheses produce a permanently erect penis which can be bent to accommodate intercourse and is flexible enough to be moved into a position of concealment. These implants usually consist of a stainless steel wire bundle encased in a bendable silicone sheath. Malleability allows the patient to bend the prosthesis into a comfortable position (Figure 12.9). The combination of silicone and stainless steel produces enough rigidity for penetration without buckling. Rear tip extenders allow surgeons to adjust the sizing at the time of operation.

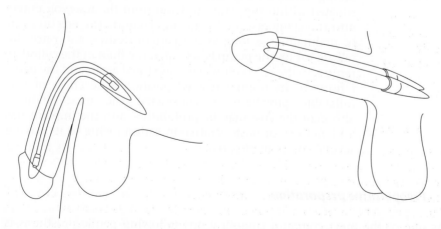

Figure 12.9   *Malleable prosthesis*

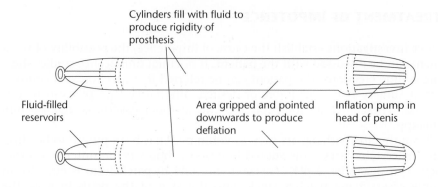

Figure 12.10 *Inflatable cylinder prosthesis*

Inflatable prostheses

There are two basic designs of inflatable prosthesis.

◆ Enclosed cylinder prostheses (Figure 12.10) consist of two enclosed inflatable units which are implanted side by side into the corpus cavernosum. To inflate the rods the end of the implant is slowly squeezed several times (this is situated at the head of the penis). Fluid moves from the reservoir and fills the cylinder to produce rigidity. To deflate the prosthesis the penis is gripped at the level of the shaft and the cylinders bent downwards. After approximately 10 seconds the grip is released and the fluid returns to the reservoir.

◆ Scrotal pump and reservoir inflatable prosthesis – this device consists of an inflation-deflation pump implanted into the scrotum, two cylinders implanted into the shaft of the penis and a reservoir containing normal saline implanted into the abdominal area (Figure 12.11). Each part is interconnected by tubing. To inflate the device the patient squeezes the pump, situated within the scrotum. Fluid from the reservoir enters into the cylinders, producing an erection. The erection can be maintained as long as the patient desires, and once the release bar on the pump is activated the fluid in the cylinders returns to the reservoir where it is stored again and the penis returns to its normal relaxed position. The effect of this inflatable prosthesis is considered the most 'natural' although the cost may be prohibitive, and the implant has a higher risk of postoperative infection owing to its having several component parts.

Preoperative preparation

As one of the most common complications following penile prosthesis is infection, work begins preoperatively to minimize this problem (Table 12.6).

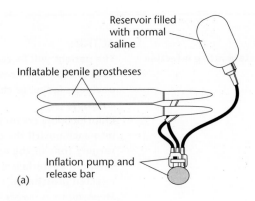

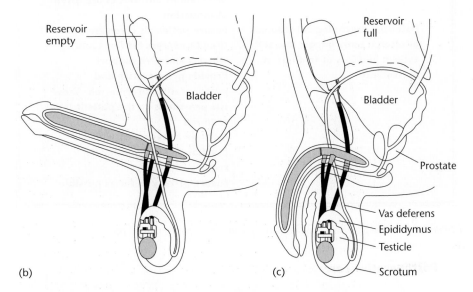

Figure 12.11   *Scrotal pump and reservoir inflatable prosthesis: (a) component parts; implanted pump with penis erect (b) and flaccid (c)*

Surgical procedure

Incisions are usually made at one of the following positions:

- penoscrotal – between the penis and the scrotum
- suprapubic – lower abdominal area

The implants are measured and cut to the correct size in theatre before insertion into the corpus cavernosum. Prophylactic antibiotics are now commonly used, e.g. gentamicin, which is injected locally into the area of insertion. The pump and reservoir are inserted into the scrotum and abdomen.

PROBLEM	ACTION
Risk of postoperative infection	**The patient will be required to have preoperative baths using povidone-iodine or chlorhexidine cleansers**
	Chlorhexidine cream is inserted into each nostril the day before surgery (one of the most common bacteria isolated from rejected prostheses, *Staphylococcus aureus* is often found in the nose)
	Shaves are carried out in theatre
	Intravenous antibiotics are given at induction
Potential psychological trauma of altered body image, low self-esteem and loss of feelings of masculinity	**Ensure patient is given enough time to express his fears and worries and give support**
	Provide preoperative and postoperative information. Show the prosthesis to the patient if required
	Arrange a session with a psychosexual counsellor if required
	Ensure privacy as far as possible

Table 12.6   Penile prosthesis implantation – preoperative specific nursing care

Postoperative care

See Table 12.7.

Potential long-term postoperative problems include:

- infection
- erosion
- pain
- displacement of component parts
- device malfunction

On discharge

Patients are advised to return to their surgeon immediately if they have any problems after discharge. Depending on the surgeon, the patient will be advised either to attempt intercourse 1 week before returning to the out-patient department or abstain until they are seen in clinic 6 weeks after discharge.

PROBLEM	ACTION
Potentially swollen and bruised penis	**Elevate penis with scrotal support or pants and pad**
	Regular analgesia should be offered
	Encourage rest
Potential inability to pass urine	**Support patient standing at the side of the bed if he is unable to pass urine while lying flat**
	Ensure adequate hydration
	Inform surgeon if patient unable to void (may require catheterization)
Potential infection and/or rejection	**Prophylactic antibiotics are given for 48 hours postoperatively**
	Wound is examined regularly for breakdown or dehiscence
	Temperature and pulse are recorded 4 hourly

Table 12.7   *Specific postoperative nursing care for penile prosthesis implantation*

Non-surgical treatment

External vacuum devices

External vacuum devices (Figure 12.12) mimic the natural process of erection by producing rigidity through vascular engorgement resulting in tumescence of the penis. Indications for use include:

- ◆ organic erectile dysfunction resulting from
    - diabetes
    - vascular disease
    - stoma surgery
    - prostatectomy
    - spinal cord injury
    - end-stage renal disease
    - medication
- ◆ psychogenic erectile dysfunction

There are several systems on the market which work on the same principle. Both battery-operated and hand pumps are available. Components include a plastic cylinder, a battery or hand pump, constriction rings, and lubrication (water-soluble).

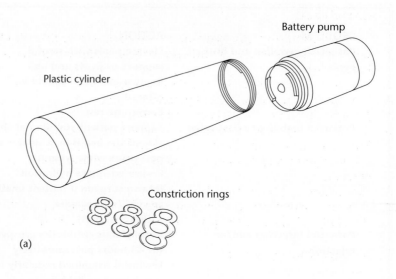

Plastic cylinder

Battery pump

Constriction rings

(a)

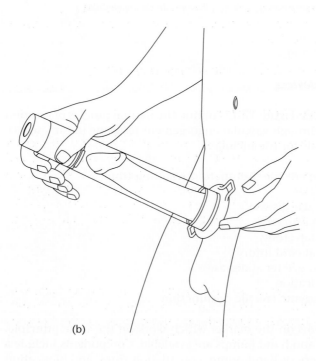

(b)

Figure 12.12 *External vacuum device (a) is placed over flaccid penis and negative pressure applied (b)*

Method of use

1. A constriction ring is placed around the open end of the cylinder.
2. Lubricant is applied around the end of the cylinder, constriction ring and base of penis.
3. The cylinder is placed over the flaccid penis.
4. The pump is activated either by hand or by battery.
5. Negative pressure – a vacuum – is created.
6. Blood is drawn down into the penis and an erection occurs.
7. The constriction ring is rolled off onto the base of the penis and the cylinder removed, trapping blood in the penis and maintaining the erection.
8. Intercourse can then take place.
9. The constriction ring is then removed – recommended time 30 minutes (ErecAid, 1992) – and the penis returns to its flaccid state.

These systems are regarded as:

- safe
- non-surgical
- painless
- relatively inexpensive
- not interfering with other treatment
- convenient – can be used as and when desired
- having a beneficial effect – in some patients may improve their natural erections

Research shows a success rate of over 90% (Price *et al.*, 1991).

Intracavernosal vasoactive agents

Until recently papaverine was the most widely used intracavernosal vasoactive agent. Unfortunately the side-effects of this therapy included prolonged erection and priapism. A comparison study by Das and Pryor (1994) between papaverine and prostaglandin E_1 (PGE_1) showed that with a 90% positive response rate with PGE_1 there were no incidences of priapism. Prostaglandin E_1 or alprostadil is a naturally occuring chemical derived from polyunsaturated fatty acids.

Effect

The effect of intracavernosal injections is to introduce high concentrations of vasoactive drugs to produce relaxation of arterial and trabecular smooth muscle. This dilates the arteries and produces relaxation of the corpus cavernosum and cavernous arteries (Hedlund and Anderson, 1985).

Indications

This method is particularly effective with patients who have:

- neurogenic impairment, e.g. spinal injury

♦   diabetes
♦   vascular insufficiency
♦   psychogenic problems

Contraindications

Contraindications include:

♦   blood disorders, e.g. sickle cell disease, leukaemia
♦   history of priapism

Dosage and administration

The injection is prepared when required (any surplus is discarded after use). Dosage will be titrated depending on response and increased until erection is achieved. The majority of patients achieve a satisfactory response with doses of PGE_1 between 10 μg and 20 μg. Doses above 60 μg are not recommended.

Administration is by 30 gauge needle. The penis is gripped in one hand with the first finger underneath the penis just in front of the testicles. The thumb is placed on top of the penis and downward tension is applied. This will expose the muscle of the penis. The injection is placed within this area (Figure 12.13). The penis is then massaged.

The erection should usually last about an hour.

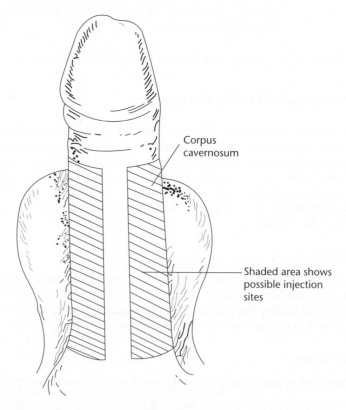

Corpus cavernosum

Shaded area shows possible injection sites

Figure 12.13 *Injection sites for intracorporal vasodilator*

Side-effects and disadvantages

1. Prolonged erection – if erection persists longer than 4 hours the patient is advised to contact the clinic as an emergency.
2. Pain at injection site – usually only transient.
3. Haematoma.
4. Cost – the drug is expensive.
5. Can only be used three times a week.
6. Needle phobia – Gould *et al.* (1992) found that some patients suffered persistent anxiety associated with self-injection and that the dislike of needles may increase, not lessen, with time.

Benefits

The temperature of the penis is consistent with normal body temperature, and overall there is more rigidity.

Psychosexual counselling and clinical nurse specialists

Both in Britain and in America the use of vacuum devices and injection therapy are now being taught by clinical nurse specialists in urology, who provide instruction to both patient and partner as necessary (Price et al, 1991). Price et al's study concluded that it is essential that men with erectile dysfunction should be given the opportunity for counselling and offered a choice of all available treatment.

Almost all erectile dysfunction has some psychological factors involved. Generally with the ageing process more intense arousal is needed, the time required to achieve erection increases, and the interval between erections is greater. Any one of these issues can have a negative impact on self-image. Both partners in a relationship are affected.

Research into the opinions of general practitioners as to the management of erectile function in the community showed that psychosexual counselling is the most common managment option for erectile dysfunction (Coyle, 1995).

REFERENCES

ALEXANDER W (1994) Diabetes, erectile impotence and the primary care team. *Diabetes in General Practice* **4**(2): 15–16.

BLANDY J (1991) *Lecture Notes on Urology*, 4th edn. Oxford: Blackwell Scientific.

BULLOCK N, Sibley G and Whitaker R (1994) *Essential Urology*, 2nd edn. Edinburgh: Churchill Livingstone.

COYLE F (1995) Erectile dysfunction: your views. *Geriatric Medicine* **25**(8): 18–27.

DAS G and Pryor J (1994) Prostaglandin E, an alternative intracavernosal vasoactive agent. *Journal of Sexual Health* **4**(5): 56–7.

ERECAID (1992) ErecAid System User Survey. Osbon Medical Systems, 1253 Broad St, Augusta, GA 30901.

FULLER J H S and Toon P D (1988) *Medical Practice in a Multicultural Society*. Oxford: Butterworth-Heinemann.

GOULD D, Switters D, Broderick G and deVere White R (1992) External vacuum devices; a clinical comparison with pharmacological erections. *World Journal of Urology* **10**: 68–70.

HAYWARD J L (1975) *Information – A Prescription Against Pain*. RCN Study of Nursing Care Series. London: Royal College of Nursing.

HEDLAND H and Anderson K E (1985) Contraction and relaxation induced by some prostanoids in isolated human penile erectile tissue and cavernous artery. *Journal of Urology* **134**: 1245–1250.

PRICE D E, Cooksey G, Jehu D, Bentley S, Hearnshaw J E and Osborn D E (1991) The management of impotence in diabetic men by vacuum tumescence therapy. *Diabetic Medicine* **8**: 964–967.

13 SCROTAL DISORDERS

Contents

The anatomy and physiology of the scrotum is described in Chapter 1. This chapter describes the nursing care of the following conditions and procedures:

- ◆ vasectomy
- ◆ vasovasostomy
- ◆ varicocele
- ◆ hydrocele
- ◆ testicular trauma
- ◆ testicular torsion
- ◆ epididymitis
- ◆ orchitis
- ◆ orchidectomy
- ◆ infertility

Under the above headings specific preoperative and postoperative nursing care as well as specific discharge advice is described.

Prior to any surgical intervention or medical treatment such as chemotherapy or radiotherapy where fertility may be affected, sperm cryopreservation is an important means of circumventing impairment; failure to advise the patient of this facility could result in litigation.

The general nursing care of patients undergoing scrotal surgery is described in three tables at the end of this chapter.

- preoperative nursing care is described in Table 13.1
- postoperative nursing care is described in Table 13.2
- discharge advice for a patient following scrotal surgery is given in Table 13.3

VASECTOMY

Vasectomy (Figure 13.1) is performed for male sterilization. The aim of the procedure is to prevent the flow of sperm through the vas deferens. Occasionally this procedure may be performed to prevent patients with epididymitis developing orchitis if fertility is not a priority.

Most commonly an incision is made in the scrotum, the vas deferens is located and approximately 1 cm of it is removed. The remaining ends are then turned back on themselves and ligated. This should prevent the tube from rejoining.

The procedure is most commonly performed under local anaesthesia in either a hospital or general practice setting. General anaesthesia may be required if the patient has had previous surgery to the area.

Specific nursing care

In most health authorities in the UK the consent form for vasectomy needs to be signed by both partners. As the procedure is essentially irreversible, it is of vital importance that both partners have been counselled prior to obtaining

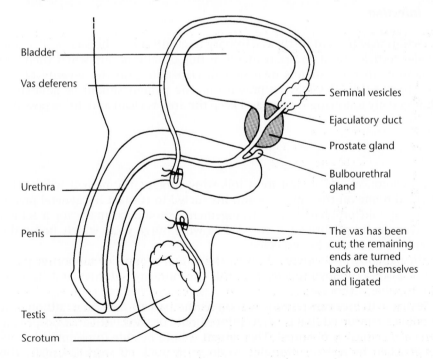

Figure 13.1 Vasectomy

their consent. Occasionally individuals encounter psychosexual problems following vasectomy. Physically, it should not affect a man's desire or capability to have sexual intercourse, but occasionally it does. In a small number of cases reanastomosis takes place, and living sperm reappear in the vas many months after azoospermia has been confirmed. It is important that this is understood by the couple, for if any unexpected pregnancy occurs, recrimination and litigation may ensue.

Following vasectomy, the couple can resume normal sexual activities as soon as they feel comfortable to do so. However, they will need to use an alternative form of contraception until semen analysis shows azoospermia. This usually takes up to 6 weeks following surgery, as living sperm remain in the vas below the point of ligation.

Despite having been counselled and then signing the consent form, many couples change their minds and do not arrive for the procedure.

Potential complications

Haematoma

To reduce the possibility of haematoma, the patient should rest quietly for approximately 1 hour following surgery. A well-fitting scrotal support and pad should be worn to provide a little local pressure. A certain degree of bruising and swelling should be expected and can be the cause of both pain and infection.

Infection

Infection may present firstly as a urinary tract infection, then as swollen and tender testicles or at the skin incision; this usually occurs when there are organisms in the patient's own semen. Depending on the severity of the infection, antibiotics may be prescribed. The patient should be advised to shower daily following surgery and keep the area as clean and dry as possible.

Discharge

If no complications are apparent following surgery, the patient will be discharged home on the same day and instructed to contact his general practitioner should problems arise. Arrangements should be made for a semen analysis to be performed 8 weeks following surgery, at which point the wound site can also be inspected.

The patient will be advised to wear the scrotal support or supportive pants for 1–2 weeks following surgery, until the bruising subsides and he feels comfortable without it.

Sexual activities can resume as soon as the patient feels able, although it should be reinforced that contraception should be used until an azoospermic semen specimen is obtained. The patient should be able to resume employment when he feels comfortable to do so; a week off work is usually the maximum required.

VASOVASOSTOMY

Vasovasostomy is the procedure used to reverse a vasectomy. The procedure may be requested owing to a family tragedy where a child has been killed or perhaps a man wants to start a family with a new partner.

Research (Howards, 1987) suggests 90% of men would have spermatozoa in their postoperative ejaculate if spermatozoa were present in fluid from the distal vas deferens at the time of surgery. In the partners of these men the pregnancy success rate was 40% to 70%. The success rate is influenced by the length of time between the initial vasectomy and the reanastomosis; the longer the time interval, the lower the success rate. The risk of failure is so great that vasectomy should not be undertaken unless both partners have fully decided they do not want any more children.

The procedure is most commonly performed under general anaesthesia. Cryopreservation of sperm is carried out at this time. A lower abdominal incision is used. The ends of the vas are found and joined together. The surgery is very delicate – whereas a vasectomy will take approximately 15 minutes to perform, this procedure usually takes 2 hours.

Specific nursing care

A full explanation of the procedure must be given. Many patients are under the misconception that the reversal of vasectomy will be as quick and straightforward as the vasectomy itself. The potential complications of wound infection, haematoma and pain will be explained as well as the fact that the success rate of the procedure is poor. To give the optimum chance for healing to occur and for the surgery to be successful, the patient should remain on modified bed rest both on the day of surgery and the first post-operative day, and get up for toilet purposes only. If all is well then the patient will be discharged on the second postoperative day.

Potential complications

Moderate or severe pain

Because the surgery is delicate and the area vascular the patient may experience a significant degree of pain and discomfort. Pain can be controlled by the administration of adequate analgesia, as prescribed. Ensuring the scrotum is adequately supported by a well-fitting scrotal support and pad (or elastic pants and pad) will also help relieve the pain.

Infection

The patient should not be discharged home with an untreated pyrexia. The wound should be checked for signs of infection such as oozing or inflammation. Dressings should be removed 48 hours postoperatively unless they require changing because of excessive oozing. Once the dressing is removed the wound can be left exposed. The patient should ensure that the area is kept as clean and dry as possible. Showers are recommended after 2 days and a daily bath after 3 days. The patient should ensure that sutures are not soaked in the bath until at least 4 days postoperatively.

Haematoma

On occasions large haematomas do develop, and it may be necessary for the patient to return to theatre for evacuation of the haematoma. A regular check should be made on the wound site and scrotal area following surgery to observe for bleeding and swelling. A well-fitting scrotal support (or pad and elastic pants) should be worn to provide both pressure to the area and also extra support and comfort.

Discharge

If all is well, patients are usually discharged home on the second or third postoperative day. Depending on the work performed by the patient, it may be necessary for him to take up to 2 weeks off work. The patient will be advised against any heavy lifting or exercise which might put strain on the area.

A scrotal support should be worn for a couple of weeks until the patient feels comfortable without it.

If the sutures are dissolvable the patient should be informed of this; if not, arrangements should be made for the sutures to be removed 7–10 days post-operatively.

Patients are advised not to have sexual intercourse for 4 weeks following surgery. An appointment should be made for the wound to be inspected 6 weeks postoperatively and for semen analysis to be performed 3 and 4 months postoperatively.

A full explanation should be given of any analgesic or antibiotics prescribed for the patient to take home. The patient is advised to keep the area clean and dry and to visit his general practitioner if any problems arise relating to the surgery.

LIGATION OF VARICOCELE

A varicocele is formed when the spermatic veins draining the testicle become varicose and distended. Varicoceles often feel like a 'bag of worms' (Figure 13.2). It is believed that these veins serve as a heat exchange mechanism, keeping the testicle cool and aiding in spermatogenesis. Infertility occurs three times more often in men with a varicocele than in the general population (La Nasa and Lewis, 1987).

The condition is usually asymptomatic and is often only found at a routine examination. Occasionally a dragging, 'aching' feeling is experienced, but the varicocele is seldom so uncomfortable that it requires supporting with a scrotal support, and very rarely requires ligation.

The operation involves opening up the inguinal canal, and all the veins except one are ligated and divided. The canal is then closed. The procedure is

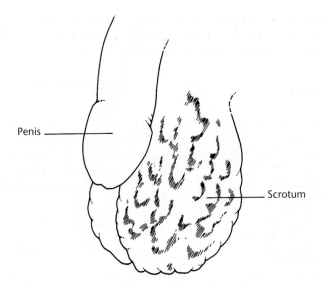

Penis

Scrotum

Figure 13.2   *Varicocele*

performed under general anaesthesia and the patient is usually discharged on the first or second postoperative day. Sexual activities can be resumed as soon as the patient feels comfortable to do so. Absence from work is usually for 1 week after discharge.

For nursing care, see Tables 13.1–13.3.

HYDROCELE

The outer covering of the testis is the tunica vaginalis. It has both a visceral and a parietal layer. Secretions from the tunica keep the two layers moist, allowing some mobility of the testes. The secretion is normally only a few millilitres. The testicle has a series of lymphatic capillaries which drain into the lymphatics of the spermatic cord. If these lymphatics become obstructed, fluid accumulates between the layers of the tunica vaginalis, resulting in the formation of a hydrocele (Figure 13.3).

There are three types of hydrocele:

1. *Primary hydrocele* – this is common in middle-aged men; the cause is unknown.
2. *Congenital hydrocele* – after birth the processus vaginalis may not be completely obliterated and peritoneal fluid is able to enter the cavity, resulting in a hydrocele. Spontaneous closure of the processus vaginalis usually occurs, resulting in the disappearance of the hydrocele. However, if by 18 months of age spontaneous closure has not occurred, the processus will have to be ligated.
3. *Secondary hydrocele* – so-called because it occurs as a result of a known cause, e.g. injury to the testicle, fibrosis of the lymphatics, or secondary to heart failure.

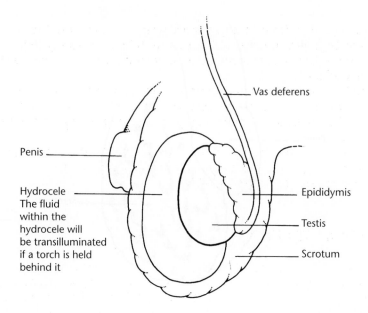

Figure 13.3 *Hydrocele*

Treatment

The treatment of hydrocele in the elderly patient is usually by aspiration of the fluid. This is performed on an out-patient basis under local anaesthesia. This method may only provide temporary relief, as the hydrocele is likely to recur.

Hydrocelectomy is performed under general anaesthesia. It is the treatment of choice when the hydrocele persistently recurs or is a source of pain and discomfort to the patient. A scrotal incision is made and the sac either drained and 'bunched' with a series of sutures (removing the potential space for fluid accumulation), or else removed completely. The procedure often leaves the patient with a large haematoma which may take several weeks to resolve. Hence the final results of surgery are not noticeable until the haematoma has resolved.

For nursing care, see Tables 13.1–13.3.

Discharge

Sexual intercourse can resume 2 weeks postoperatively if the patient feels comfortable. A scrotal support should be worn until the haematoma resolves and the patient feels comfortable without it. The length of time off work following surgery is usually 2 weeks after discharge from hospital.

SPERMATOCELE

Tiny cysts may develop in the sulcus between the epididymis and testis. They are thought to be diverticula in the collecting tubules of the vasa efferentia. If these enlarge, they form multiple translucent cysts, causing the epididymis to become thin and stretched. The cysts contain clear, watery fluid and also dead sperm. When many sperm are present within the cysts, they are known as spermatoceles.

Spermatoceles can be left untreated, unless painful. Before surgery is peformed to remove a spermatocele, the patient must be informed that it may result in infertility as the surgery may cause the vasa efferentia to be interrupted.

The procedure is performed under general anaesthesia and the patient is generally discharged on the first or second postoperative day.

For nursing care see Tables 13.1–13.3.

TESTICULAR TRAUMA

The testicles are frequently damaged as a result of sporting injuries. The injury usually causes a split in the visceral layer of the tunica vaginalis, resulting in a large, painful haematocele. If left untreated over a period of weeks the haematocele will gradually subside. However, prior to this, the pressure exerted on the testicle as a result of the haematocele may squeeze it flat, resulting in permanent atrophy of the testicle and loss of spermatogenic function. If medical advice is not sought immediately by the patient, it is important that the possible loss of spermatogenic function as a direct result of the injury is explained prior to surgery.

The testicle should be explored as soon as possible after such an injury. An incision is made in the scrotum, the blood clot is removed and the tear in the visceral layer of the tunica vaginalis repaired. Some of these injuries and haematoceles turn out to be tumours of the testicle – an additional reason for not delaying exploration of the testicle.

The procedure is performed under general anaesthesia and the patient discharged on the second postoperative day. The patient is advised to abstain from sexual intercourse for 1–2 weeks and not to resume sporting activities for 3–4 weeks until the area is healed and comfortable.

For nursing care see Tables 13.1–13.3.

TESTICULAR TORSION

Testicular torsion can occur in both normal and undescended testicles where there is excessive mobility of the testes – allowing the testes and epididymis to rotate on its mesentery, resulting in first the venous drainage and later the arterial supply being obstructed (Figure 13.4). This leads to infarction of the testicle and requires urgent treatment. If the blood supply is compromised for longer than 6 hours it is likely that complete infarction of the testicle will result.

The patient experiences sudden acute pain in the testicle owing to vascular obstruction. Occasionally referred pain is felt in the inguinal or abdominal area. The testes are tender to touch. Within 1–2 hours the testicle will appear red and become swollen, accompanied by oedema.

The torsion can be corrected by untwisting the testicle, rotating it first one

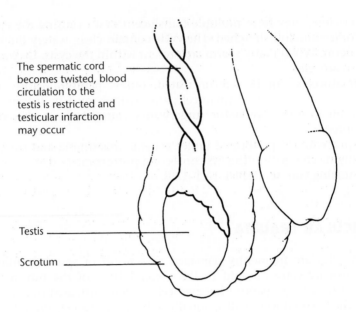

The spermatic cord becomes twisted, blood circulation to the testis is restricted and testicular infarction may occur

Testis

Scrotum

Figure 13.4 *Testicular torsion*

way and then the other. A distinct click will be felt and the patient will experience immediate relief when the torsion is corrected.

Surgical correction of the torsion is performed under general anaesthesia. An inguinal scrotal incision is made. The torsion is corrected and the viability of the testicle assessed. If infarction has occurred then orchidectomy is the treatment of choice. If the testicle is viable, it should be fixed to the excised edges of the tunica vaginalis and inner layer of the scrotal skin. This will lessen its mobility and guard against recurrence. If the other testicle feels equally mobile, it should be fixed at the same time. This procedure is called orchidopexy.

Specific nursing care

The patient will be admitted as an emergency for urgent transfer to surgery. Prior to surgery, bed rest should be maintained and adequate analgesia administered as prescribed. The possibility of reduced infertility due to testicular infarction or orchidectomy should be explained.

For general nursing care, see Tables 13.1–13.3.

EPIDIDYMITIS

Acute epididymitis

Acute epididymitis is usually the result of bacterial infection, caused by one or two principal groups of pathogens. These are:

1. Sexually transmitted organisms, e.g. *Chlamydia trachomatis* or *Neisseria gonorrhoea*, either alone or in combination.
2. Non-sexually transmitted organisms – this type of infection is often associated with urinary tract infection and prostatitis, and common causative organisms are Enterobacteriaceae and *Pseudomonas*.

Acute infection of the epididymis is rarely seen prior to the age of puberty, but after that occurs in all other age groups. The infection may reach the epididymis via the blood stream or via the perivasal lymphatics. In addition, retrograde spread from the prostatic urethra and seminal vesicles can occur, a process that may be enhanced by the hydrostatic pressure associated with voiding forcing infected urine into the ejaculatory ducts and through the vas deferens to the epididymis.

Genitourinary tuberculosis is also a potential cause of acute epididymitis, and remains common in areas where pulmonary tuberculosis remains a significant problem. However, in many cases no causative organism or underlying problem can be found.

Treatment

The condition is usually treated with a combination of:

◆　　bed rest
◆　　a well-fitting scrotal support
◆　　appropriate analgesia, as the testicle can become extremely painful
◆　　scrupulous scrotal hygiene
◆　　appropriate antibiotic therapy, provided a causative organism can be identified

The nursing care of these individuals will centre upon the above priorities, as well as attempting to provide a supportive environment, where the potential embarrassment of the patient is minimized.

The most common complication of epididymitis is orchitis or epididymoorchitis which may result in atrophy, sterility from fibrosis, and destruction of the tubules and ductal system (McConnell, 1987).

Chronic epididymitis

Chronic epididymitis usually results from a severe attack of acute epididymitis that has been followed by repeated further attacks of less severity. When this happens, the vas becomes 'beaded' and shortened and the epididymis nodular and hard. The pathological changes in chronic epididymitis may cause an interruption to the vas, thus influencing the fertility of the patient. Tuberculosis (TB) remains an important cause of chronic epididymitis.

Treatment

Treatment of this condition is by appropriate antibiotic therapy, particularly if TB is the cause. Occasionally a vasectomy may be performed if fertility is not a priority.

In terms of nursing management, the care is similar to that for cases of acute epididymitis, though this will vary according to the severity of the patient's discomfort.

ACUTE ORCHITIS

Viral infections account for most acute infections of the testis (e.g. rubella, infectious mononucleosis, mumps). Mumps orchitis occurs in 16–20% of adult males who contract the infection, but is rarely seen prior to puberty (Blandy, 1989). The diagnosis of acute orchitis can be difficult, as the symptoms are similar to those of testicular torsion. To exclude the possibility of torsion, exploration of the testicle is required, under general anaesthesia.

Treatment

Acute orchitis is usually treated conservatively, using a combination of:

- bed rest
- a well-fitting scrotal support
- suitable analgesia

Some units advocate steroid therapy, to reduce the degree of subsequent testicular atrophy. There is debate over the effectiveness of this strategy.

Depending on the degree of testicular atrophy resulting from the infection, patients may require counselling regarding reduced fertility; if the condition is bilateral, sterility may result.

ORCHIDECTOMY

Orchidectomy is the removal of the testicle. It may be unilateral or bilateral, depending on the reason for removal. Cryopreservation of sperm should be discussed with the patient and organized prior to surgical intervention.

Bilateral orchidectomy

The bilateral procedure is performed in patients with advanced prostatic cancer. Prostatic tumours are generally testosterone-dependent and their growth is therefore retarded when the amount of circulating testosterone is reduced. This can be achieved either by the oral or intramuscular administration of synthetic oestrogen, or by the use of testosterone antagonists, such as cyproterone acetate. Surgically, testosterone production can be reduced by bilateral orchidectomy. A scrotal incision is made and the testicles removed. A dressing and scrotal support are then applied. The length of hospital stay is usually 4 days.

For general nursing care, see Tables 13.1–13.3.

Specific nursing care

The specific nursing care required by the patient is the provision of comfort and support to enable the patient to come to terms with his altered body image.

The reduction of circulating testosterone is likely to reduce the patient's sexual desire and also his ability to achieve both erection and orgasm. Sterility will occur, and it is likely that such patients will suffer a loss of perceived masculinity. The nurse should allocate time to listen and provide comfort to the patient and his family. The positive aspects of treatment can also be emphasized (e.g. the patient will probably have considerable pain reduction following surgery).

Unilateral orchidectomy

Unilateral orchidectomy may be required following testicular torsion if the testicle is found to be infarcted. It may also be necessary following testicular trauma, where the testicle has been compressed by a haematoma causing testicular atrophy.

The most common reason for performing unilateral orchidectomy is the presence of testicular tumours. Patients who are suspected of having testicular tumours will undergo surgical exploration of the scrotum. If malignant tissue is found then unilateral orchidectomy will be performed. The procedure is performed under general anaesthesia through an inguinal incision. Testicular biopsies are not performed for suspected neoplasms, since there is risk of spreading malignant cells to healthy tissue. Most testicular tumours are prone to metastatic spread and additional treatment is therefore often required. This is dependent upon the type of tumour (see Chapter 10).

The average length of stay following unilateral orchidectomy is 5 days. However, this will depend upon the follow-up care required.

For general nursing care, see Tables 13.1–13.3.

Specific nursing care

The specific role of the nurse with regard to nursing care is to provide a supportive environment for the patient and to correct any inaccurate notions he may have regarding his illness. The nurse will need to provide psychological support and comfort for the patient and his partner. The patient will have to come to terms with an altered body image (e.g. he may feel less sexually attractive owing to the idea of having only one testicle and therefore being different from other men). Surgical implantation of a gel-filled silicone prosthesis can be performed at a later date. It should be reinforced that although the patient will have a lower sperm count, he will still be fertile and his ability to have an erection and orgasm will not be affected.

If radiotherapy or chemotherapy are required, fertility will probably be impaired for a number of years, as the treatment has an adverse effect on spermatogenesis. If lymphadenectomy is performed the patient may suffer from ejaculatory failure, depending on the extent of surgery. It is of vital importance that patients are allowed time and space in which to express their fears and anxieties over their diagnosis, treatment and prognosis. The patient will require frequent follow-up examinations so that any recurrence can be detected early and treated.

INFERTILITY

Male fertility

Male fertility depends on the production of viable sperm in the testes and their passage through the vas deferens to the seminal vesicles where other components are added to manufacture seminal fluid. Fertility also depends on the ability of the male partner to maintain an adequate erection (to enable penetration) and the ability to ejaculate. Problems may arise at any point in this process, resulting in subsequent infertility.

Testis

Each lobe of the testis contains seminiferous tubules, surrounded by Leydig cells. The Leydig cells produce testosterone. They are dormant until puberty and stimulated by the pituitary gland situated in the hypothalamus.

Spermatogenesis

Spermatogenesis begins in the seminiferous tubules under the influence of follicle-stimulating hormone (FSH) produced by the pituitary gland. The basilar membrane of the seminiferous tubules is lined with two types of cells: spermatogonia and Sertoli cells. Spermatogonia undergo growth and multiplication to become primary spermatocytes, secondary spermatocytes and finally spermatids.

The Sertoli cells provide nutrients for the spermatids. They engulf the spermatid and begin a metamorphosis which produces viable spermatozoa.

When growth is complete, sperm are released into the lumen of the seminiferous tubule and rapidly transported to the epididymis through the ductal system. As they progress through the ducts, sperm increase in vitality and vigour, undergoing further maturation. (Sperm removed from the tail rather than the head of the epididymis are more fertile.) If the sperm are not ejaculated they degenerate and are absorbed.

Spermatogenesis is continuous – the whole process takes approximately 74 days for completion. It is sensitive to heat, occurring at temperatures a few degrees lower than body temperature. The dartos muscle within the scrotum contracts or relaxes in response to varying external temperatures, thus allowing the temperature of the testis to be regulated. Men with uncorrected cryptorchidism remain sterile, because the intra-abdominal temperature is incompatible with successful spermatogenesis.

Viable sperm must be transported from the testis through the penis to the female reproductive tract so that fertilization can take place. The vas widens into a broad ampulla as it ascends the pelvic cavity. The ampulla and seminal vesicles meet to form the common ejaculatory duct. The seminal vesicles produce a fluid rich in nutrients which provides for the sperm until fertilization. At ejaculation, the seminal vesicles contract and seminal fluid is forced into the common ejaculatory duct and into the prostatic urethra, where the prostatic gland also discharges its fluid. The prostatic fluid is alkaline and believed to reduce the acidity of the seminal fluid and vaginal secretions. (The motility and viability of the sperm are greatly reduced in an acid solution.) Sperm are thus more motile in a neutral or slightly alkaline solution.

The bulbourethral glands add further fluid to the semen, which then acts as a lubricant and fluid medium for the sperm.

At ejaculation the muscle layers of the prostate gland contract rhythmically, forcing prostatic fluid into the prostatic urethra. The bladder neck muscles also contract, closing the internal urethral orifice. Powerful rhythmic contractions then result in the semen being forced along the length of the erect penis. To deposit the semen in the vagina the penis must be erect. This change is due to the engorgement of the corpora cavernosa and corpus spongiosum (see Chapter 12).

Treatment of infertility

Infertility is the inability to cause conception after 1 year of regular, unprotected intercourse. It affects 15% of all couples; a third of cases are due to male-related problems such as a low or absent sperm count or impotence. A further third of cases are due to female-related problems, and the remaining third are due to problems existing in both partners (Baun, 1987).

Infertility should be regarded as a joint problem; initially both partners should be investigated. Occasionally it is found that couples do not know the fertility cycle and have not been having intercourse at the appropriate time. Other psychosexual difficulties may be identified.

Infertility is more commonly a problem later in a women's reproductive life, increasing after the age of 30 years and becoming more serious after the age of 35. Although the age of the male partner appears not to be a problem there is increasing interest in examining the sperm of older and younger men and its effect on the quality of the pregnancy (G. Bahadur, personal communication, 1996). Another issue is that of declining sperm counts in relation to the quality of the environment, which has implications for the survival of the human race.

Fertility treatment in the UK is regulated by the Human Fertilisation and Embryology Act 1990. Issues such as gamete donation and the use of dead partners' sperm are covered by the Act. The Act makes provisions to regulate and monitor treatment centres and to ensure that research using human embryos is carried out in a responsible way. This is done by means of a licensing system. The Human Fertilisation and Embryology Authority

(HFEA) is an independent body set up to carry out the work required by law. The HFEA is responsible for regulating and licensing clinics which provide in vitro fertilization (IVF) or any treatment involving donated sperm or eggs. To obtain a licence a clinic must comply with the Human Fertilisation and Embryology Act 1990 and with the HFEA's code of practice. All clinics must keep to these standards, but the type and range of services they offer may differ widely. Counselling and patient consent is an integral part of all patient activities. Three distinct types of counselling should be provided: implications counselling, support counselling and therapeutic counselling.

Investigation of infertility

On the couple's first visit to the infertility clinic a fertility questionnaire is normally completed by the doctor together with both partners. A full physical examination of the male partner, as well as semen analysis, will be performed. The questionnaire investigates the following topics:

1. Previous marriage and pregnancies
2. Time attempting to conceive – any pregnancies?
3. Frequency of intercourse (weekly) – erection, penetration, ejaculation.
4. Knowledge of fertility phase? (day 14 in menstrual cycle).
5. Previous investigation and treatment.

The full investigation should include:

◆ Past history of the male partner – the following aspects are discussed:
  general health
  operations
  hernia (may cause obstruction of the vas)
  undescended testicles (should be corrected before age of 4 years)
  varicocele (elevated testicular temperature)
  mumps (if before 15 years of age, testicular damage rare)
  epididymitis, urinary infections
  diabetes
  recent illnesses
  chemotherapy
  deep X-ray treatment
  general health
  frequency of shaving (may indicate pituitary failure)
  emotional problems
  smoking habits (atheroma in arteries may cause erectile dysfunction)
  alcohol intake (if high may cause decreased libido)
  current drugs
◆ Past history of the female partner – the following details are discussed:
  age
  menstrual history

◆ previous pregnancies
previous operations
previous illnesses
family history
previous treatment

◆ Investigations of female partner – the following are discussed or performed as appropriate:
biphasic temperature chart
progesterone levels
tubal patency
cervical mucus
postcoital test

◆ Examination of male partner – the male partner is examined for:
height
weight
hair distribution
physique
breasts (the patient may have Klinefelter's syndrome, a chromosome abnormality where there is an extra X chromosome. These patients have long limbs, small testes, gynaecomastia and female distribution of hair. They are usually infertile)
abdomen may show presence of scars
undergarments (tight/loose)
penis: uncircumcised, external meatus
testis (right and left)
varicocele
epididymis
vas
prostate and seminal vesicle

◆ Investigations of male partner – the following tests are performed:
seminal analysis (2 samples)
blood test for levels of follicle-stimulating hormone, lutenizing hormone, testosterone, prolactin
vasogram
buccal smear
chromosomes
testicular exploration/biopsy

Testicles

The scrotal contents are examined. The size and consistency of the testis are noted. Fertility is usually suppressed when both testes are 3 cm or less. The epididymis and vas deferens are felt and any abnormality noted. Rectal examination is performed, as any thickening or tenderness of the prostate or seminal vesicles may suggest infection. The patient is examined in the standing position for the presence of any varicocele. These are important as they may raise the testicular temperature, causing impairment of spermatogenesis.

Penis

Phimosis may be present – a pinhole meatus can interfere with ejaculation and necessitate circumcision (see Chapter 12).

Peyronie's disease is the development of fibrous plaques within the corpus cavernosum. This results in curvature of the erect penis, which may prevent vaginal penetration (the patient will require a Nesbitt's procedure; see Chapter 12).

Impotence may be a cause of infertility. Psychosexual counselling or surgical intervention may be required, dependent on the cause (see Chapter 12).

Seminal fluid analysis

Seminal fluid analysis is important in the study of infertility but has its limitations. The specimen should be produced by masturbation into a clean, wide-mouthed container after 3 days of abstinence. It should be examined as soon as possible (within 1–2 hours) by an experienced technician. One reading in isolation is insufficient; several samples should be examined over a period of 3 months.

The volume of ejaculate may vary. The normal range is 2–5 ml. Volumes of far less than this have been known to produce conception. If the volume of ejaculate is less than 0.5 ml, retrograde ejaculation or the absence of the seminal vesicles should be excluded.

Normal sperm concentration

The normal sperm concentration is 60–160 million per ml. It is only when the sperm count is less than 20 million per ml that infertility is likely to be due to a lack of spermatozoa. Azoospermia refers to a complete absence of sperm. Oligospermia refers to a sperm count of less than 20 million per ml and requires further investigations.

The percentage of motile spermatozoa is important and should be more than 40% at 1 hour. The quality of movement is important and the progressive movement is assessed objectively. Patients whose sperm have a persistent lack of progressive motility have a poor prognosis.

The morphology of spermatozoa is varied and even in a normal semen specimen there will be many morphological abnormalities. The prognosis is poor when most of the sperm are abnormal.

The complete evaluation of semen includes the assessment of the viscosity, pH measurement, microscopic examination for pus cells and the mixed erythrocyte agglutination reaction test for antisperm antibodies. Antisperm antibodies in the blood serum should be tested if there is any indication of sperm antibodies in the semen.

Additional investigations

Endocrine assessment of the infertile male is essential in men with azoospermia or severe oligospermia. In these patients, plasma FSH, luteinizing hormone (LH) and testosterone levels are measured. The presence of any circulating anstisperm antibodies is detected.

A postcoital test is valuable in the assessment of the infertile male, and also assesses factors of the partner. This test is only of value when carried out at the time of ovulation. An in vitro penetration test and crossed penetration test with donor sperm and cervical mucus may also provide useful information on the behaviour of sperm.

Surgical treatment

Ligation of varicocele

This procedure is only performed when other causes of infertility have been excluded, particularly in the female partner.

Treatment of undescended testicles

The chances of improving fertility are remote, but testicular biopsy may diagnose carcinoma in situ. Orchidopexy should be performed in patients below the age of 6 years.

Vasovasostomy, epididymovasostomy

Sperm retrieval

If there are severe spermatic defects, sperm retrieval is possible by mid-epididymal sperm aspiration (MESA) or testicular epididymal sperm aspiration (TESA).

Azoospermia and its treatment

Azoospermia may be due to:

1. *Primary failure of the testes to produce spermatozoa* – these patients usually have small testes and a raised FSH level; no treatment is possible.
2. *Obstruction.* If obstruction is present the patient will require surgical exploration to determine the level of the block. This is only done on patients with a normal sized testis (4–5 cm) and those without a gross elevation of plasma FSH level. Testicular exploration is carried out under general anaesthesia. The epididymis is inspected for evidence of obstruction; vasography is performed to exclude vasal obstruction, and the testes are biopsied.

If an obstruction is seen an epididymal bypass operation can be performed. The nursing care is similar to that for vasovasostomy. Vasal obstruction can also occur following inexpert herniorrhaphy in childhood. Ten per cent of men with obstructive azoospermia have vasal or varying degrees of epididymal aplasia. Various techniques have been described for collecting spermatozoa for performing artificial insemination. Those collected from the head of the epididymis are infertile, but those collected from the tail have been known to fertilize human oocytes in vitro.

The most common cause of azoospermia at the present time is previous vasectomy. The main advantage of overcoming obstruction is to enable the couple to achieve conception in privacy and avoid intrusive techniques to the woman.

Oligospermia and its treatment

Patients with defective spermatogenesis (small testes and high FSH levels) are unlikely to respond to treatment. Any hormonal deficiencies should be identified and treated.

Other factors that depress spermatogenesis include drug treatment (e.g. sulphasalazine) and hyperthermia in a patient with viral infections. For these reasons the sperm concentration should be monitored over a 3-month period before coming to any firm conclusion. Obstructive oligospermia can be treated with surgery, and infection treated with antibiotics.

Drug therapy

1. *Poor motility of sperm* – occasionally high doses of ascorbic acid can improve motility.
2. *Infection* – genital tract infections are a recognized cause of infertility and should be treated with appropriate antibiotics; the presence of alkaline semen and pus cells should alert the clinician. Semen, prostatic secretions and urinary cultures are necessary to confirm the diagnosis.

Hormone therapy

A few men may benefit from hormonal treatment (McNally, 1987; Sckol, 1987).

1. If the patient has low levels of FSH and LH, he is treated with human chorionic gonadotrophin and human menopausal gonadotrophin or gonadotrophin-releasing hormones.
2. If the patient has normal body build and normal testes, azoospermia, a low FSH level and testicular biopsy shows spermatogenic arrest at the spermatocyte stage, he is treated with gonadotrophin replacement therapy.
3. Men with androgen insensitivity, who have high FSH, high LH and high testosterone levels, are treated with high doses of androgens.
4. Oligospermia, with low FSH levels and impaired spermatogenesis, is treated with tamoxifen or clomiphene citrate.

Patients with oligospermia should be given the following practical advice:

- wear loose underwear
- avoid hot baths
- avoid regular heavy drinking
- take exercise and try to maintain a level of health and fitness
- do not use a lubricant with spermicidal action
- cut down on smoking

Antibody problems and their treatment

Antisperm antibodies may be detected in both peripheral blood and seminal plasma. Immunoglobulin G antibodies are related to circulating antisperm antibodies. Immunoglobulin A antibodies are related to the shaking movement of spermatozoa entrapped in cervical mucus. Treatment with high doses of methylprednisolone (as much as 96 mg daily) results in a success rate of around 30%.

Nursing care

Nursing care focuses on the psychological aspects of infertility. The nurse should be aware that the patient with infertility has been under considerable emotional stress for a prolonged period. The main objective of the nurse is to provide a supportive environment.

After full investigation it is possible to give couples an estimate of their chances of conception and what treatment is likely to alter their prospects.

Other treatment options

The following treatment options are available at HFEA licensed clinics:

Donor insemination

If a woman can not conceive because of problems with the male partner, or if the male partner has an inherited disease, it may be suggested that the couple consider artificial insemination using donated sperm.

In vitro fertilization

In vitro fertilization using the couple's own eggs and sperm may be appropriate if infertility is caused by the woman's blocked fallopian tubes, for example.

In vitro fertilization using donated sperm can be used if the male partner is infertile, or if the woman has (for example) ovulation problems, donated eggs or embryos can be used.

Gamete intrafallopian transfer

If it has been identified that there is nothing wrong with the woman's fallopian tubes, or infertility is unexplained, gamete intrafallopian transfer (GIFT) using donated eggs or sperm may be offered. It involves retrieving eggs from the woman, mixing them with sperm and quickly replacing up to three of them in the woman's fallopian tubes. If necessary the treatment can be carried out with donated sperm or eggs.

Intracytoplasmic sperm injection

Intracytoplasmic sperm injection (ICSI) means that men with very poor quality sperm or a low sperm count (fewer than 1 million per ml) will be able to father a child. However, this technique is not widely available on the National Health Service and costs £2,000 to £4,000 (1996 UK price).

Counselling and patient consent is an integral part of all patient activities. Some couples will choose to continue treatment no matter how improbable the likelihood of conception; some will choose to adopt children; others will decline further treatment and accept their infertility.

PATIENT'S PROBLEM OR NEED	EXPECTED OUTCOME FOR PATIENT	ACTION
Potential anxiety due to hospitalization and impending surgery	Patient will state he feels safe and informed about operation and will experience no excessive anxiety	1. Identify cause of anxiety by interviewing patient and provide opportunity for him to ask questions 2. Provide information about preoperative preparation using diagrams if necessary to make things clear. Inform patient where incision will be made 3. Explain about transfer to and from theatre; what to expect postoperatively with regard to dressings, discomfort and provision of analgesia and length of hospital stay (Egbert et al, 1964) 4. Check prior to theatre whether patient still wishes to go through with surgery 5. Ensure doctor has obtained written consent before administration of premedication
Correct identification of patient	Correct patient will go to theatre with correct documentation	1. Ensure medical notes, drug chart, X-ray and results are on ward and (a) are available at time of premedication, and (b) accompany patient to theatre 2. Check patient identity band against theatre request slip 3. Accompany patient to theatre
Potential injury from or loss of jewellery, dentures, contact lenses	No injury from, damage or loss of personal belongings will occur	1. Lock valuables away if patient wishes, according to hospital policy 2. Tape or remove jewellery – explain reason for doing this 3. Remove dentures, contact lenses and any prosthesis, if present 4. Ask if any teeth are loose or crowned, and record

Potential postoperative infection (e.g. urine, wound)	No signs of infection will be present	1. Take patient's temperature preoperatively, report pyrexia if present 2. Observe for any skin complaint, soreness or rash around scrotal area 3. Test urine for any abnormalities, send midstream urine specimen if indicated 4. Shower patient prior to surgery (Stokes, 1984) 5. Provide patient with clean theatre gown to change into following bath or shower
Risk of vomiting and aspiration of stomach contents	Patient will not vomit or aspirate	1. No food for 6 hours and no fluids for 4 hours prior to general anaesthesia (Hamilton Smith, 1972) 2. Ensure premedication is given as prescribed
Risk of incontinence owing to loss of voluntary muscle control while unconscious; potential bladder damage due to full bladder	Patient will remain continent	1. Ensure bowels have been open at least 24 hours prior to surgery (this will also reduce the chance of patient straining to have his bowels open postoperatively) 2. Give patient opportunity to void before premedication
Difficulty in sleeping	Patient will state that he has had a comfortable night's sleep	1. Provide environment conducive to restful sleep for individual 2. Give night sedation if prescribed and if patient wishes
Ensure skin area is prepared prior to surgery	1. Infection will not occur 2. Discomfort will be reduced when dressing is removed	1. The hair will have to be removed from the area where the incision is to be made. To reduce infection risk this should be done in theatre (Alexander et al, 1983) 2. A wide area should be shaved to reduce the chance of adhesive tape dressings being stuck to hair, which would be painful to remove
Perform baseline recordings of pulse and blood pressure prior to general anaesthesia	Postoperative pulse and blood pressure will compare favourably	1. Perform pulse and blood pressure 2. Report any abnormalities

Table 13.1   *General preoperative nursing care for patients undergoing scrotal surgery*

PATIENT'S PROBLEM OR NEED	EXPECTED OUTCOME FOR PATIENT	ACTION
Potential problems with breathing due to anaesthesia and surgical intervention	Airway will remain clear	1. Observe and ensure clear airway 2. Stay with patient until able to maintain own airway 3. Ensure suction and oxygen available 4. Observe and record respirations after 15 min, 30 min, 1 h, 2 h and 4 h. Report abnormalities 5. Administer oxygen as prescribed
Potential shock	Signs of shock will not be present	1. Observe and record pulse and blood pressure after 15 min, 30 min, 1 h, 2 h and 4 h. Observe for falling blood pressure, rising pulse 2. Observe wound site for oozing, bleeding, haematoma, swelling of scrotum 3. Report excessive oozing. Patient to remain on bed rest for at least 2 hours immediately postoperatively 4. Be aware of signs of shock 5. Change dressing as required
Potential difficulty maintaining body temperature in immediate postoperative period	Temperature will be 35.5–37.5°C	1. Observe and record temperature after 15 min, 30 min, 1 h, 2 h and 4 h. Report if outside these parameters 2. Ensure patient is not left exposed 3. Use 'space blanket' if temperature falls below 35.5°C
Potential pain or discomfort due to surgical intervention	Pain or discomfort will be controlled to a level acceptable to patient	1. Assess degree of discomfort experienced by use of verbal and non-verbal communication (Seers, 1987) 2. Position patient comfortably, ensure correct size scrotal support in situ and that it is positioned comfortably with a dressing pad to absorb any oozing from wound site 3. Give analgesia as prescribed and assess effectiveness
Potential nausea and vomiting	Patient will not feel nauseated, will not vomit	1. Observe for signs of nausea 2. Administer antiemetic as prescribed and monitor effect

		3. Supply with mouthwash, vomit bowl and tissues
		4. Commence on oral fluids and light diet as tolerated
Potential inability to eliminate urine and/or faeces normally	Patient will pass urine by 12–18 hours postoperatively	1. Explain to patient that he probably will not feel the urge to pass water for about 6–12 hours postoperatively, depending on amount of fluid intake
		2. Assist with adjusting and applying new dressing after passing urine
		3. Ensure that patient does not strain to have his bowels open
		4. Administer aperient as required as prescribed if necessary and monitor its effect
Potential difficulty meeting personal hygiene needs postoperatively	Patient will state that he feels comfortable	1. Assist with postoperative wash
		2. Ensure items available for regular oral care if patient not tolerating fluids
		3. Assist as necessary with hygiene needs, maintaining maximum independence of patient
Care of wound site, potential infection	Infection will not develop	1. Record temperature 4-hourly, report any significant pyrexia
		2. Observe wound site for oozing inflammation, large haematoma
		3. Re-dress wound site as necessary, clean with normal saline if required and apply dry dressing wool pad, then scrotal support
		4. Daily shower from day 2 postoperatively, bath from day 4. Ensure wound is dried afterwards (hairdryer may be useful)
		5. Antibiotics as prescribed (if indicated)

Table 13.2   General postoperative nursing care following scrotal surgery

PATIENT'S PROBLEM OR NEED	EXPECTED OUTCOME FOR PATIENT	ACTION
To be adequately prepared for discharge home	Patient will feel safe and secure with regard to his discharge home	1. Patient will be advised not to do anything that would cause straining around the wound site, and to perform activities being aware of his own limitations 2. In most cases sporting activities can resume 2 weeks postoperatively. In the case of vasovasostomy or orchidectomy, a 4–6 week resting period is required 3. The patient should not do any heavy lifting 4. Sexual intercourse can resume 1–2 weeks after discharge (4 weeks in case of vasovasostomy) 5. Patient advised to observe wound site daily for any changes, or signs of infection – oozing, inflammation, swelling, redness. If area appears infected, then patient advised to either contact his general practitioner (GP) or telephone the hospital and speak to his doctor or ward staff. Antibiotics may be required 6. Sutures should dissolve 7–20 days postoperatively, if dissolvable. If not, then arrangements will be made prior to discharge for the sutures to be removed by the GP 7–10 days postoperatively 7. Daily showers are recommended after 2 days and baths from day 4 8. It may be necessary to take analgesia home. The nurse will explain how frequently these should be taken. If they are not sufficient to control the pain then patient is advised to contact GP or hospital. Patient advised to continue to wear the support or supporting pants for 1–2 weeks

	9. **Antibiotics may be prescribed if the wound appears inflamed and the patient has a slightly raised temperature prior to discharge home. The nurse will explain how frequently to take the tablets and whether they should be taken before or after food, as well as any other relevant information**
Supplies of dressings	10. **The patient should be given a week's supply of dressings for discharge home. A spare scrotal support of the appropriate size, or elastic pants should be supplied**
Follow-up appointment	11. **Prior to discharge a follow-up appointment should be made for 6 weeks postoperatively, unless further specific treatment is required**
To drive a motor vehicle	1. **Driving should not be undertaken for at least 2 weeks postoperatively owing to possible strain on the scrotal area (for example caused by an emergency stop)** 2. **The patient is advised to check his driving insurance documentation as it may require him not to drive for 4 weeks postoperatively**
To return to work	**The patient should know his own limitations. If he performs strenuous work which requires heavy lifting it may be necessary to take 2–3 weeks off work; otherwise 1–2 weeks**

Table 13.3 *Discharge advice for patient following scrotal surgery*

REFERENCES

ALEXANDER J W *et al*. (1983). The influence of hair removal methods on wound infection. *Archives of Surgery* **118**: 347–352.

BAUN N (1987) Introduction: male infertility. *Postgraduate Medicine* **81**(2): 191.

BLANDY J P (1991) *Lecture notes on urology*, 4th edn. Oxford: Blackwell Scientific.

BLANDY J P and Moors J (1989) *Urology for Nurses*, 3rd edn. Oxford: Blackwell Scientific.

EGBERT L D *et al*. (1964) Reduction of post-operative pain by encouragement and instruction of patients. *New England Journal of Medicine* **170**: 285.

HAMILTON SMITH S (1972) *Nil by Mouth*? London: Royal College of Nursing.

HOWARDS S S (1987) Microsurgery for male infertility. In: *The Male Factor in Infertility: Pathophy-*

siology, Evaluation and Treatment. American Fertility Society, 20th Annual Postgraduate Course, Sept 26–27, pp 21–42.

LA NASA J A Sr and Lewis R W (1987) Varicocele and its surgical management. *Urology Clinics of North America* **14** (1): 127–135.

McCONNELL J D (1987) The role of infection in male infertility *Problems in Urology.* **1** (3): 467–475.

McNALLY M R (1987) Male infertility: endocrine causes. *Postgraduate Medicine* **81** (2): 207–213.

SEERS K (1987) Perceptions of pain. *Nursing Times* **83** (48): 37–39.

SCKOL R Z (1987) Pharmacological treatment of infertility. *Problems in Urology* **1** (3): 461–466.

STOKES K (1984) Showering before surgery, shaving before surgery. *Nursing Times* **80** (20): 71.

FURTHER READING

KARLOWICZ K A (1995) *Urologic Nursing Principles and Practice.* London: WB Saunders.

SCOTT R T and Russell L (1983) *Urology Illustrated*, 2nd edn. Edinburgh: Churchill Livingstone.

STURDY D E (1986) *An Outline of Urology.* Bristol: Wright.

REASSIGNMENT SURGERY

Contents

'Sexual body image is probably more to do with what we believe we are than in the physical attributes we possess' (Price, 1986)

WHAT IS TRANSSEXUALISM?

A transsexual is an individual who feels an overwhelming need to function and live in the opposite sex to which he or she is born biologically. A female–male transsexual feels that she is a man trapped inside a woman's body. A male–female transsexual feels that he is a woman trapped inside a man's body. The factors that make up sexual identity are set out in Table 14.1.

The World Health Organization (1992) and the American Psychiatric Association (1994) both identify criteria considered essential to procure a diagnosis.

Prevalence

Transsexualism is a relatively uncommon condition, but is all-important to the person in whom it exists. There are approximately 25,000 transsexuals in Britain, of whom 40% are female to male. When considering the recorded rate of transsexualism, one must be aware that many of these individuals live out their lives without ever declaring their transsexualism, and thus exact incidence and prevalence are difficult to establish (see for example, Thomas, 1993).

> *Psychological*
> **Gender identity (sense of being male or female)**
> **Social sex role (masculiniity or femininity)**
> **Public sex role (living or dressing as a male or female)**
> **Sexual orientation (homosexual, heterosexual, transsexual)**
> **Sex of rearing (brought up as a male or female)**
>
> *Biological*
> **Genetic (presence or absence of Y chromosome)**
> **Gonadal (histological structure of ovary or testes)**
> **Hormonal function (circulating hormones)**
> **Interior genital morphology (presence or absence of male or female internal structures)**
> **External genital morphology (presence or absence of male or female genitalia)**
> **Secondary sexual characteristics (body hair, breasts, fat distribution)**

From Walters and Ross (1986)

Table 14.1   *Components of sexual identity*

Aetiology

In 1954 Harry Benjamin, a pioneer in transsexual research, coined the term 'gender role disorientation', which is now commonly called gender dysphoria – a disturbance of gender identity. Transsexualism, it is argued, is a symptom of this underlying disorder. Two main theories attempt to explain transsexualism:

1. The gender and sexual identity of an individual are dependent on physical identification at birth and the subsequent rearing and socialization ('sex of rearing') (Moir and Jessel, 1991).
2. The gender and sexual identity of an individual are biological in nature and dependent on hormonally induced differentiation of the brain at a critical period of intrauterine development.

Onset

The onset of transsexuality may be either:

1. *Primary* – occurring during the first 10 years of life when the child begins to feel that he or she is different, identifying as a member of the opposite sex. This feeling remains constant throughout adolescence and into adulthood.
2. *Secondary* – transsexuals may always have been aware of some gender disturbance throughout life, but manage to suppress it until it is brought to the fore by problems such as divorce, ageing, death or failure.

A realization phase, when the child becomes aware of his or her identification with the opposite gender, then leads to an attempt at cross-dressing. This is usually followed by an attempt to assume a gender identity consistent with the biological sex (i.e. a formal denial of the individual's transsexualism). This may include taking an overtly masculine or feminine job (e.g. bricklaying in the case of a male) and the formation of heterosexual relationships which may end in marriage, which often fails to succeed owing to the suppression of transsexualism.

Medical advice may be sought for symptoms such as depression, anxiety or sexual dysfunction which are all indirectly related to the transsexualism of the individual.

Presentation

Two possible courses of action are open for the individual diagnosed as transsexual:

1. To accept their life according to their biological sex.
2. To seek gender reassignment.

Biological sex is determined by an individual's chromosomes and therefore it is not possible to have a 'sex change' in the true meaning of the phrase (this fact has legal consequences for the transsexual, discussed later in this chapter). What can be achieved are different aspects of gender reassignment – namely social, hormonal and surgical. If successful, these represent a reasonable external attempt at 'sex change'.

Before embarking on a scheme of management it is important to assess the individual's commitment to the proposed new identity. For example, is the problem really lifelong and fundamental, or may it possibly be transient? Is the individual fully aware of the extent of the readjustment that will be required? Such questions have to be faced and discussed in detail. If the ultimate goal of the transsexual is gender reassignment surgery, then referral by a general practitioner to a gender identity clinic (GIC) or a psychiatrist specializing in gender issues is desirable. The main function of the GIC is to establish that the individual is genuinely transsexual before embarking on the complicated procedure for changing gender roles.

Transsexual management begins with the encouragement of appropriate behaviour patterns for the adopted sex. The booklet 'Standards of Care' (Benjamin, 1953) insists on a period of 2 years continuous 'cross-gender living' to establish that the individual can function within the preferred gender. This first-hand experience of living, working and dressing in the chosen role is very important in proving commitment.

Cross-dressing for females is made easier by the bisexual clothing available. It has been shown that if one is given a silhouette or back view of a person to look at, the majority of people will automatically say that the silhouette is male. The male gender is applied to most people until proved otherwise. Cross-dressing for males may be more difficult owing to the larger body frame, masculine voice and beard.

Hormone therapy can be prescribed by the individual's general practitioner on the advice of the consultant psychiatrist specializing in gender issues (though many transsexuals may already be taking hormones, illicitly purchased or obtained from friends). For females, the male hormone testosterone may be prescribed. This can be given in tablet form, e.g. Restandol which is taken daily usually in divided doses. Alternatively, it can be given by monthly intramuscular injections, e.g. Sustanon, or by testosterone implant. As a result of hormone therapy, the following physical changes may occur:

- voice deepens
- increase in body and facial hair
- menstruation is suppressed
- body weight increases because muscle mass increases and subcutaneous fat deposits decrease
- clitoral enlargement
- libido increases

Hormone therapy will not increase body size (bone structure) unless it is taken before puberty.

For males the female hormone oestrogen is given (e.g. Premarin, ethinyloestradiol). This will:

- decrease and soften body hair
- soften and improve facial skin
- promote growth of breasts (gynaecomastia)
- cause testicular atrophy
- promote changes in body contours by laying down subcutaneous fat with a subsequent reduction in muscle bulk
- cause reduction in libido
- cause cessation of erections

Hormone therapy will not alter the tone or pitch of the male voice. For most male or female transsexuals, one of the biggest problems is hiding facial hair growth. Oestrogens will make a subtle difference to beard growth, but cyproterone acetate (an antiandrogen) may be needed to retard growth further. Many individuals spend thousands of pounds on facial electrolysis, which is not available as a National Health Service treatment.

Hormone therapy cannot change the original body structure, especially in relation to hands, feet and height. Thus, a small woman becomes a small man; a large man becomes a large woman.

Legal issues

For successful cross-gender living, it is usually necessary for transsexuals to change their name either by statutory declaration or by deed poll. The services of a solicitor will be required to do this.

After a change of name, an individual will be in a position to change every official record *except* the birth certificate. These records include:

- National Insurance record
- income tax

- driving licence
- medical card
- passport
- electricity, gas and phone bills
- insurance policies
- examination records

Birth certificate

The Registrar General has the power to order a complete entry to be altered if satisfied that there has been an error of fact or substance in relation to a birth. The entry is a record of the facts at the time of the birth. As long as a transsexual's sex is determined by biological criteria only at the time of birth, the Registrar General does not have the power to make an alteration regarding gender. British courts maintain that gender is determined at birth – a view that has recently been upheld by the European Court. In the future this may change as attitudes towards transsexual identity become more sympathetic. The inability to alter the birth certificate means that the following are affected.

Marriage

A female to male or male to female transsexual who has undergone surgery cannot marry. In English law, marriage is regarded as a relationship between a man and a woman. Marriage between a female transsexual and her male partner can be prevented by the law using biological criteria. A female transsexual will regard a biological and psychological female as a member of the opposite sex but they cannot marry as the law regards them both as female. However, a male transsexual living as a woman can marry a female transsexual living as a man. Many transsexuals go abroad to marry where birth certificates are not required for marriage.

Prison

Should transsexuals commit crimes in this country they could be sent to a prison determined by their original gender. A female to male transsexual could be sent to a female prison. At the discretion of the prison doctor hormone therapy may be discontinued.

Pensions

Under existing legislation in the UK, which is currently being reviewed, a female to male transsexual should retire at 60 years old. A male to female transsexual would not be entitled to a state pension until 65 years old.

Life insurance

Transsexual status must be declared on life insurance policies. Failure to do so may result in non-payment of benefit. It has come to the author's attention that a major insurance company doubled a client's premium on admission of gender dysphoria, on the advice of their medical officer.

Employment

The Sex Discrimination Act 1975 and the Equal Pay Act 1970 prohibit discrimination on the grounds of sex in places of employment. However, sex refers to the original biological sex, therefore discrimination against transsexuals is not unlawful under these Acts. Many employers are becoming sensitive to issues surrounding their transsexual employees and are seeking help and advice from professionals working in this field.

Social issues

The transsexual must accept the possibility of permanently losing family and friends when they are informed of forthcoming changes. People will react differently, unfortunately often with anger, disbelief, guilt, shame and embarrassment. Counselling for the transsexual's family may be necessary. Of course, some transsexuals are fortunate to retain the support of family and friends. Many transsexuals find help and support from specialized organizations and make friends with other transsexuals who understand the difficulties and can thus offer advice regarding achieving a more successful cosmetic appearance.

In many cases, in order to accomplish a successful social reassignment transsexuals may be forced to move away from home in order to start afresh in their new identity.

To be considered for surgery it is essential that the individual is either in employment, a full-time student or undertakes regular voluntary service. However, the transsexual may have difficulties in securing appropriate employment. Where the employer is sympathetic and work is appropriate to either gender then a problem may not arise; on the other hand, it may be necessary to seek alternative employment.

SURGICAL TREATMENT

Criteria qualifying transsexuals for surgical treatment include:

- age – surgeons may insist on an age minimum and maximum, e.g. 21–58 years
- successful endocrine masculinization or feminization
- 1–3 years of total cross-living and working in the gender of choice
- success in social, psychological, employment and sexual spheres
- freedom from psychosis or significant sociopathy

Female to male gender reassignment surgery

Female to male gender reassignment surgery consists of:

- bilateral mastectomy (this may well be done without intention to have further surgery)
- hysterectomy and salpingo-oophorectomy
- phalloplasty (construction of penis)

Bilateral mastectomy

Bilateral simple mastectomy is performed, preserving the nipples.

Preoperative management

Management of this procedure varies considerably between surgical departments. It is now commonly undertaken by surgeons specializing in breast augmentation and reduction, which gives improved cosmetic results. Individuals are admitted as a male to the male ward, or to a single room if requested (and one is available). Preoperative nursing assessment is undertaken using the model of nursing practised within the area. A full explanation is given regarding surgery and informed consent obtained.
Investigations include:

- full blood count
- group and cross-match 2 units of blood

Postoperative care

Postoperative care is as for any patient following general anaesthesia and surgery.

Specific nursing care

A pressure dressing is strapped across the chest. This remains in position for approximately 48 hours and helps reduce swelling and bruising. A vacuum drain is in situ and is removed when there is minimal drainage. Sutures are usually dissolvable and therefore will not require removal.

Complications

- *Scarring* – if scarring is present it can often be hidden by chest hair growth.
- *Haematoma* – return to theatre may be necessary for drainage.
- *Necrosis of nipple* – the nipple blackens and sloughs.
- *Infection* – if signs and symptoms of infection occur a wound swab should be taken and sent for microbiological culture, and appropriate antibiotic treatment prescribed if indicated.

Hysterectomy and salpingo-oophorectomy

Hysterectomy and salpingo-oophorectomy involve the surgical removal of the uterus, fallopian tubes and ovaries.

Preoperative management

Preoperative nursing assessment is undertaken using the model of nursing practised within the area. A full explanation is given regarding surgery and informed consent obtained.

Investigations include:

- full blood count
- group and cross-match 2 units of blood

Postoperative care

As for any patient following a general anaesthesia and abdominal surgery.

Many female to male transexxuals do not proceed beyond the above two procedures, particularly in the UK.

Phalloplasty

In the UK the procedure to construct a phallus has been modified over the years. Techniques include:

- Gillies' phalloplasty (Figure 14.1) – this involved several stages of surgery and repeated admissions to hospital over a period of approximately 12 months:

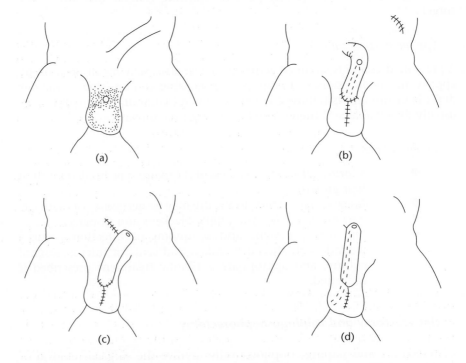

Figure 14.1 *Gillies' phalloplasty*

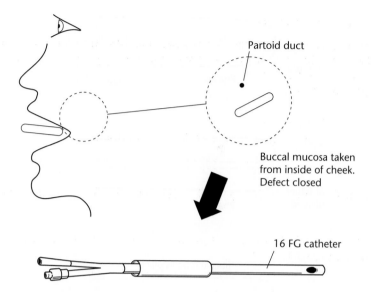

Partoid duct

Buccal mucosa taken from inside of cheek. Defect closed

16 FG catheter

Figure 14.2 *Buccal phalloplasty: buccal mucosa is taken from the inside of the cheek, and formed into a tube over a 16 FG catheter. (D Ralph, personal communication, 1996)*

stage 1 is formation of the neourethra
stage 2 is the formation of the tube flap
stage 3 is detachment of the pedicle from the iliac crest
stage 4 is detachment of pedicle completely to form the phallus (Gillies and Millard, 1957)
Gillies' phalloplasty is no longer used.

◆ Clitoral phalloplasty – a one-stage procedure. Abdominal flaps are raised from abdominal skin; the existing urethra is extended to the tip of the clitoris and clitoral skin is then used to extend the urethra futher.

◆ Pubic phalloplasty – a two-stage procedure involving phalloplasty and urethroplasty. A clitoral-based suprapubic flap and a pedicled labial neourethra are used.

◆ Buccal phalloplasty – a recent technique, primarily used to repair stricture in the pubic phalloplasty. Buccal mucosa is taken from inside the cheek, avoiding the parotid duct, and formed into a tube over a 16 FG catheter. The stricture is divided and the buccal tube placed in the phallus (Figures 14.2 and 14.3). More recently the buccal tube has been used as a primary procedure with the phallus created as in the pubic or clitoral phalloplasty.

The aim of surgery is to produce a phallus that is functional in that the 'male' can stand to void. The construction of the male urethra is a complex aspect of this surgery and there is the risk of both stricture and fistula formation. Nothing like the erectile function of the normal penis can be achieved, but at future surgery it is possible to implant Silastic penile prostheses which will then allow for penetration during sexual intercourse.

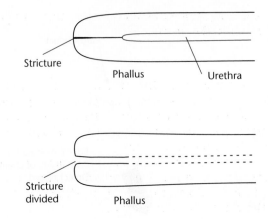

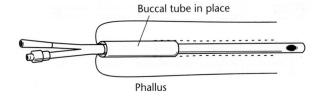

Figure 14.3 *Buccal phalloplasty: the stricture is excised and the buccal tube inserted. (D Ralph, personal communication, 1996)*

Preoperative management

Preoperative nursing assessment is undertaken using the model of nursing practised within the area. A full explanation is given regarding what the patient can expect preoperatively and postoperatively. Informed consent is obtained. Surgery will have been discussed at length prior to admission at an outpatient consultation.

Investigations include:

◆ full blood count
◆ group and cross-match 2 units of blood

Postoperative care

Postoperative care is as for any patient following general anaesthesia and surgery.

Specific nursing care

Pain should be well controlled so as to promote mobility. A continuous opioid infusion is useful for the first 48 hours.

Wound

One or more vacuum drains should remain in situ until drainage is minimal. Prophylactic antibiotics are given according to local protocols. The wound is observed for signs of infection. It is particularly important to notice any discolouration, e.g. darkening along the suture line, as there is a potential risk of breakdown of the wound due to necrosis.

Catheters

The urethral catheter acts as a stent within the neourethra and is left in situ for up to 3 weeks. It is important that the catheter is well supported to avoid traction which could damage the neourethra. There is also a risk of urinary tract infection, therefore the individual must be encouraged to maintain an adequate fluid intake (2–3 litres in 24 hours).

A urethrogram is performed prior to removal of the catheter; this is done in the radiography department. Contrast dye is inserted via the catheter and the patient asked to void. Any leakage from the neourethra is demonstrated. If there is no leakage the catheter can be removed.

Complications

Complications include:

- infection
- fistula
- necrosis of phallus
- stricture of the neourethra
- expectations not realized

The patient undergoing gender reassignment surgery is vulnerable and needs considerable psychological support. Just being there and having the time and interest to listen and talk with the individual is very important, for both the patient and the nurse.

Male to female gender reassignment surgery

In addition to surgical reassignment of the genitalia, many male to female transsexuals will have had surgery such as:

- orchidectomy
- rhinoplasty
- thyroid chondroplasty (shaving of the Adam's apple)
- breast augmentation
- genoplasty (reducing jaw line)
- vaginoplasty (construction of vagina)
- penectomy (removal of penis)
- clitoroplasty (construction of clitoris from tip of penis)

These operations may be obtained on the NHS on the referral of the psychiatrist, though many transsexuals choose private treatment to avoid long waiting lists for non-emergency operations.

Surgical reassignment of genitalia

Patients are preferably admitted to a single room on a mixed urology ward. Preoperative nursing assessment is undertaken using the model of nursing used within the area. A full explanation of the procedure is given to allay any worries and provide a rationale for care. Informed consent is obtained using a special consent form which specifies that the patient consents to the removal of his penis and testicles, and realizes that this will not change his biological sex but will allow him to live more comfortably in his chosen role (a sobering thought for anyone not committed to this type of surgery).

Investigations and preparations include:

◆ full blood count – urea and electrolytes
◆ group and cross-match 2 units of blood
◆ shaving of hair as close to the time of surgery as possible, or in the theatre itself

Preoperative care

The preoperative care for male to female gender reassignment surgery is directly related to the prevention of certain postoperative problems. The patient is admitted 2 days prior to surgery and commenced on fluids only. An enema is given to completely empty the bowel on the day before surgery and the patient will be given nil by mouth for 6 hours prior to surgery.

Hormone therapy must be discontinued 1 month prior to admission. Anti-embolic stockings and/or prophylactic heparin should be given. A bath and a shave from umbilicus to mid-thigh should be carried out by the patient and checked by a nurse. It must be remembered that the transsexual is usually very embarrassed about his penis and testes, so the nurse must exercise tact here. Prophylactic antibiotic therapy is commenced on the day prior to surgery.

Surgical procedure

The operation takes 4–5 hours with the patient in the lithotomy position. The spermatic cords are transfixed and the testicles removed. The skin covering the penis and its underlying fascia is undermined and the penis is pulled out of its skin. The skin is kept intact and later pushed 'inside out' to become the lining of the neovagina. The penis is pulled upwards, and with a urethral catheter in situ, is amputated at its roots. Dissection is carried out upwards and backwards from the root of the penis into the pelvic peritoneum, in order to create a space for the neovagina. Care must be taken not to dissect too close to the rectum as this can result in a rectovaginal fistula.

The scrotal sac is dissected to form the labia, and skilled surgeons are able to construct a neoclitoris from the tip of the penis. The neovagina is sutured in place and packed with ribbon gauze. Two wound drains are then inserted. A second outer pack is applied to the vaginal and perineal areas and a tight T-bandage applied.

Postoperative care

Postoperative care is as for any patient following general anaesthesia and surgery; specific nursing problems related to the nature of the operation include:

1. *Partial prolapse of neovagina* – the neovagina is tightly packed with ribbon gauze to promote healing. Bed rest is strictly maintained for 5 days, and all food is also withheld for 5 days to prevent any bowel movement which might cause a neovaginal prolapse. Clear fluids only are allowed and nothing which will act as a bowel stimulant (e.g. cigarettes or coffee) is given. These 5 days are very difficult for the patient, and the temptation to sneak out of bed for some food may be too much for some. The nurse must provide reassurance and try to divert the patient's attention from food wherever possible.

2. *Potential shock and haemorrhage* – an intravenous infusion is usually given for the first 24 hours, after which time the patient should take clear fluids. Routine postoperative observations are made. Special care is taken to check the bleeding from the wound site. The vagina is packed for 5 days and a pressure dressing in the form of meniscectomy wool with two tight T-bandages is applied. If oozing occurs the wool may be changed. The two wound drains are removed after 48 hours. The inner vaginal pack must not be removed.

3. *Potential infection of wound area* – the urethra is amputated during surgery and as a result may swell considerably. A urethral catheter is passed before surgery commences and remains in situ for 5 days afterwards. In some units chymotrypsin is given orally to reduce swelling at the urethral meatus. When the urethral catheter is removed, a guiding suture is left in place in case the patient develops urinary retention, necessitating the passing of a further catheter. Patients should be warned that for some months postoperatively they may experience 'spraying' of urine on voiding, owing to the surgical refashioning of the urethral meatus.

4. *Potential closure of neovagina* – the internal pack stays in place for 5 days and is moved only by an experienced nurse or the surgeon. When the pack and the catheter have been removed the patient must be taught to dilate the vagina. The dilator is twisted into position gently, after lubrication with K-Y jelly, and retained for 10 minutes. It is necessary for the patient to use a Perspex dilator three times a day. This is carried out for several months until the surgeon is satisfied that sexual intercourse can be initiated. While the patient is having regular sexual intercourse the need to dilate is avoided.

5. *Potential risk of deep vein thrombosis and pulmonary embolism* – this is increased by pelvic surgery, bed rest and excess of the hormone oestrogen. Active and passive exercise of the limbs and deep breathing exercises are important in the prevention of these life-threatening problems. Correctly fitted thromboembolism deterrent stockings (TEDS) should be worn, and subcutaneous heparin given.

6. *Anxiety* – the patient is usually very anxious to see the new vagina. It is important that the patient is prepared for the swelling, which may make it unsightly for the first few weeks. The stitches in the refashioned labia are removed on day 7, prior to discharge, and the patient may need reassurance that the neovagina will have a 'normal' appearance. In fact, after about 6 weeks when pubic hair has regrown, the results are usually very good. Some patients worry greatly about the depth of the vagina: this is usually 15–20 cm, which should be satisfactory for sexual intercourse. Further surgery may be required to increase the length of the vagina. The vagina can be augmented using colon to form a

colovaginoplasty. There may be some anxiety about the process of dilating, which will need a tactful and understanding approach from the nurse.

Discharge

The patient is usually discharged on the seventh postoperative day, after removal of the sutures. The patient is instructed to use a douche (or shower) daily and a povidone-iodine pessary is used once a week for 10 weeks. The patient is advised to avoid constipation because of the risk of prolapse, and to continue the dilation (in the event of a prolapse, a colovaginal repair may be undertaken using a piece of colon to form the vagina).

The patient may restart hormone treatment 2 weeks after surgery, which is usually a great relief as facial hair may have started to regrow. Patients are advised not to do any heavy lifting for 6 weeks and to avoid sexual inter-course until after their outpatient appointment. Following surgery, some patients may continue to see their psychiatrist.

Some patients may need to have follow-up surgery such as vaginal lengthening, refashioning of the urethra or labial reduction, but most appear happy with the results and in the author's experience seldom require further surgical treatment.

Once the site is healed and has been seen by the surgeon, the patient is free to have sexual intercourse. The use of K-Y jelly is recommended as there is no natural lubrication within the neovagina. Many patients are able to reach orgasm as nerve endings are, whenever possible, left intact during surgery.

CONCLUSION

The reluctance of some surgeons to become involved in gender reassignment surgery is understandable, as it can be perceived as very mutilating to an otherwise healthy body. There is also the question of whether surgery should be performed on the National Health Service or regarded in the same light as private cosmetic surgery, which would probably render the surgery out of reach for most transsexuals.

There remains a general lack of social awareness and tolerance of the many problems encountered by transsexuals, who are unfortunately regarded by many as social oddities. Public confusion between transsexuality and homo-sexuality is common. Far more media attention has been given to transsexuals in recent years. Loss of civil liberties (Gooren, 1993; McMullen and Whittle, 1994) is still of great concern to those involved in transsexual groups. There is no reason, legally, socially, psychologically or medically why any transsexual who has changed gender role should receive any less respect and understanding than any other individual. Female to male trans-sexuals were virtually unheard of in the media until relatively recently. Often in an attempt to pass as 'normal', the transsexual may somewhat overem-phasize masculine or feminine characteristics (e.g. a male to female transsex-ual may overapply makeup), and sadly, this may then allow them to be 'read' (exposed), leading to embarrassment. However, it may also be said that, in the author's experience, there are many transsexuals who have no difficulty in promoting an extremely credible gender image.

A high degree of nursing professionalism is the right of every individual requiring nursing care. Individuals undergoing gender reassignment require a great deal of emotional and psychological support. Transsexuals are often very willing to talk about their problems, sometimes to anyone who comes to listen, and they will often do so in graphic detail. Nurses must be comfortable with their own sexuality in order to help transsexuals cope with theirs. Junior nurses may need the help of a more experienced nurse when dealing for the first time with individuals undergoing gender reassignment. If the nurse's feelings regarding gender reassignment interfere and are detrimental to the patient's care, then the nurse should not be put in the position of caring for such a patient. However, nurses who are willing to be open-minded may well find that caring for a patient having reassignment surgery is both an enlightening and a rewarding experience.

REFERENCES

AMERICAN PSYCHIATRIC ASSOCIATION (1994) *Diagnostic and Statistical Manual of Mental Disorders*, 4th edn. American Psychiatric Association.

BENJAMIN H (1953) Transvestism, transsexualism. *Journal of Sex Research* **5** (2): 13.

GILLIES H and Millard D R (1957) *The Principles and Art of Plastic Surgery*, vol. 1, pp. 370–71. London: Butterworth.

GOOREN L J G (1993) Biological aspects of transsexualism and their relevance to its legal aspects. *Proceedings of the 33rd Colloquy on European Law: Transsexualism, Medicine and the Law.* Strasbourg: Council of Europe.

McMULLEN M and Whittle S (1994) *Transvestism, Transsexualism and the Law.* London: Gender Trust.

MOIR A and Jessel D (1991) *Brainsex.* London: Mandarin.

PRICE R (1986) The range of factors affecting body image. *Nursing Times* **82** (39): 30–32.

THOMAS B (1993) Gender loving care. *Nursing Times* **89** (10): 50–51.

WALTERS W and Ross M (eds) (1986) *Transsexualism and Sex Reassignment.* Oxford University Press.

WORLD HEALTH ORGANIZATION (1992) *International Classification of Disorders.* Geneva: WHO.

PAEDIATRIC UROLOGY

15

Contents

INTRODUCTION

The major difference in nursing care between general surgical and urological patients is probably the inevitable presence of various drainage tubes. Training nurses to care for children who are encumbered with an assortment of catheters takes time and patience but can be very rewarding. It is important that the nurse knows the different types of catheter available, the reasoning behind a particular choice, the anatomical position, whether the catheter should or should not be draining – and why. It is vital to teach nurses the best way of securing catheters to prevent accidental removal and drainage failures (e.g. kinking of tubing), particularly as children are very determined and inquisitive and do not always understand the consequences of their actions.

Parents of children with congenital abnormalities require support, understanding, information and teaching to enable them to come to terms with their child's condition and help them face the future with courage and hope – a future that often seems to them to be an endless round of waiting, appointments, investigations, hospitalizations and periods of despair. It is often essential to have parents or carers resident in hospital prior to the discharge of their child to ensure that they are confident and competent to look after any appliances or long-term drainage systems such as suprapubic catheters or nephrostomy tubes. Some of the conditions are so rare that the family receives little or no assistance from the community – not because people do not want to provide it, but simply through ignorance. This can be a frightening situation for parents, particularly if they live a long distance from the hospital.

The management of infants and children with genitourinary abnormalities has been revolutionized by several factors. These include:

- ◆ the introduction of clean intermittent self-catheterization by Lapides in the 1970s (Lapides *et al.*, 1972)
- ◆ new surgical techniques which concentrate on creating a continent urinary diversion using bowel to augment or replace the bladder
- ◆ improvements in paediatric anaesthesia permitting earlier surgical intervention
- ◆ advances in antenatal ultrasonography, radiological and urodynamic investigations
- ◆ well-informed and motivated nursing staff

The genitourinary system is the most common site of congenital abnormalities. The delicate and embarrassing nature of genitourinary problems has enormous implications in the psychological, emotional, physical and social development of children. The paediatric urological nurse may care for these children in a variety of settings – during the initial presentation when the child may be acutely ill, during investigations, in the outpatient clinic, before, during and following surgery; nurses must therefore have a working knowledge of the complexities of different conditions to fulfil their responsibilities to educate, advise and care for these children and their families.

EMBRYOLOGY OF THE GENITALIA

The majority of paediatric genitourinary conditions are due to congenital abnormalities; therefore it is important to understand the normal development of the internal sexual organs and external genitalia.

The early fetus has the potential to develop both male and female internal sexual organs (Figure 15.1). The müllerian duct can develop into the uterus, fallopian tube and upper vagina. The wolffian duct can develop into the vas deferens, seminal vesicles and ejaculatory ducts. The müllerian duct appears to develop normally in the absence of any oestrogenic or hormonal stimulation; however, the development of the wolffian duct is stimulated by testerone which is secreted by the fetal testis. A second hormone is secreted by the fetal testis – a large molecular weight protein – which causes regression of the müllerian duct. The continuation of an 'androgen milieu' leads to the development of male external genitalia. Prior to this differentiation the external genitalia are the same regardless of genetic sex (Figure 15.2).

The testosterone from the fetal testis probably needs to be converted by 5-alpha reductase into dihydrotestosterone for the continuing normal development of male external genitalia. The testis descends from its original position in the abdomen to its final position in the scrotum by the seventh or eighth month. This descent is also dependent on the normal development of the scrotum and on other hormonal mechanisms not yet identified.

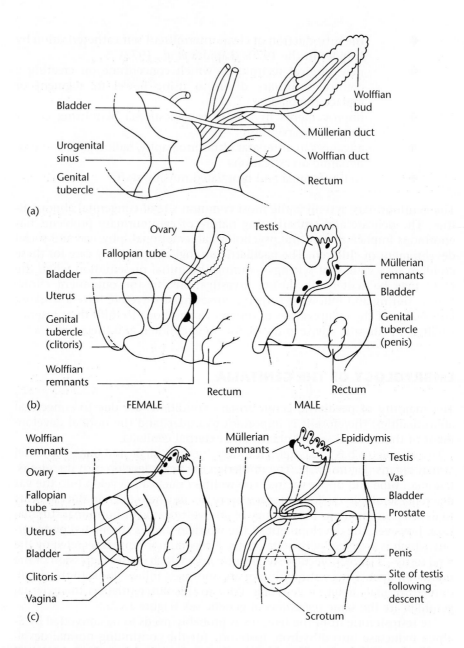

Figure 15.1 *Fetal sexual development, transverse view: (a) undifferentiated, 8–10 weeks; (b) differentiation at 12–16 weeks; (c) fully developed sexual organs*

ABSENT OR ABNORMAL DIFFERENTIATION OF THE KIDNEYS

Renal agenesis

The incidence of a child being born with no kidneys is approximately 1 in 3,000, and the child is either stillborn or may only survive for a few days. As well as the absence of kidneys, the ureters, bladder and urethra may be

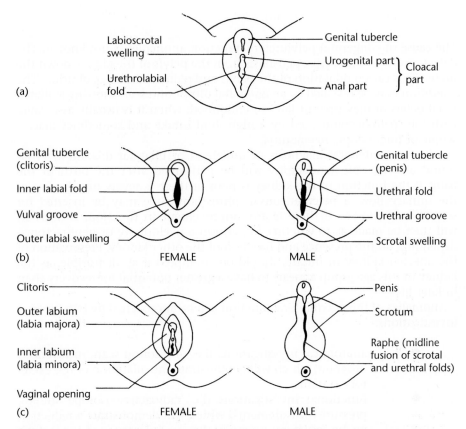

Figure 15.2 *Fetal sexual development, anterior view: (a) undifferentiated, 8–10 weeks; (b) differentiation at 12–16 weeks; (c) fully developed sexual organs*

affected. The child has the typical Potter's facies of low-set ears, flattened nose and wide-set eyes as well as hypoplastic lungs owing to the absence of fetal urine.

Unilateral renal agenesis is more common, affecting between 1 in 500 and 1 in 1,000 of the population. The absence of one kidney may go unnoticed unless the child is being investigated for renal trauma or urinary tract infections. Treatment should only be necessary if the kidney has associated anomalies.

Fused (horseshoe) kidneys

Fusion of the two kidneys across the midline occurs most commonly in males, with an incidence of 1 in 600 to 1 in 1,800. Usually the discovery of a horseshoe kidney in a neonate is associated with other congenital abnormalities; however, complications may occur later in life with obstruction, calculi or reflux.

Pelviureteric junction anomalies

The cause of congenital pelviureteric junction anomalies is not known. The defect results in ineffective peristalsis from the pelvis of the kidney down the ureter. This causes dilatation of the pelvis and reduced drainage of urine. The condition may be revealed by an antenatal ultrasound scan showing a dilated renal pelvis or may present later in childhood, when it is usually associated with loin pain accompanied by a high fluid intake and sometimes macroscopic or microscopic haematuria.

Following antenatal diagnosis of unilateral or bilateral dilatation, ultrasound and isotopic renography will be performed after the birth of the baby. If the function of the kidney is poor or there is severe impairment of the urinary flow, a percutaneous nephrostomy tube may be inserted for several weeks to see if there is any improvement in function. A decision will then be made as to whether to perform a pyeloplasty or nephrectomy, depending on the presence and function of the other kidney. Preservation of the affected kidney in infants should be attempted if at all feasible, as the kidney in this age group appears to have a greater potential for recovery than in later life.

Anomalies of the pelviureteric junction can be approached by two types of investigations:

- ◆ anatomical investigations (i.e. ultrasound scan, intravenous urogram) which will demonstrate the dilatation of the excretory system
- ◆ functional investigations (i.e. radioactive isotope studies, pressure measurements) which will demonstrate a reduction of the ipsilateral function, deficient clearance of the isotope and a possible increase of pressure in the renal pelvis

If the differential function of the affected kidney is less than 10% and the other kidney shows good function and no obstruction, then a nephrectomy may be considered. If the function of the affected kidney is reasonable then a pyeloplasty is preferred.

Pyeloplasty involves the refashioning or widening of the pelvis of the kidney at the junction of the ureter and the excision of the abnormal pelviureteric junction. Depending on the anomaly and the surgeon's preference, a transanastomotic stent will be left in situ for up to 10 days to avoid leakage through the anastomosis; some patients will have a urethral catheter and/or a suction wound drain. The order of removal of these tubes and drains depends on the surgeon's preference.

Complications following a pyeloplasty include urine leakage, haemorrhage, clot retention and stenosis at the anastomosis site, either in the immediate postoperative period or in the long term. For this reason follow-up is by means of ultrasound scans and isotope renography at 3 months, 6 months and 1 year postoperatively.

URETERIC CONDITIONS

Duplication of the ureter

There are various forms of ureteric duplication which, depending on the complexity, will depend on the severity of the child's symptoms and treatment. Duplication of the pelvis of the kidney and ureter are more common in girls and are frequently bilateral.

The simplest form is duplication of the pelvis of the kidney with partial duplication of the ureters (Figure 15.3). Problems associated with this form of duplication include a 'yo-yo' or 'see-saw' movement of urine from one pole to the other, leading to stasis of urine and associated infections. If investigations such as isotope renography show that severe renal scarring has taken place then a heminephrectomy may be considered – usually removing the upper pole.

Complete simple duplication is where two ureters enter the bladder separately (Figure 15.4). Where this occurs the upper pole ureter always enters the bladder below that of the lower pole. Vesicoureteric reflux is common, especially into the lower pole, and if recurrent severe urine infections are a problem then a heminephrectomy may be performed.

Symptoms of urine infections with or without outflow obstruction, especially in girls, may lead the surgeon to discover an ectopic ureter with a ureterocele (Figure 15.5). This abnormality occurs seven times more frequently in females and in 10% of cases is bilateral. A ureterocele is a bulbous dilatation at the terminal submucosal end of the ureter, which may be large enough to cause outflow obstruction. In girls, prolapse of the ureterocele may occur and the abnormality may be visible on perineal examination.

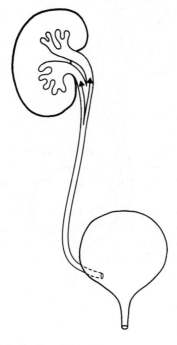

Figure 15.3 *Simple partial duplication of the ureter*

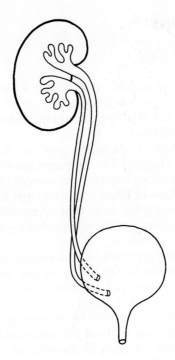

Figure 15.4 *Simple complete duplication of the ureter*

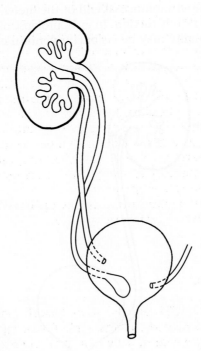

Figure 15.5 *Ectopic ureterocele*

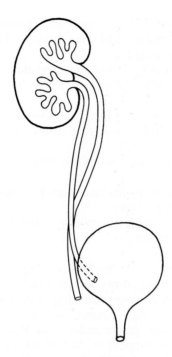

Figure 15.6 *Ectopic ureter opening outside the bladder*

Treatment will depend on the severity and complexity of the abnormality and will vary from endoscopic incision of the ureterocele to excision of the ureterocele by open surgery with or without partial nephrectomy.

Ureteroceles may also occur without ureteric duplication and treatment is similar, with either endoscopic incision or formal excision of the ureterocele.

Another way in which a child may present with a duplex urinary system with ectopic ureters is by persistent incontinence in females and chronic epididymitis in males. In females this is due to one of the ectopic ureters opening into the urethra below the sphincter, or into the vagina or vulva. The child presents with a history of continuous wetting, despite normal voiding, and having never been 'dry'. Rarely in boys, problems of recurrent epididymitis may be caused by an ectopic ureter draining into the posterior urethra, vas, seminal vesicle or ejaculatory duct.

Treatment is by partial nephrectomy – removing the pole of the kidney that is draining into the affected ureter (Figure 15.6).

Vesicoureteric reflux

Urinary tract infections (UTI) are the second most common infections in children. Investigations carried out on a child following a UTI may reveal a congenital abnormality which may need surgical intervention.

Vesicoureteric reflux (VUR) is the abnormal backflow of urine from the bladder into the ureters and/or the kidneys. Between 30% and 50% of children presenting with a UTI have urinary anomalies, the most frequent being VUR. At birth and in infancy the oblique angle at which the ureters enter the bladder may not be well developed; during normal growth of a child, the base of the bladder and trigone mature and the submucosal tunnel of the ureters may lengthen and so reflux ceases.

An accepted grading system for reflux was formulated by the Birmingham Reflux Study Group (1983) who classified reflux as follows:

VUR grade I   – backflow into the lower ureter(s)
VUR grade II – backflow filling but not distending ureter(s) and pelvi-calyceal system
VUR grade III – backflow filling and mildly distending ureter(s) and renal pelvis
VUR grade IV – backflow filling and moderately distending ureter(s), renal pelvis and calyces
VUR grade V   – backflow filling and grossly distending ureter(s) and pelvi-calyceal system

Diagnosis and grading is generally made following a micturating cystoure-throgram (MCU); other investigations include plain abdominal X-ray, ultra-sonography and static radioisotope scanning. Controversy surrounds the issue of MCU because of its invasive nature and the attendant risk of infec-tion – however, it remains the 'gold standard' for diagnosis.

Treatment of VUR is either surgical or medical with the aim of preventing or limiting renal damage. Recent studies have confirmed that medical man-agement is preferable in low-grade VUR (grades I to III). Surgery is indicated in grades IV and V and in lower grades if there are breakthrough infections or worsening reflux. It is generally accepted that there is a 70% chance of spontaneous cessation, but a 95% chance of surgical cure. When making a decision on treatment options the condition of the child and social circum-stances should be considered along with the grade of reflux.

Conservative treatment uses antibiotics commonly prescribed to treat acute infections – trimethoprim, nitrofurantoin, co-trimoxazole and co-amoxiclav – and are usually prescribed as a single, nightly dose. Treatment continues until the reflux resolves or for a maximum of 5 years, the rationale being that the condition is likely to resolve spontaneously and that renal scarring is secondary to infection, not to reflux itself. Careful monitoring into adult-hood is necessary as there is a high risk of the development of hypertension owing to reflux nephropathy. Follow-up studies indicate that approximately 10% of children with renal scarring develop hypertension after 10–20 years.

Surgical treatment is usually in the form of reimplantation of the ureter(s) in a non-refluxing manner using a variety of different techniques, e.g. the Politano–Leadbetter procedure (Politano and Leadbetter, 1958) and the Cohen operation (Cohen, 1977). The less invasive endoscopic procedure of injecting Teflon paste subepithelially around the ureteric opening into the bladder (O'Donnell and Puri, 1986) initially had good results but problems occurred with migration of the substance out of the bladder. Recently other products – Macroplastique and Uroplastique – have become available and it appears so far that migration of the colloid is less likely. The success rate of open surgery is between 80% and 90%; much depends on the grade of reflux. A recent study into the success rate for Teflon injection is 90%, although repeated procedures may be necessary to achieve this figure.

The postoperative management of a child undergoing ureteric reimplantation will depend on the degree of ureteric dilatation and, as a consequence, whether ureteric plication is necessary as well. If the reimplantation is straightforward the child will have a Pfannenstiel incision and usually a suprapubic catheter. Haematuria is likely for 2–3 days and the catheter is left on free drainage for 7–10 days. The catheter is then clamped and voiding re-established. When residual volumes (checked via the suprapubic catheter) are small, the catheter is removed.

If plication has taken place, ureteric stents are usually inserted as well as a suprapubic catheter. Because of the lengths of catheter tubing outside the body and the importance of maintaining free drainage through the stents, these children are often confined to bed to reduce the risk of accidental removal of the stents. These ureteric stents are kept in situ for 7–10 days, and 24 hours following removal the suprapubic catheter is clamped, voiding re-established and the catheter removed as described above. Frequency and urgency of voiding is not uncommon in the postoperative period.

Follow-up continues to be important after surgery but the nature of the surveillance changes, with fewer urine specimens required and less frequent radiological investigations.

BLADDER EXSTROPHY AND EPISPADIAS

Bladder exstrophy and epispadias, although rare, are the most common forms of a group of congenital abnormalities affecting the lower abdominal wall and urinary tract, caused by a failure of midline fusion of the ventral wall of the urogenital sinus and associated structures. The incidence is approximately 1 in 40,000 to 1 in 50,000 live births, with a female to male ratio of 1:3 or 1:4. In all cases there is a gap between the pubic bones. In epispadias (the simplest form) the bladder is formed, though often of a small capacity, but the bladder neck is usually incompetent and the angle at which the ureters enter the bladder generally inadequate to prevent reflux. There are abnormalities of the genitalia. In males these include a short, broad penis with the urethral meatus opening onto the dorsal surface of the penis and upward chordee. In females there is a bifid clitoris and a short, wide urethra.

Bladder exstrophy is a more severe anomaly where the bladder lies open, like a red ulcer, on the abdominal wall with the ureters discharging urine onto the exposed urothelium. Epispadias always accompanies exstrophy and males may also have undescended testes. In females there is a cleft clitoris, separated labia or an absent vagina. There are often associated hernias – umbilical or inguinal – skeletal abnormalities and rectal prolapse. The most severe form is cloacal exstrophy. In this condition the exstrophied bladder is separated into two lateral portions, each containing an ureter, by an exstrophy of the bowel. In this group the genital tract and development is rudimentary. The clinical features presented by this group of patients are numerous and demand all the skill and expertise of the urological surgeon and the support and ingenuity of the multidisciplinary team. The problems include:

- an open bladder plate with a small capacity bladder once closed
- urinary incontinence

- chronic or recurrent urinary tract infections
- reflux
- pyelonephritis
- renal failure
- an increased risk of malignant changes
- 'waddling' gait due to skeletal abnormality
- abnormal genitalia
- psychosocial and psychosexual dysfunction
- subfertility in males

As the general health and life expectancy of the adult exstrophy patient have improved, fertility issues have assumed increasing significance. While females have normal fertility potential, pregnancy occurs in only 18–22% of couples where the male partner has either exstrophy or epispadias. The reason for this is multifactorial and can include any combination of cryptorchidism, erectile dysfunction, retrograde ejaculation, epididymal or vasal obstruction, urethral strictures and dysfunctional urethral transport of semen.

Very little has been published about the psychosexual and psychosocial implications of children with bladder exstrophy. However, a pilot study at Johns Hopkins Hospital in Baltimore involving 42 children and adolescents with this condition found that exstrophy patients tended to demonstrate more severe behavioural and developmental problems than children with other abnormalities. They exhibited significant self-esteem and body-image distress (Carr, 1995). Genital satisfaction and body image are negatively influenced by surgery, scarring and frequent examinations of genital and perineal areas – not just by medical and nursing staff but also by parents or carers and the child. These examinations are often accompanied by pain or discomfort when associated with surgery or invasive procedures. All these events may dissuade children from exploration of their genitalia as areas of curiosity and pleasure. Many of these fears are 'normal' fears also expressed by their 'normal' peers, but the intensity with which they are expressed is significant.

The management of these children represents a major reconstructive problem and their long-term health is largely related to the efficiency of the urinary system. The option of no treatment is unrealistic, socially, physically and psychologically. Until the late 1970s urinary diversion via an ileal conduit, colonic conduit or ureterosigmoidostomy was the treatment of choice. Late complications of these operations included stomal and conduit stenosis, ureterointestinal stenosis, reflux and deteriorating renal function, metabolic disturbances and malignant changes. Since then the preference has been to provide these patients with an internal continent urinary diversion in the form of bladder substitution (e.g. Kock's pouch) or augmentation using detubularized bowel segments.

Current management favours staged repair with the multiple aims of restoring the integrity of the abdominal wall, correcting the external genital appearance and function, achieving urinary continence but above all protecting the upper tracts from reflux and preserving renal function.

Bladder closure

Bladder closure is best undertaken at birth but can be delayed until the infant is older. If surgery is delayed the skin needs careful cleansing and protection from excoriation with barrier creams. Moist, sterile pads are applied to the exstrophied bladder to absorb the urine, and should be changed frequently. Closure within 24 hours is usually done without osteotomy as the pelvic ring is extremely malleable; these babies are usually nursed postoperatively with their legs bandaged together in a 'mermaid' fashion for approximately 6 weeks. Closure after 24 hours, or if the separation of the symphysis pubis is greater than average, should be combined with some form of osteotomy to facilitate closure of the anterior abdominal wall and reduce the risk of dehiscence (Gearhart, 1993). Several approaches are currently used, and depending on the choice the child may return to the ward with external fixation, in the form of bilateral horizontal pins protruding through the anterior abdominal wall, a bilateral 'spica' plaster cast with the hips held in internal rotation, or traction (skin or skeletal) if the bone is soft or no internal fixation is used. The pins and cast are removed following a check X-ray after 5–7 weeks. The duration of traction depends on the age of the patient, varying from 2–3 weeks in an infant to 4–6 weeks in a child.

Most bladder exstrophy babies are born at full term and, like all babies, are totally dependent on their parents for all their needs. Nursing neonates is a great responsibility at all times, particularly when they are sick. Changes in the infant's condition are often sudden and require immediate intervention. The skills and judgement of the nursing staff must be highly developed. Inevitably the parents of a baby born with a congenital abnormality will be shocked and distressed and will need a great deal of support to enable them to cope. Initially they will require basic educational information regarding how these anomalies develop and reassurance that no act nor omission on their part contributed to the problem; this information should be provided by medical and nursing staff experienced in the condition. Later, other members of the team will support and counsel the parents. It is important to remember that parents are unlikely to absorb more than a fraction of all they are told, and consequently will ask the same questions repeatedly – the need for consistency in answering their questions cannot be overemphasized.

Parents may need support while they go through a grieving process for the loss of their 'perfect' baby. Every effort must be made to promote bonding of parent and child, and nurses require an insight and knowledge of this special relationship in order to foster it. Some indicators that this process is failing are prolonged reluctance by the parent to hold or participate in the baby's care, a sudden decision to bottle-feed, poor compliance with care, and delayed naming of the baby. Parents will need to be taught and encouraged to look after their baby and the nurses must remember that they are important role models in this process. The baby is likely to spend 24 hours in the intensive care unit following surgery to enable close monitoring and rapid intervention should any problem arise.

Specific complications following surgery are wound dehiscence, stenosis of the bladder neck and reflux. Although the bladder has been closed, the bladder neck will still be open, incontinence will persist and the epispadias will still be present.

Epispadias closure

All male epispadias cases will require surgical repair to some degree. In the female the external deformity is small and hardly requires any treatment; however, if treatment is necessary it can be delayed and done in conjunction with later surgery. It is possible to undertake the bladder neck and penile repair at the same time; however, some males do have urinary control and it is preferable to delay bladder neck surgery until this can be established. The penile repair can be performed earlier to achieve a more normal appearance.

The preferred method of treatment is a simple anatomical reconstruction at the age of either 9–15 months or 3–3½ years. The aim is to straighten the penis with a single-stage repair, by resecting the chordee, reducing the terminal meatus, providing a urethra of uniform, satisfactory calibre and providing an adequate cosmetic result in respect of the length, direction and strength of the urinary stream, and resting position of the penis ('angle of dangle').

For 3 months prior to surgery the infant may be given a monthly injection of testosterone 50 mg to provide an adequate size of penis. Massage of the phallus with testosterone cream for several weeks prior to surgery to enlarge the penis has also been tried with limited success. The surgery and complications are similar to hypospadias repair and the nursing care is virtually the same. The compressive dressing is maintained for 7–10 days.

Following epispadias repair the child still has an incompetent bladder neck with little or no sphincter control, resulting in persistent incontinence.

Bladder neck reconstruction

Bladder neck reconstruction should be delayed until incontinence is proved to be present; consequently it is usually undertaken after 4 years of age. The most common surgical repair is the Young–Dees reconstruction and it is generally combined with the external genital repair in females and ureteric reimplantation to correct reflux, if necessary.

Preoperative investigations are likely to include ultrasound scans, urodynamic studies to assess the bladder capacity, pressures and function, a urethral pressure profile designed to measure the pressure at the internal and external sphincter, and assessment of renal function including radioisotope studies. During this time it is worthwhile reminding parents that reconstruction is not an exact science and depends on many factors, including the skill and experience of the surgeon; consequently it is possible that the child will still be incontinent, or alternatively will be unable to void adequately and may need to self-catheterize postoperatively. This information will be discussed with the parents during outpatient appointments and any physical or mental difficulty with using catheterization explored and minimized.

Nursing care is the same as that prior to any major surgical procedure. It is particularly important to ensure that the child has a bowel motion before the operation as constipation will lead to straining in the postoperative period which may compromise the reconstruction.

Specific postoperative care includes the following:

1. Maintaining the patency of urinary drainage systems. The patient will always have a suprapubic catheter in situ and may have a urethral catheter as well. Following reimplantation of the ureters there will be one or two ureteric stents (depending on whether the reimplant was unilateral or bilateral). If bilateral stents are present, nurses should be aware that there is unlikely to be any drainage from the bladder catheters, in which case gentle bladder washouts or irrigation may be necessary to remove clots from the bladder and keep the catheters patent; this does not commence for the first 24–36 hours. The ureteric stents are removed first (after 10–14 days) followed by the urethral catheter (if present) 24 hours later. The suprapubic catheter is clamped, to allow voiding, and is only removed when voiding has been re-established.
2. Females may have a vaginal pack in situ which can be removed after 24–36 hours. Vulval toileting will help promote comfort.
3. Bed rest is recommended for 10–14 days and the child needs to be entertained and occupied.
4. A high fluid intake is necessary to maintain patency of the catheters; this may necessitate giving intravenous fluids but this should be discontinued as soon as the child is tolerating oral fluids.
5. Intravenous antibiotics are usually prescribed for the first 24–72 hours. These are sometimes followed by a course of oral antibiotics although these may not commence until after the removal of the catheters.
6. Constipation must be avoided. It can be difficult to persuade children to eat enough roughage, although most like grapes and other fruit, and it may be necessary to give a laxative or suppository if there has been no bowel movement by day 3.

Following this operation 20–30% of patients achieve continence. For those who do not there are several options and these should be fully discussed with the family. The choices include:

◆   further surgery to tighten the bladder neck, which will almost definitely mean the child will need to learn, and do, clean intermittent catheterization (this is often the best option for females). It may be possible to tighten the bladder neck with the less invasive endoscopic procedure of injecting a colloid substance such as Uroplastique around the bladder neck (as described for the correction of ureteric reflux).

◆   bladder augmentation, which may also require the child to self-catheterize, either urethrally or via a Mitrofanoff stoma.

◆   the placement of an artificial urinary sphincter; this option may be negated by the prohibitive cost – over £3,000 (1996 UK price).

There is a further choice for males which is to wait until puberty and prostatic development, which may increase outflow resistance sufficiently to achieve continence.

Apart from continuing incontinence (usually secondary to a small bladder and inadequate outflow resistance), other complications include bladder neck obstruction leading to urinary retention and, potentially, hydronephrosis.

Bladder augmentation

Following bladder neck surgery many children remain incontinent with a debilitatingly small bladder capacity, which is often further reduced by the bladder neck reconstruction, necessitating bladder augmentation.

The optimal material for augmentation should be readily available, result in a low-pressure reservoir, allow complete, controlled and spontaneous voiding, and prevent further (or new) problems arising. The ureter is the ideal tissue for this purpose but unfortunately an extra ureter or megaureter is not often available. Virtually all segments of the gastrointestinal tract have been used in bladder augmentation and diversion: colon, ileum, ileocaecal segment and stomach. However, numerous complications resulting from the use of bowel are reported, including metabolic disturbances, intestinal malabsorption, impaired growth, increased risk of malignancy and spontaneous perforation. The more common complications include excessive mucus production, urinary tract infections and stone formation. There appear to be fewer complications with a gastrocystoplasty (Nguyen, 1994), but metabolic disturbances still occur – albeit of a different nature – and there is a potential to develop haematuria or dysuria syndrome. There is also a risk of developing a peptic ulcer in the gastric portion of the cystoplasty.

Alternative solutions such as autoaugmentation, synthetic substances and collagen-rich tissue to provide a scaffold for regeneration of bladder tissue, tissue engineering and prosthetic bladders composed of silicon rubber, hold promise for the future (McKenna, 1995). For the present, enterocystoplasty remains the most common form of bladder augmentation. Preoperative preparation includes:

1. The physical and psychological preparation of the child and family, which entails giving detailed information regarding the need for careful and effective bowel clearance and about the numerous catheters, tubes and drains likely to be present postoperatively, including their function and duration of need, and providing the child and family with an opportunity to discuss their own fears and worries.
2. Different surgeons have their own preferences on methods of bowel preparation, but it usually includes aperients, enemas and washouts. The use of intestinal antibiotics to sterilize the bowel is not recommended today but is still favoured by some surgeons. A diet low in roughage followed by 1–2 days of a fluid-only diet immediately prior to surgery is often recommended, but it is important to remember that children do not have the same reserves as adults and prolonged starvation is not recommended. A suitable regimen is sodium picosulphate (Picolax) titrated for the age and condition of the child, on two occasions prior to surgery. During this period of preparation the induced diarrhoea adds to the child's discomfort.
3. Warnings about the presence of mucus in the urine should be reiterated, as parents find it worrying if they are not prepared for it.

Specific postoperative care includes:

1. Parenteral fluid administration – electronically controlled infusion systems or burette type administration sets with a safety valve and Luer

connectors should be utilized routinely for all paediatric patients to ensure accurate administration of small volumes of fluid, prevent accidental 'overloading' and reduce the risk of accidental disconnection.

2. Nasogastric decompression until bowel sounds return or the child passes flatus.

3. Wound drainage. The quantity and type of drainage should be measured, assessed and recorded. The drain is removed – as instructed by the surgeon – when there has been no further drainage for 24 hours.

4. Control of postoperative pain. The most effective and comfortable method of achieving this in the initial postoperative phase is by continuous infusion of opioids. These can be administered just as effectively – and more safely – by the subcutaneous route, rather than intravenously. In older children patient-controlled analgesia (PCA) systems are effective. Nursing staff need to be vigilant in observing and monitoring the child for signs of excessive sedation, transient muscular spasm and twitching and respiratory depression, and should know exactly what to do should this occur – slow or stop the infusion, notify the doctor and prepare to administer an antagonist (naloxone) according to local policy. Other analgesics such as co-proxamol, diclofenac and paracetamol are effective as the child's condition improves.

5. Maintaining the patency of urinary catheters (usually both suprapubic and urethral). Owing to the presence of mucus these catheters are liable to become blocked. Gentle 'milking', intermittent washouts or continuous irrigation with small volumes of saline can be used. If continuous irrigation is required the fluid is instilled via the smaller catheter (usually the urethral catheter) and urine, debris and clots drained out via the larger (suprapubic) catheter; this must be carefully monitored to ensure there is no build-up of irrigation fluid in the bladder. Urinary drainage via the catheters is generally maintained for 3–4 weeks; the urethral catheter is removed first and the suprapubic catheter clamped to allow voiding to be re-established. Residual urine volumes are monitored via the suprapubic catheter and when these are proved to be insignificant the suprapubic catheter is removed. If residual volumes continue, clean intermittent catheterization commences and the suprapubic catheter remains until this is well established.

6. Encouraging a high oral intake of fluid (1–2 litres daily depending on age) is very important, and should be continued throughout life.

7. The child and parents should be taught how to wash out the bladder as mucus production may compromise bladder emptying, particularly if the child will need to do clean intermittent catheterization. The issue of routine bladder washouts is controversial, with some surgeons advocating regular (weekly or even daily) washouts and others unconvinced of their value. A regular daily intake of cranberry juice has been shown to decrease mucus production and reduce the incidence of urinary tract infection (Rosenbaum et al., personal communication; Rodgers, 1991; Sobata, 1984). It has a bitter taste and many children refuse to drink it, but it may be made more palatable by dilution and the addition of sweeteners; alternatively, cranberry capsules are now available.

Families need to be given supplies of catheters and washout equipment on discharge and details of how to obtain further supplies on prescription. They will also require detailed written advice for trouble-shooting, although they are encouraged to maintain close links with the hospital.

The complications of bladder augmentation have already been enumerated so the need for stringent follow-up appointments should be recognized. Consultants will have their own regimens; these should include annual ultrasound scans and X-rays of the kidneys, ureters and bladder, radioisotope renal scans, urodynamic studies and blood tests.

Artificial urinary sphincter

The artificial urinary sphincter (AUS) made its debut in 1972 and has proved to be of immense benefit in the management of urinary incontinence in patients with neuropathic bladder. It has not been approved for general use but preliminary trials with other groups of patients have shown it has value.

Prior to implantation it is essential to establish that the incontinence is due to an incompetent bladder neck and not detrusor instability. If the latter is present it must be demonstrated that the instability can be controlled – either pharmacologically or by other methods. Outflow must be unobstructed and the patient able to void efficiently. The bladder should be of a good capacity and normal compliance. Urodynamic studies can provide this information. Renal function needs to be assessed and any significant vesicoureteric reflux must be corrected before the device is implanted. The tissues at the proposed site of implantation must be well vascularized as there is a risk of erosion and incomplete urethral occlusion in the presence of poor-quality tissue.

Careful assessment of the patient's physical, psychological and educational ability is necessary. The child needs to have sufficient intelligence, motivation and manual dexterity to operate the device. It is important to explain the risks and limitations, as well as the advantages, of the device. Ideally the procedure should be postponed until after puberty so that children do not need to have the device revised as they grow (and any increased resistance provided by the prostate in males will have occurred), but this may not be acceptable socially and developmentally.

The most important factor governing success or failure is infection. There should be no instrumentation of the lower urinary tract for 48 hours pre-operatively. A midstream urine specimen should be sterile – surgery used to be deferred in the presence of an infection although with the use of antibiotics this is less likely. Skin and hair cleansing with a bactericidal solution (such as chlorhexidine) is recommended for 36–48 hours prior to surgery and the rectum should be empty. These patients should be first on the theatre list.

The artificial sphincter is composed of three parts: the cuff, which comes in eleven sizes; the pressure-regulating balloon, in four sizes; and the pump (Figure 15.7). The components are joined by tubing.

Postoperatively, the child is unlikely to have any drainage tubes in situ, but should be given intravenous antibiotic therapy for 72 hours. The care is similar to that described for simple orchidopexy. There is a period of persistent incontinence postoperatively as the tissues need to be allowed to heal completely before the device is activated. Activation occurs 4–8 weeks following surgery and is usually an outpatient or 'ward attender' procedure. Patients need to be reminded of this preoperatively.

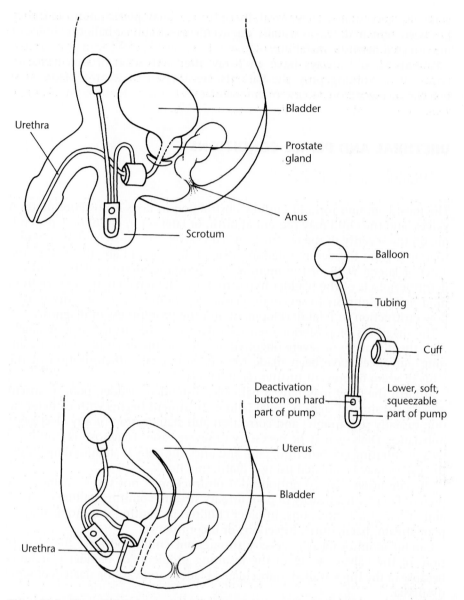

Urethra

Bladder

Prostate gland

Anus

Scrotum

Balloon

Tubing

Cuff

Deactivation button on hard part of pump

Lower, soft, squeezable part of pump

Uterus

Bladder

Urethra

Figure 15.7 *The artificial urinary sphincter (a) and its positioning in the male (b) and female (c). To operate the sphincter, locate the pump and grasp the tubing above it, thereby immobilizing it; with the other hand, squeeze the lower, soft part of the pump until it is flat. The cuff is now open and micturition can occur. The cuff reinflates automatically within a few minutes*

The AUS is a mechanical device with the potential for malfunction of any component. Blockage of the tubing may be caused by kinking, air bubbles, fluid leakage and incorrect 'tailoring' of the tubing at insertion. Erosion may occur owing to improper cuff sizing, incorrect balloon selection and infection. Meticulous preoperative preparation reduces the risk of infection, but nurses should be alert to the potential. Patients must be advised to seek early treatment at all times if they suspect an infection – infection of the device generally necessitates its removal. Incontinence may persist after the device has been activated; this is usually due to incorrect cuff or balloon choice or uncorrected detrusor instability.

Patients should always have an X-ray after activation of the device to ensure it is working properly. Patients are advised to wear a Medic-Alert bracelet or medallion in case of emergencies.

URETHRAL AND PENILE CONDITIONS

Posterior urethral valves

The most common form of outflow obstruction in boys is posterior urethral valves, and the child may present at birth, or later on in childhood, depending on the severity of the obstruction. The valves are sail-shaped membranes that arise from the verumontanum, extend distally and are attached to the anterior lateral walls of the urethra. The prostatic urethra dilates, and the detrusor muscle of the bladder hypertrophies. The renal changes range from mild hydronephrosis to severe dysplasia, depending on the severity of outflow obstruction in fetal development and the promptness of diagnosis.

The diagnosis of posterior urethral valves may be suspected antenatally with the discovery of severe oligohydramnios on maternal ultrasound scanning. Advances have been made towards antenatal catheterization of the fetus in utero to prevent further renal damage.

At birth the baby may have a palpable, distended bladder, poor or absent urinary stream and signs of renal failure. Treatment begins with catheterization (usually suprapubic) and correction and stabilization of any electrolyte imbalance. Dialysis may be necessary in severe cases. Diagnosis is confirmed by a micturating cystourethrogram, and once the baby is stabilized medically the valves may be ablated using a diathermy hook.

The condition may go unnoticed if obstruction is not severe. Babies may present later with a history of poor urinary stream, vomiting, failure to thrive and urinary tract infections. In older children presenting symptoms may be poor stream, haematuria, infections or incontinence.

Careful monitoring is necessary throughout childhood after the 'disruption' of the valves owing to the resulting problems of bladder instability because of the thick-walled, trabeculated bladder and varying degrees of renal dysplasia.

Male hypospadias

Hypospadias is one of the most common congenital abnormalities, occurring in approximately 1 in 500 live male births. At around 10 weeks of fetal development a urethral groove develops in the genital tubercle. This deepens and closes over to form the urethra. Hypospadias results from incomplete closure of the groove, with the urethral meatus terminating on the ventral surface (underside) of the penis. Chordee (longitudinal bands of fibrous tissue in the corpus spongiosum tethering the penis in a downward, flexed curve) is often present and can be mild, moderate or severe. Other associated conditions include cryptorchidism and intersex; upper tract anomalies appear to be no greater than in the general population. Hypospadias represents a spectrum of deficiency (approximately 65% are of the anterior variety), consequently there is no single repair suitable for all forms. Table 15.1 shows a classification according to the position of the urethral meatus prior to surgery and common repairs in use today.

Hypospadias is usually detected at birth during routine inspection, and symptoms vary according to the degree of severity. These may include:

◆   difficulty with micturition
◆   retention of urine (if meatal stenosis is severe)
◆   a thin stream
◆   altered position for voiding – sitting (penoscrotal and perineal) or holding the penis upwards (mid-shaft), which can cause embarrassment and psychological distress
◆   potential difficulties with penetration during sexual intercourse when severe chordee is present

The aim of hypospadiac surgery is to straighten the penis by releasing the chordee, reduce the terminal meatus, construct a hairless urethra of uniform, satisfactory calibre and provide a cosmetically acceptable penis by creating a symmetrical glans and shaft with normalization of voiding and erections (Greenfield, 1972; Kaplan, 1992; Keating and Duckett, 1989).

The timing of surgery is very important. Shultz et al. (1983) described the optimal psychological window for hypospadias repair as being between 6 months and 18 months to minimize the emotional effects of surgery. The surgeons in the authors' unit prefer to operate when the infant is 9–18 months, and if this 'window' is missed wait until the child is over 3 years old. Surgery should be completed before the child starts school (5 years).

CLASSIFICATION	SURGICAL REPAIR
Glanular	Meatal advancement and glanuloplasty incorporated (MAGPI)
	IPGAM (reverse MAGPI)
	Mathieu (meatal-based) flap
Distal shaft	Mathieu flap
	Pedicle preputial patch and tube
	Onlay island patch
Mid-shaft	Duckett's repair
	Transverse preputial island graft
Penoscrotal and perineal	Buccal mucosal graft (this involves obtaining a strip of mucosa from either the cheek or inner lip, tubularizing it and anastomosing it to the viable urethra); the original surgery used bladder mucosa for this procedure

Table 15.1 Classification of hypospadias repair

Some of the psychological factors that need consideration are:

- ◆ the bonding of parents and child, which may be impaired by the baby not being 'perfect'
- ◆ genital awareness and sexual orientation; Stoller (1968) described 'core gender identity' as developing between the ages of 2 years and 4 years
- ◆ the child's own body image

Multistaged repairs were standard in the 1960s and 1970s and are still used today – for the more difficult and 'redo' repairs – but contemporary preference is for the single-stage repair which offers patients the benefits of simplification of treatment and a single general anaesthetic, and surgeons the opportunity to utilize virgin tissue, devoid of scars and disruption of the normal blood supply. Difficulties experienced in operating on young children include the risks of anaesthesia and the size of the penis; advantages include the fact that the younger child is more easily managed and appears to have less memory of the operation through subsequent development.

Successful management is contingent upon adequate preoperative parental teaching and meticulous attention to detail in postoperative care: hence nursing staff have a vital role to play. In some centres in the USA hypospadias surgery is routinely done on a day-care basis with no reported adverse affects. However, in Britain the preference is still for hospitalization for several days except in the simplest of repairs.

Nursing considerations in the preoperative period should include:

1. Psychological preparation. It is important to warn parents and the child that the penis may look bruised and swollen following removal of the dressing and that the appearance will resemble that of a circumcised penis.
2. Obtaining and sending a midstream urine specimen (as well as routine ward urinalysis) as any infection will jeopardize healing.
3. Obtaining a flow rate recording (if the child is old enough to co-operate) for objective comparison postoperatively.
4. Ensuring that appropriate blood samples have been obtained (the penis has a very good blood supply, therefore there is a potential for haemorrhage postoperatively).

Postoperative care

The specific postoperative care includes the following:

Catheters

Ensure all urinary catheters and stents are patent and draining. Virtually all patients will have some form of urinary diversion as premature voiding is undesirable and may lead to wound dehiscence and fistula formation. (When collecting patients from theatres, the nurse should ensure that catheters are draining before leaving the recovery area.) If the child has voluntary bladder control, urinary drainage is generally via a self-retaining balloon catheter draining into a bag; in the infant drainage is generally via a 'dripping stent' (a thin Silastic tube placed through the neourethra and into the bladder), which is secured by one stitch to the glans penis and drains continuously into a double nappy. A recent variation of this is the 'voiding stent', where the proximal end of the tubing lies outside the external urinary sphincter, allowing intermittent voiding. These latter methods appear to decrease bladder spasms. Urinary diversion continues for an average of 3–14 days depending on the extensiveness of the repair and the assessment of healing by the appearance of the penis following removal of the dressing. (Following a bladder mucosal graft, patients will have a suprapubic catheter as well as an urethral catheter, and the latter will be removed first.) Catheters should be adequately secured to the child's abdomen (not the leg) to reduce the risk of friction to the anastomosis. Gentle 'milking' of the catheter may be necessary, especially if there is significant haematuria, to maintain patency, but this can increase bladder spasms so should be avoided if possible (bladder washouts may be necessary in the case of bladder mucosal grafts). The drainage bag must always be situated lower than the bladder and tubing must be observed at regular intervals to prevent kinking and obstruction. The child often complains of the urge to pass urine – even though the catheters are draining freely – and the nurse will have to provide much reassurance (having first ascertained that drainage has not been compromised).

Great care must be taken when removing catheters to prevent damage to the neourethra. If a balloon catheter is used it is essential that the balloon is completely deflated prior to removal (too strenuous deflation of the balloon can lead to ridging of the material which could make removal more traumatic), and that any retaining sutures are cut. If there is any resistance encountered on withdrawing the catheter the procedure should be halted and the doctor notified. Following removal, observation of urinary output is essential; leakage or dribbling from the meatus or suture line, the angle, strength and fluidity of the stream should be noted and reported to the surgeon. A flow rate recording should be obtained (the first void following catheter removal does not usually reflect an accurate assessment). Reassurance is necessary as the child is often frightened or reluctant to pass urine.

Bleeding

The patient should be carefully observed for signs of bleeding. It is important to monitor and record vital signs postoperatively with particular reference to signs of shock. Most patients will have some form of compression dressing in place which fulfils three functions: assisting with haemostasis and containment of oedema; immobilization of the penis and drainage tube; and protection of the suture line. In the simpler repairs an occlusive, self-adherent dressing such as Tegaderm or Opsite is commonly used. Parents are often distressed and frightened by seeing the state of the penis beneath the dressing and need much reassurance. Surgeons claim this dressing is easily removed but nursing staff would not necessarily agree – such dressings can be very difficult to remove at the prescribed time, even after bathing. This type is generally removed after 2–5 days.

The other commonly used dressing is Silastic foam – this is provided in a quick-setting, liquid form which is poured into a mould surrounding the penis. After setting the mould is removed and the dressing secured to the skin with adhesive tape such as Elastoplast. This is easier to remove after the child soaks in a bath for about 30 minutes. There is usually a retaining suture in the tip of the glans which is secured to the outside of the dressing, and it is very important to remove this suture prior to removing the dressing. Foam dressings are generally removed after 7 days although the range is 5–10 days. The child and parents should be reminded that although the penis may look very swollen and bruised initially, this will resolve spontaneously and the final appearance may not manifest itself for several weeks.

Pain relief

Children undergoing penile surgery are usually given caudal anaesthesia as for circumcision. Most children obtain adequate postoperative analgesia from diclofenac or coproxamol initially, followed by paracetamol.

Fluids

Adequate fluid intake (1–2 litres per day) is essential to ensure the catheters drain freely and do not block; this can tax the patience and ingenuity of even the best of paediatric nurses. The child may require an intravenous infusion initially but this should be discontinued as soon as oral intake is established. The nurse should ensure that fluids are balanced so the child will still eat and not be filled up with inappropriate drinks.

Diet

A well-balanced diet is necessary to promote healing. Children in hospital often lose interest in eating; the food may not be visually appealing and is prepared differently; they may be eating more sweets and crisps than usual as a form of compensation.

Constipation

Prevention of constipation is important to prevent straining, excessive tension on the sutures, increased incidence of bladder spasms and compromised urinary drainage. Systemic measures such as a mild laxative (e.g. lactulose) or local measures such as suppositories should be given if the child has not had a bowel movement by day 2 or 3. Explanations and reassurance are again necessary as the child is often frightened that passing a stool will be painful.

Bladder spasms

Bladder spasms are due to irritation from the catheter and can lead to forcible expulsion of urine via the neourethra with serious adverse affects. Spasms are difficult to control and cause much distress to both child and parents. Anticholinergics (e.g. oxybutynin), muscle relaxants (e.g. diazepam) and opiates (more commonly used in the USA) may be helpful.

Infection

The routine use of antibiotics is controversial, with some surgeons denying their value, some restricting their use to patients with open urinary drainage (dripping stents) and others who prescribe them routinely particularly after catheter removal. It is important to anticipate the potential problem of infection following instrumentation of the urinary tract and monitor the child's temperature regularly, notifying the medical staff if it is elevated above 37°C.

Mobility

Restricting mobility (by confining the child to bed) promotes healing by helping to prevent accidental removal of drainage tubes; it is recommended for all but the simplest repairs and should continue until the dressing is removed. Attention to general hygiene needs to be maintained appropriately during this period and parents are usually anxious to assist after being shown what to do. Boredom is a potential problem and should be prevented by providing games, toys, videos and supervised play.

Wound hygiene

The genital area should be kept clean and dry; daily or twice daily baths are encouraged following removal of the dressing, depending on the state of the wound. It is particularly important to keep the urethral meatus free of any scabs which could obstruct the flow of urine and cause wound breakdown and fistula formation. The child may find the use of a hairdryer more comfortable than a towel for drying the genital area. Some surgeons like to apply an antibiotic ointment to the urinary meatus to help prevent infection and keep the meatal skin supple.

Discharge

Prior to discharge, parents should be given a date and time to attend the outpatient clinic (usually after 6 weeks). They should be given written and verbal information regarding potential problems and whom to contact should they occur (the hospital or general practitioner). It is essential that children are prevented from playing with 'ride astride' toys such as bicycles and rocking-horses for a few weeks after surgery, and they will probably find loose clothing (boxer shorts and track suits) more comfortable than tight trousers.

Complications

Complications following hypospadiac surgery include the following:

1. Fistula formation – the frequency is as high as 30% in some centres. 'Pinhole' fistulae may close spontaneously and this may be encouraged by teaching the child to occlude the fistula with his finger while voiding. Even comparatively large fistulae may heal spontaneously. Surgical repair may be necessary but should not occur for at least 3 months to ensure complete healing.
2. Persistent chordee will need further surgery.
3. Meatal stenosis and retraction (this is seen infrequently in the single-stage repair).

4. Urethral diverticula and strictures – usually due to postoperative infection or stenosis of the neourethra/meatus, sometimes due to poor surgical technique.
5. Poor cosmetic results and potential sexual problems in later life. Some studies and reports suggest that with hypospadias there is a sense of inferiority, poor body image and poor or late onset of sexual activity. Other reports refute this. The potential problems should be recognized so early intervention can be provided if necessary.

Female hypospadias

In female hypospadias the vulva appears superficially normal, but on closer inspection the urethral meatus is abnormally positioned on the anterior wall, a short distance within the vaginal introitus. Minor degrees of this abnormality are relatively common and require no treatment. Severe deformities are rare and usually complicated by urinary obstruction, a trabeculated bladder and urinary reflux; other cases may include bifurcation of the vagina and a degree of vaginal outlet obstruction. These cases will require surgical repair.

Circumcision

Circumcision is a minor surgical procedure involving the removal of the foreskin hooding the end of the penis, thereby exposing the glans. The foreskin is there to protect the glans. In the neonate and infant the exposed glans can be damaged by ammonia from wet nappies leading to dermatitis, meatal ulceration and meatal stenosis.

Circumcision is a controversial issue in that it is rarely performed on the basis of medical need and frequently performed for religious, cultural and social reasons. Medical indications for performing circumcision include:

◆ phimosis – the inability to fully retract the foreskin because it is too tight
◆ paraphimosis – retraction of the foreskin behind the glans with an inability to replace it
◆ balanitis – irritation and infection under the foreskin
◆ posthitis – inflammation of the prepuce

It should be noted that all the above conditions are actually quite rare. As long ago as 1949 a British physician, Gairdner, noted that 'the prepuce is still in the course of developing at the time of birth'. In fact, the foreskin is fully retractable in only about 4% of boys at birth; at 6 months of age, about 15%; at 1 year, about 50%; and it is not until about 3 years of age that 90% of boys will have a fully retractable foreskin, consequently any attempt at retraction prior to age 3 years should be actively discouraged.

Claims that circumcision decreases the incidence of penile and cervical cancer and reduces the incidence of prostatic cancer are not completely verified by research studies. Variables such as personal hygiene habits, frequency of intercourse, age of onset of sexual activity, numbers of partners, sexual hygiene and contraceptive use need to be considered as well.

The strongest medical argument favouring circumcision is its ability to reduce childhood urinary tract infections which may necessitate hospitalization and scar delicate young kidneys which could potentially lead to renal failure. Urinary tract infections can also lead to meningitis and generalized septicaemia (sometimes fatal). However, infant urinary tract infections are still rare – occurring in 1–4% of male babies – and complications of circumcision do occur in approximately 2–10% of all cases.

Circumcision is definitely contraindicated in infants born with congenital anomalies such as hypospadias, epispadias or megalourethra where the foreskin may be needed for reconstruction of the defect. It is also contraindicated in prematurity, infants who are unwell and those with a known family history of bleeding disorders.

Leaving controversy aside, the operation is ideally suited to day-case surgery (as described under orchidopexy). Other care specific to penile surgery is as follows.

Specific nursing care

Caudal anaesthesia

Caudal anaesthesia has a dual purpose in that it provides effective pain control in the initial postoperative phase without recourse to strong analgesic drugs such as pethidine, and the vasoconstriction provides a relatively blood-free field for the surgeon in an area that has an excellent blood supply. The child (if old enough to understand) and parents should be advised of the risk of headache and dizziness if he gets up too quickly after surgery; he should be encouraged to lie flat for about 6 hours. He is likely to complain of loss of function or sensation of the lower limbs and may experience some discomfort and 'pins and needles' as the caudal anaesthetic wears off; gentle massage may promote comfort. The nurse should observe the lower limbs for colour, sensation, warmth and movement in the immediate postoperative period. The first time the child gets up he should be accompanied by a parent or the nurse as a safety precaution.

Risk of haemorrhage

Primary or reactionary haemorrhage (due to vasodilation or a slipped suture) could occur immediately and up to 48 hours after surgery; parents should be advised of how, where and at what compression to apply direct pressure, the use of a cold compress, and to call the general practitioner immediately, day or night. (Parents may be advised to call the ward, depending on local policy.)

Secondary haemorrhage can occur as a result of infection; parents should be advised to look out for fever, local discharge, increased pain or discolouration, and to call their general practitioner if they are worried. The use of cold packs should be carefully monitored and supervised to prevent more damage occurring. The nurse should inspect the penis for bleeding prior to discharge.

Difficulty with micturition

The child should pass urine before being discharged. He should be observed for signs of discomfort; the nurse can palpate the abdomen to assess the degree of retention and should notify the doctor appropriately. Several steps can be taken to encourage the child to void: change of position and mobilization; the application of warm packs to the abdomen; analgesia; the sound of running water; a warm bath, although this may be contraindicated immediately postoperatively; and increased oral fluids. Parents should be advised to contact their doctor or the hospital if pain and difficulty persist longer than 12 hours.

Swelling

The best treatment for swelling is to reduce activity, advise the careful and supervised use of cold packs, and ensure the child wears loose clothing (boxer shorts and track suits).

Complications

Postoperative complications can be divided into several categories, namely anaesthetic, immediate and delayed. Haemorrhage is the most common and may be caused by inadequate haemostasis, coagulation disorders or aberrant blood vessels. Wound infection is another fairly common complication and it is possible for the localized infection to develop into something much more serious, such as partial necrosis of the penis or a generalized septicaemia – usually staphylococcal in origin – which can be fatal.

Surgical trauma is less common, but even experienced and competent surgeons have been known to remove too much penile skin and yet this operation is often performed by junior medical staff with little experience and inadequate supervision.

Other complications include accidental laceration of penile and/or scrotal skin; incomplete circumcision resulting in the formation of adhesions and secondary penile deformity; accidental amputation of the glans; secondary haemorrhage, and retraction of the penis subcutaneously because of contraction, healing and fibrosis of the circular wound.

Delayed complications are usually related to the newly circumcised penis being in frequent and prolonged contact with urine and faeces. The raw, bruised and bleeding glans can easily become inflamed and infected, with subsequent development of fibrotic and scarred tissue. Meatal stenosis is accompanied by dysuria, urinary frequency and enuresis.

As well as anatomical and structural complications there are also psychological considerations which may or may not become significant until the child is older. Different opinions exist as to the importance of the foreskin in relation to sexual pleasure and although sexual satisfaction is highly subjective and individualized, body image and a sense of self is crucial in the development of healthy relationships.

The principles and importance of personal and sexual hygiene can and should be taught to parents and children and a programme of education could be initiated by health-care professionals in the interest of public health and preventive medicine. Once the child is past the age of 3 years and it is established that the foreskin can be withdrawn, retraction of the prepuce, cleansing and careful replacement of the foreskin during bathing should become just as routine as cleaning behind the ears or brushing the teeth.

ABNORMALITIES OF THE TESTES

Undescended testes (cryptorchidism)

The testis begins in the gonadal ridge of the fetus, high in the abdominal cavity and behind the peritoneal cavity, and by the time of birth it should have descended into the scrotal sac via the inguinal canal which forms the channel between the abdomen and the scrotum. By 3 months of fetal life the testes should lie close to the inguinal region and by 7 months they should have passed down through the inguinal canal into the genital swelling which then fuses to form the scrotum. On completion of testicular descent the inguinal canal is closed off by fusion of the processus vaginalis; if this fusion does not occur there is a risk of fluid from the abdominal cavity collecting in the scrotum creating a hydrocele.

The absence of one or both testes from the scrotum requires careful examination by palpation in order to differentiate between true cryptorchidism (failure of or arrested descent of the testis), ectopic testis (where the testis has emerged from the external inguinal ring but has not entered the scrotum) and retractile testis (where the testis can be found in the groin at the external inguinal ring but can be gently manoeuvred into the scrotum).

The complications of undescended testes include:

◆ inguinal hernia
◆ torsion
◆ infertility
◆ psychological effects
◆ malignancy

The aim of treatment is to secure the testes sufficiently early to allow maximum functional potential.

Orchidopexy

The optimum age for a child to undergo orchidopexy – the operation to bring the testis down and secure it in the scrotum – is 2–3 years. Unfortunately the diagnosis is often not made until the child is much older; these children should have surgery as soon as practical and prior to puberty.

There is very little required in the way of specific preoperative preparation prior to a simple orchidopexy; however, if there is a possibility of a laparatomy being performed, blood should be obtained and sent to the laboratory for routine haemoglobin estimation and 'group and save' – the nursing staff should check that this has been done.

A child with no other health problems undergoing a simple orchidopexy may be a suitable candidate for day-case surgery; this should be encouraged providing that the social circumstances are appropriate. It is vital to ensure that the child and parents are adequately prepared prior to the admission, either during the initial outpatient appointment or on a preoperative ward visit. Written information should be provided for reference as it may be some months before the child is called for surgery. The benefits of a preoperative ward visit, particularly for those patients having day surgery, cannot be over-emphasized; for the child and family it helps to reduce anxiety through familiarization with the ward environment and the opportunity to express their fears and worries regarding the diagnosis, the surgery and the post-operative care. These fears may include the possibility of delayed develop-ment, a lifetime of hormonal therapy, the fear of malignancy and reduced fertility. Nursing staff should be prepared to provide information about causes, available treatments and the ultimate effect on reproduction; they should therefore familiarize themselves with the facts regarding the indivi-dual's condition and reinforce what they have already been told by medical staff. Nursing staff are better able to assess the family's ability to cope with the postoperative care following a meeting of this type and can mobilize community support as necessary.

The specific preoperative and postoperative advice should include the following:

- Fasting prior to surgery – parents should be advised of the exact time to stop their child eating and drinking (no solids or milk for 6 hours and no clear fluids for 2 hours prior to surgery).

- Arrival time on the ward and whether or not the child should have a bath at home.

- Control of postoperative pain. Paracetamol is usually suffi-cient to keep a child comfortable following orchidopexy. Parents should be advised of the appropriate dose and fre-quency of administration.

- The risk of haemorrhage. Reactionary haemorrhage can occur up to 3 hours postoperatively; this is caused by vaso-dilation of the small veins in the scrotal skin. Rarely, patients may need to return to theatre for cautery to these veins, but the bleeding will usually stop spontaneously. The scrotum should be inspected prior to discharge and parents advised to contact their own doctor or the hospital (according to local policy) if they notice any bleeding or discolouration of the scrotum. They should be reassured that the bruising will disappear, although it may take a week or two.

- Scrotal oedema – swelling is not uncommon following sur-gery and restricting mobility for several days postoperatively is helpful in reducing swelling and pain. Parents should be advised to put away 'ride astride' toys such as bicycles and rocking-horses and prevent their child from playing with these for about 2 weeks postoperatively. Play with siblings and others will need to be supervised for a week or two; this should not prevent the toddler or preschool child returning to playgroup or nursery after a week or so providing the staff are aware of the recent surgery and are happy to provide the extra vigilance necessary. The child may find snug-fitting underpants more comfortable than boxer shorts as these provide more support.

◆   Stitches – there will be a small groin incision (usually secured with dissolvable sutures subcutaneously and two or three sterile skin closure strips) and a couple of stitches on the underside of the scrotum; these do not require removal. The incisions are usually left uncovered and the skin closure strips can be removed after about 5 days, by the child or parents.

◆   General hygiene – the groin and scrotal incisions should be observed and kept clean and dry for a couple of days, after which the child can start bathing again. If there is any swelling, increased local tenderness or discharge from the incisions the general practitioner should be notified as it may indicate an infection that requires antibiotic therapy.

Ward staff should liaise with the general practitioner and the health visitor prior to the child's discharge and the parents should be aware of whom to contact should any problems arise, day or night.

Specific nursing care

The child who has undergone a laparotomy and orchidopexy will need to stay in hospital for a longer period (generally 5–7 days) if there has been significant handling of the bowel while locating the testis. The general principles surrounding any patient following abdominal surgery will apply.

1. Parenteral fluid administration is needed to maintain adequate hydration. A burette type administration set with a safety valve and Luer connectors should be used routinely for all paediatric patients to ensure accurate administration of small volumes of fluid, prevent accidental 'overloading' and reduce the risk of accidental disconnection.

2. Wound drainage (vacuum type) will be present, to prevent haematoma formation. This is removed, according to the surgeon's instructions, when there has been no drainage for 12–24 hours – generally by day 3.

3. Nasogastric decompression may be used, although the routine use of nasogastric tubes following abdominal surgery is being questioned and reassessed. Children tend to find the nasogastric tube the most uncomfortable 'accessory' and are always more cheerful following its removal; however, inserting a nasogastric tube in an alert child is an unpleasant postoperative procedure requiring all the skills of persuasion, patience and dexterity that the paediatric nurse possesses, and the advantages and disadvantages must be assessed very carefully.

All cannulae and tubing should be firmly secured to the patient's skin. If the child is old enough to understand, the need for each item should be explained – using appropriate language and diagrams – as this helps the child to tolerate them. The use of restraints to prevent 'fiddling' and dislodgement (either accidental or intentional) is discouraged, divertional therapy is recommended.

Early mobilization is encouraged to reduce the risk of complications.

Prior to discharge, the child should be given a date and time to attend the outpatient clinic in 6–12 weeks.

Testicular torsion

Torsion of the testis is caused by twisting of the spermatic cord and blood vessels. It is not an uncommon condition and may occur in childhood at any age, most often around puberty (Blandy and Moors, 1989). The testis will only be viable for 6–8 hours if its blood supply is impaired, therefore this is considered a surgical emergency. The surgeon may attempt to untwist the torsion manually after prescribing a strong analgesic (such as pethidine). The nurse should stay with the child following administration of the injection and help to calm, distract and reassure him. Surgical exploration is essential even if the attempt is successful and the initial pain is relieved. If the diagnosis is confirmed the opposite testicle must be explored as the same underlying condition that allowed the torsion to occur initially is often present.

Nursing care is similar to that described for the child undergoing orchidopexy.

Hydrocele

The normal space around the testicle contains a trace of fluid which allows it to move within the scrotum and helps protect it against minor injury. This fluid increases in certain conditions – lack of fusion of the processus vaginalis, obstructed testicular lymphatic drainage, testicular disease and malignancy. Most hydroceles are idiopathic.

Treatment initially consists of 'tapping' the hydrocele – aspirating the fluid using a small plastic cannula. This is a minor procedure and can be done as an outpatient procedure with the child sedated. If the fluid collection recurs quickly, the child will need a small operation to close the processus vaginalis, or treatment of the underlying cause.

Testicular tumours

Malignant testicular tumours account for not more than 1% of all solid tumours in infancy and childhood. Table 15.2 is a simplified classification of testicular tumours found in children based on Mostofi's (WHO) classification, giving the incidence and recommended treatment (Mostofi and Price, 1983). There is no way to distinguish benign testicular tumours from malignant ones by clinical investigation and biopsy is contraindicated because of the danger of tumour spillage, consequently these patients should be prepared for orchidectomy – the excision of the testis, vas and vascular pedicle. If there is any evidence of lymphatic spread of the tumour a radical retroperitoneal lymphadenectomy will also be done. The preoperative investigations may include ultrasound and CT scanning, urography, lymphography,

CLASSIFICATION	INCIDENCE	TREATMENT
Tumours of germ cell origin Embryonal carcinoma	Most common testicular tumour in infancy and childhood (approximately 50%) and usually confined to the age group up to 4 years. Metastases develop readily (approximately 30%).	Orchidopexy and bilateral retroperitoneal lymph node dissection: prophylactic chemotherapy is controversial though generally recommended only in patients with metastases. Three out of ten children die from metastases, usually within 2 years of surgery
Seminoma	Found only in older boys and comprises less than 5% of the testicular neoplasms in this age group: up to 10% of this group have metastases when diagnosed	Orchidectomy followed by irradiation of the para-aortic and iliac area: chemotherapy recommended only when metastases are present; mortality about 10%
Teratoma	Accounts for approximately 30% of testicular tumours in children. Majority of patients are under 4 years old. The tumour may be congenital and metastases are rare	Orchidectomy; retroperitoneal lymph node dissection and postoperative chemotherapy are less indicated in children than in older patients
Mixed germ cell tumours Tumours derived from specialized gonadal stroma Rare or unclassified testicular tumours	Relatively frequent (20% of all testicular tumours). Metastases are extremely rare	Orchidectomy
Metastatic (secondary) testicular tumours	There is a higher incidence of secondary tumours in children than in adults	Orchidectomy and bilateral retroperitoneal lymph node dissection, irradiation and chemotherapy

Table 15.2 Classification of testicular tumours

chest X-ray and the collection of serum for measurement of tumour markers and hormonal status.

The focus of nursing care revolves around providing psychological and emotional support during this very difficult period as well as physical preparation and care of the child. The nurse should explain the investigations in language the child understands, and be available to assist as necessary. Some of the investigations are unpleasant and time-consuming so the child may require sedation. The dye used in some of the radiological investigations may stain the skin and the urine; this resolves spontaneously after a few days, but the child and family should be warned about this.

Chemotherapy is unpleasant and the preferred regimen of drugs is subject to frequent change. This therapy should only be given under the direct supervision of a well-trained, specialist team. The side-effects include bone marrow suppression, loss of hair and severe vomiting, although this can be controlled by drugs.

Testicular cancer today can nearly always be cured, and knowing this can be of enormous help to children and families in providing the encouragement they need in the months of treatment that may be necessary.

REFERENCES

BIRMINGHAM REFLUX STUDY GROUP (1983) Prospective trial of operative versus non-operative treatment of severe vesicoureteric reflux: two years observation in 96 children. *British Medical Journal* **287**: 171–174.

BLANDY J P and Moors J (1989) *Urology for Nurses*. Oxford: Blackwell Scientific.

CARR M C (Ed.) (1995) Fertility, sexuality and gender identity in exstrophy and cloacal exstrophy patients. *Dialogues in Paediatric Urology* **18**(10).

COHEN S J (1977) The Cohen reimplantation technique. *Birth Defects* **13**: 391–395.

GAIRDNER D (1949) The fate of the foreskin: A study of circumcision. *British Medical Journal* **2**: 1433.

GEARHART J P (Ed.) (1993) Osteotomy and the bladder exstrophy patient. *Dialogues in Paediatric Urology* **16**(1).

GREENFIELD S P (Ed.) (1992) Mathieu hypospadias repair. *Dialogues in Paediatric Urology* **15**(10).

KAPLAN G W (1992) Reconstruction of hypospadias and epispadias. *Dialogues in Paediatric Urology* **15**(10).

KEATING M A and Duckett J W (1989) Current status of hypospadias repair. *Paediatric Urology* Boston: 94–114.

LAPIDES J, Ananias C D, Silber S J and Lowe B S (1972) Clean intermittent self catheterization in the treatment of urinary tract disease. *Journal of Urology* **107**: 458–461.

McKENNA P H (Ed.) (1995) Current and future options in nonbowel augmentation cystoplasty. *Dialogues in Paediatric Urology* **18**(1).

MOSTOFI F K and Price E B (1983) Tumors of the male genital system. Washington, DC: Armed Forces Institute of Pathology.

NGUYEN D H (Ed.) (1994) The use of stomach in the urinary tract: an update. *Dialogues in Paediatric Urology* **17**(9).

O'DONNELL B and Puri P (1986) Endoscopic correction of primary vesicoureteric reflux: results in 94 ureters. *British Medical Journal* **293**: 1404–1406.

POLITANO V A and Leadbetter W F (1958) An operative technique for the correction of vesicoureteric reflux. *Journal of Urology* **79**: 932–941.

RODGERS J (1991) Pass the cranberry juice. *Nursing Times* **87**(48): 36–37.

SOBATA A E (1984) Inhibition of bacterial adherence by cranberry juice: potential use for the treatment of urinary tract infections. *Journal of Urology* **131**(5): 1013–1016.

STOLLER R (1968) Sex and gender. On the development of masculinity and femininity. London: Hogarth.

FURTHER READING

BRAREN V (1990) Post-op instructions for circumcision care. *Journal of Urological Nursing* **9**(2): 896–897.

DUCKETT J W and Snyder H McC (1985) Use of the Mitrofanoff principle in urinary reconstruction. *World Journal of Urology* **3**: 191–193.

FRANCO I (ed.) (1995) Surgical alternatives in neurogenic bladder management. *Dialogues in Paediatric Urology* **18**(5).

GIBBONS M (1995) Urinary problems after formation of a Mitrofanoff stoma. *Professional Nurse* January: 221–223.

HEALTH NEWS (1993) The circumcision debate. *Health News* **11**(3): 6–7.

McFARLANE K (1993) Primary vesicoureteric reflux in childhood. *Paediatric Nursing* **5**(8): 20–22.

MOURIQUAND P D E et al (1995) The Kropp-onlay procedure. *British Journal of Urology* **75**: 656–662.

ROBERTS J A (1990) Is routine circumcision indicated in the newborn? An Affirmative View. *The Journal of Family Practice* **31**(2): 185–188.

ROSELLA J D (1994) Testicular cancer health education: an integrative review. *Journal of Advanced Nursing* **20**(4): 666–671.

SNYDER H M (1991) To Circumcise or Not. *Hospital Practice* **26**(1): 201–207.

SUMMERS E (1995) Vital Signs . . . testicular cancer. *Nursing Times* **91**(25): 46–47.

THOMPSON R S (1990) Routine circumcision in the newborn: An Opposing View. *The Journal of Family Practice* **31**(2): 189–196.

TURNER D (1995) Testicular cancer and the value of self-examination. *Nursing Times* **91**(1): 30–31.

16 PSYCHOLOGICAL EFFECTS OF UROLOGICAL PROBLEMS

Contents

NURSING ADULTS WITH UROLOGICAL PROBLEMS

Innovative urology – implications for the patient

The new advances in minimally invasive therapy have many implications for the patient. Perhaps the most noticeable effect of endourology is that the length of hospital stay is reduced. In some instances, hospitalization may be replaced by a visit to the day surgery unit or the uro-radiology department for treatment.

It has long been recognized that prolonged hospital stay can lead to detrimental effects for the patient – see for example Wright (1974) and Dyson (1978). However, a short stay may not afford much time to prepare patients psychologically for their treatment.

When patients enter the urology department it may be their first experience of hospital care. Their expectations may be very different from the reality. People often have misconceptions, gleaned from horror stories in the tabloid press, or indeed from individuals who enjoy recounting their bad experiences. Conversely, patients may have high, or unrealistic expectations that the surgery will cure all problems. With the addition of the other significant stressors that the patient may be experiencing – for instance, the pain of renal colic, the shock of a newly diagnosed malignancy or the fear of the planned change in body image – one may be faced with a very vulnerable patient. By building a trusting relationship the nurse can identify and try to resolve the emotional and psychological needs of the patient, both real and potential.

To provide a quality service for patients all these issues need to be considered. The surgery may be less invasive but the psychological impact for the patient may not alter. Boore (1978) and Haywood (1975) illustrated the importance of preoperative information. The development of preadmission clinics is in part a response to the reduction in the length of hospital stay for the patient. The nurse is able to provide preoperative information and address any anxieties. Patients appear reassured by their visit and are relieved at the prospect of meeting a familiar face on admission to hospital.

Psychological issues in urological nursing

Incontinence

There are several definitions of urinary incontinence, but as Faugier (1988) pointed out, it is commonly seen as 'loss of control'. The International Continence Society defined incontinence as 'the involuntary loss of urine so severe as to have social and/or hygienic consequences' (Bates, 1979). Inherent in this definition is the idea that the severity or importance of the problem as perceived by the sufferer. This is important to consider when making a nursing assessment.

Incontinence remains a taboo subject and this is in part due to deeply engrained myths and beliefs. Mitteness (1990) found that the public has only a vague understanding of the causes and parameters of incontinence. Commonly held beliefs include the idea that it is an inevitable part of ageing, or a consequence of childbirth (Cheater, 1991). As a result only a small percentage of incontinence is reported. Norton et al. (1987) found that 60% of their sample delayed their presentation for over a year. This may be partly explained by denial to friends, family or self. People often feel embarrassed and guilty about such a loss of control of a complex but basic bodily function learnt in earlier years.

A qualitative study by Ashworth and Hagan (1993) of the effects of urinary incontinence on a group of young women highlighted three main areas to which the group paid particular attention. These were the vague and difficult to grasp nature of their problem, the effect on their self-image and the impact of the problem on their lives. Thus patients may be harbouring feelings of embarrassment, shame and even guilt about their problem. A sensitive approach to the problem is required, as is reassurance by the nurse that their incontinence will be treated as a legitimate problem.

Disfigurement

Surgery that causes disfigurement of the patient can be likened to the grieving process (Kübler-Ross, 1973). In urology there are several conditions to consider; for example, malignancy of the genitalia may in extreme cases lead to penectomy or orchidectomy. Malignancy and other pathology affecting the bladder may lead to formation of a stoma (ileal conduit).

Formation of an ileal conduit

Stoma surgery challenges many of the values and beliefs instilled in childhood. As toddlers we were rewarded if we made it to the toilet in time, but accidents were not viewed so positively. Incontinence is seen as regression or bad behaviour, reinforcing the idea that it is something to feel guilty, ashamed or embarrassed about (Faugier, 1988).

The patient with an ileal conduit will no longer have control over urination. The activity which used to be a private one will be discussed openly by medical and nursing staff. The urine which was formerly expelled out of sight, down the toilet, is now permanently visible. The fear of leaking bags and of lack of attraction within a sexual relationship are all common anxieties (Salter, 1996).

The support of nursing staff and the stoma care nurse, in both the emotional adjustment and practical management of the stoma (see Chapter 11), will help the patient to adapt. The patient may exhibit changes in behaviour in a struggle to come to terms with an altered body image. Reassurance that such a response is not uncommon will help them through the process.

Body image

Individuals bring with them a personal body image which is an intrinsic part of their being. Once they become a patient their body image will inevitably be challenged. Body image, as defined by Price (1990), is what we think and feel about our body. A body image model devised by Price (1990) illustrates the 'tension' and 'balance' needed to satisfy a person's body image. Individuals are seen to possess a dynamic personal image of their body and this comprises three central components (Figure 16.1). The model is intended to

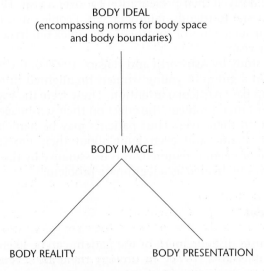

BODY IDEAL
(encompassing norms for body space
and body boundaries)

BODY IMAGE

BODY REALITY   BODY PRESENTATION

Figure 16.1   *Body image model, adapted from Price (1990)*

provide a framework for nurses in assessing, planning and implementing care for those undergoing procedures that could damage the individual's body image and concept of self.

Price views the nurse as the prime mover in the team best qualified to assist patients in re-establishing a satisfactory body image. The nurse has most contact with the patients, attending to their physical and psychological needs in an holistic framework.

The three components of body image

Body ideal 'Body ideal' concerns our view of what we think our body should look like, and how it should behave. Price uses the term 'body ideal' because we continuously check ourselves against society's ideal figure. An individual's cultural background influences this perception of an ideal image. Components of a person's body ideal include body size, contours, strength, control and body ageing. A patient awaiting surgery may feel their 'body ideal' is challenged by anxiety, and a reduced level of awareness (premedication).

Body presentation 'Body presentation' is the way in which we present ourselves and is influenced by body ideal. Other important contributing factors include social trends and fashions, portrayed through the media and advertising industry. Components of a person's body presentation include posture, dress and action. Surgery can have a significant effect on the patients' body presentation, for example the removal of jewellery, make-up, dentures and other prostheses preoperatively, together with the postoperative intravenous lines, catheters and drainage bags, wound drains, nasogastric tube and oxygen mask which the patient may require.

Body reality 'Body reality' refers to the body as it really is. It differs from body ideal in that it is a mirror image of self, with no trick lighting. Components of a person's body reality include height and scars. Considerations for the surgical patient include wearing a theatre gown, thromboembolic deterrent stockings and identification bands. Postoperatively the patient may have a wound site, shaved hair or a stoma.

Summary Of the three components of body image, individuals have least control over their body reality. A person has to compete hard if they wish to live up to an ideal body image and tend to have most control over their body presentation. The nurse should make note of the patient's body presentation on admission to hospital and note changes thereafter, to assess how an individual is adjusting to changes in body image. If patients are aware that the nurse is supporting them to this end, it will help to reduce their vulnerability. It is important to recognize the very real body image needs of the patient undergoing comparatively routine urological surgery. For the nurse, it may be part of an average day at work, but for the patient it may be a very new and daunting prospect.

The factors influencing the surgical patient's body image will be changeable, and may alter rapidly in response to their recovery from the operation. The nurse should be able to respond quickly in a calm, efficient and informative manner. It is vital that we warn patients and close relatives of potential expectations in an attempt to allay anxieties.

Altered body image

When an individual becomes a patient all three components of body image may be challenged and this will make it difficult to sustain control when the patient faces an alteration of body image. Under these circumstances people will employ any number of coping mechanisms. Platzer (1987) identified a number of negative coping strategies:

- ◆ Denial and displacement – the person avoids the issue at hand, often steering the conversation and choosing to focus on other issues, over which they have more control.
- ◆ Projection – the individual projects their own anxieties through another person. For example, 'my wife can't cope' or 'my friend went through a similar experience and was unable to deal with things'.
- ◆ Reaction foundation – patients' behaviour is exactly opposite to how they feel, often to avoid fuss or attention on the area which they are finding difficult. This can range from remarks such as, 'No, really I'm fine', to a more extreme response when the behaviour may seem quite inappropriate. An example would be of a patient who is being overtly sexual following surgery which has rendered him impotent.
- ◆ Regression – the person becomes more dependent than is necessary. Often they can be demanding, unable to take control of their own basic needs and requirements which would not cause a problem in normal circumstances.
- ◆ Rationalization and intellectualization – these give the appearance of coping. This behaviour occurs when the individuals have insight into how they are supposed to be coping and are able to 'turn on' this behaviour, but in fact are not coping in that fashion at all.
- ◆ Depersonalization – the individual takes themselves out of the experience so that they do not have to deal with the circumstances. For example, 'I can cope with this if I think of myself as just another number'.

While in the short term these may be perfectly adequate coping mechanisms, long-term they may prevent the patient from being able to make personal adjustments and adaptations to their change in body image.

How can the nurse help?

As nurses our role is to support patients through their experience with a view to reducing their vulnerability. Price (1986) emphasized that supporting is not about propping up, it is about augmenting strengths and returning patients to mastery of their body.

Another element of supporting is ensuring the patient is well informed. Wilson-Barnett (1980) reflected that by sharing nursing and medical knowledge of perceived expectations then the patient's coping strategies are more effective. Patient information leaflets and booklets can contribute greatly to this support. The Royal College of Surgeons' information booklet for patients

Surgery on the Prostate (Devlin, 1995) for example, gives a comprehensive overview of what the patient can expect.

Applying the nursing process

The nurse is in a prime position to assist patients through the process of a change to their body image. Perhaps the most important step is the first, i.e. making a good assessment. If the nurse is able to gain the patient's confidence and lay the foundations of a trusting relationship, this can reduce many of the initial anxieties.

Planning care   Planning care for body image is about setting individual priorities, choosing approaches and setting long-term and short-term goals. The planning for body image changes cannot be separated from the planning of other care for the patient – the two should be integrated (Price, 1990).

- ◆ 'Body reality' requirements include planning for nutritional support, maintaining a safe environment, etc.
- ◆ 'Body ideal' is best achieved by acknowledging the old body ideal, learning about new limitations and identifying a new body ideal.
- ◆ 'Body presentation' is managed by preserving patient's dignity within a changing body image, for example concealing drainage bags.

Delivering care   Delivering care involves carrying out the planned care in a supportive framework when patients are unable to care for themselves. The intention is to restore patients to a position in which they can take control over the change in their body image. This requires a sensitive approach, and the knowledge and skills to carry out the care, and teach the patient self-care. Furthermore, nurses must recognize their own limitations and refer to other members of the care team as appropriate.

Evaluation   Price suggested that it is wise to evaluate both long-term and short-term goals together. Evaluation of improvements in body image are very subjective. A patient who continues to express dissatisfaction with an altered body image may well be displaying positive coping strategies. This should be noted, fed back to the patient and viewed with encouragement.

What are positive coping strategies?

Salter (1988) suggested that we may be able to consider a patient to be coping positively when the altered body image is no longer an all-consuming problem in the person's daily life. The patient is equipped with the necessary 'resources, devices, philosophies and social skills that enable him to deal with the daily problems arising out of an altered body image' (Salter, 1988) – that is, he appears to be independent.

Body image changes and nursing models

One way of contributing to the positive adaptation to an altered body image is to use a nursing model that requires assessment in the self-concept mode, such as the Roy adaptation model (Roy, 1976). Two levels of assessment are made: firstly, whether the behaviour is adaptive or maladaptive; secondly, to identify the stimuli causing the behaviour. Stimuli that lead to adaptive behaviour are to be encouraged. Conversely, those which contribute to maladaptive behaviour should be addressed.

Sexuality

Body image is an integral part of an individual's sexuality (McKenzie, 1988). Woods (1975) stated that 'sexuality pervades human beings, influencing their self-images, feelings and relationships with others'. Sexuality is part of a person's total personality, encompassing biological, psychological and social aspects. If as nurses we grasp the fundamental concepts of sexuality then as individuals we will be more able to reflect on our values and challenge any prejudices that may exist.

Biological aspects

Biological aspects cover the physical components of sexuality and include:

◆ the reproductive system and sexual organs
◆ the secondary features of sexual development, such as breast development or hair growth
◆ erectile function, menstruation and contraception

The close proximity of the urinary system to the reproductive organs means that any urological intervention can significantly affect the individual's sexuality. Norton (1982) studied the effect of incontinence on a sample of 55 women and found it had affected their relationships.

Psychological aspects

Psychological aspects include body image (see above). Gender preferences are also important, whether the person is attracted to the same sex, the opposite sex, or both.

It is important not to assume heterosexuality when making a nursing assessment. Andrews (1988) talked about 'de-genderizing' the language. It is far more sensitive to ask the patient, 'Do you have a partner?' rather than, 'Are you married?' The latter option may unleash a whole barrage of emotions for a patient who may have been recently widowed. If the patient has recently split up from a relationship, or is having difficulties within a relationship, they may share this information with you. The nurse could then follow with a question such as, 'How are you feeling about the break-up/relationship now?' The patient may go on to talk openly about it, or not. A patient who feels that their privacy is respected may feel more comfortable about approaching the nurse with any further anxieties.

Social aspects

Social aspects include the values of a specific culture, gender roles and stereotypes. Within a given culture there is a socially approved sexual behaviour for both sexes. Brink (1987) explored these issues. In westernized culture, a heterosexual relationship is the dominant accepted sexual pattern. However, within heterosexuality there are acceptable and unacceptable behaviours. For example, sexual intercourse between heterosexuals when one member is non-consenting is not socially valued.

♦   Cultural issues: every culture exerts an enormous pressure on individuals to conform to accepted norms. Homosexuals, bisexuals and transsexuals continue to be less positively valued, and often fall victim to stigma and judgement in day-to-day life. This is a particular issue for patients with gender dysphoria, and a sensitive approach to their needs on a main ward is required.

♦   Cross-cultural issues: living in a multicultural society, nurses can expect to confront some cross-cultural issues in their careers. One extreme example is female circumcision: in certain cultural groups, it continues to be practised and is an accepted norm. It is a valuable exercise for nurses to explore the arguments and ethical debates surrounding these matters. Should such an issue ever arise, the nurse will then be able to respond in a more informed manner.

Approaching sexual issues – the need for introspection

As nurses, we should aim to work non-judgementally within the individual's frame of reference (Brink, 1987). If we ourselves feel uncomfortable with someone's sexual orientation then we must first recognize this in ourselves and avoid using 'blocking' techniques (McLeod Clark, 1981) as a coping strategy; for example, avoiding questions by keeping 'busy'. We could alleviate our own anxiety about the topic by becoming better informed.

Peer support may be useful, and using nursing hand-over time to explore such issues can often be very supportive, and particularly useful in enlightening student nurses and fulfilling our position as role models to them. The use of value clarification exercises to explore values and moral questions within a teaching programme or privately can also be an effective method of reflecting on personal beliefs and moral values.

♦   *Example 1*: a patient recovering from a radical prostatectomy has been rendered impotent as a result. While you are assisting him with a wash he is overtly sexual with you in conversation. How does this make you feel?

♦   *Example 2*: a patient of the same sex makes a sexual remark directed towards you while you are assisting them with a wash. How does this make you feel?

Both of these scenarios may make you feel uncomfortable. The nurse's response to the situation will be affected by the socially accepted sexual norm and also by a personal sexual preference.

An understanding of the effects of an altered body image will help the nurse to recognize that this may be a response when the patient feels that their sexuality is being threatened. In both examples the patients' needs are the same. A supportive response might be to say, 'You are making a lot of sexual remarks. Some people in your situation worry about their sexual functioning. Is this something that is on your mind?' Responding in this way will then allow the patient to explore such issues, if they feel they want to. If a person is embarrassed to discuss sexual issues, we are reinforcing this by ignoring such comments. All patients have a sexual orientation, including the elderly who are often forgotten. Nursing models tend to include sexuality as a feature, for example Roper et al (1985). Jacobson (1974) pointed out that we have a duty to address the issue when – or even before – it arises. A private environment, spending time with the patient and good communication skills will all help the patient feel more at ease.

People's understanding of their anatomy varies considerably, as does their vocabulary of sexual terminology. It is important to be clear, and avoid euphemisms, for example using the word 'fellatio' when talking about oral sex. Check you have understood what the patient has said by reflecting back to them their concerns. One approach could be, 'From what you have said you seem to be concerned about A, B and C . . . ?'. The patient will not be angry if you have misinterpreted them initially, if you are then able to clarify their concerns.

Erectile dysfunction

Many patients undergoing urological procedures are faced with the prospect of erectile dysfunction. The widely accepted definition of erectile impotence is the inability to obtain or sustain a penile erection sufficient for intercourse. It is an underreported problem traditionally viewed as a man's problem, but considered also to affect the man's partner. It can affect the man's self-esteem and put tremendous pressure on his physical relationships.

It is important that the patient is aware of the potential risk and able to give informed consent for the surgery. The patient also needs to know that alternative help is available, such as the vacuum device, intracavernosal injection therapy and penile prostheses (Chapter 12). Likewise, women who experience difficulty with sexual intercourse should be offered advice about devices to enhance their physical satisfaction (Davis, 1990).

The emergence of nurse-led erectile dysfunction clinics is in part a response to a great demand for the service. In this innovative period, the literature is scant as to the qualitative outcomes of such clinics. However, the initial positive feedback from patients indicates that nurses are knowledgeable, skilled practitioners able to provide a holistic approach to the problem.

The underlying skills required of the nurse are a sensitive approach to issues, in a non-hurried fashion, with attention to the patients' dignity and privacy at all times. It is fundamentally about building a trusting rapport with the patient and supporting them and their loved ones through an experience, and providing them with the skills to reach a point of adaptation and acceptance of their situation.

NURSING ADOLESCENTS WITH UROLOGICAL PROBLEMS

As adolescent care becomes an established area both in medicine and surgery, nursing adolescent patients becomes an important issue in patient care today

(Department of Health, 1991; Audit Commission, 1993). More and more paediatric consultants are now transferring their patients to adolescent consultants. Adolescent oncology and orthopaedic units are becoming well-established. The nursing care of adolescents has become an area in urology which requires exploration and research.

Children with long-term urological abnormalities are vulnerable to psychological trauma in their adolescence. The intention of this chapter is to highlight the importance of these problems, and to help nurses involved in the care of adolescents to have a knowledge and understanding of this age group and their long-term adaptation to urological problems.

Congenital urological abnormalities, such as bladder exstrophy and epispadias (see Chapter 15), are major conditions where affected patients can suffer from total incontinence of urine and abnormal-looking genitals from birth. These problems require many hospital admissions and major reconstructive surgery from a very early age. It is known that early hospitalization can cause behavioural disturbances in later life (Douglas, 1975; Quinton and Rutter 1976; Rodin, 1983). Surgery may continue into puberty and late adolescence, with a slow and sometimes unsuccessful outcome until the patient is 'dry' and able to empty the bladder by means of voiding or self-catheterization. Meanwhile, these children attempt to live their lives as normally as possible. Dealing with the accompanying problems of wetness at school age, wearing nappies and pads when other children of the same age are able to control their bladder, can be the cause of much stress and anxiety for children, teachers and parents. Normal development is restricted, such as playing with other children for long periods of time (Fradd, 1988; Peterson, 1989). They can be teased and called names both at home and in school. Everyday enjoyable pastimes children want to engage in, such as games, sports, camping trips and staying overnight with friends, are an added source of stress for the child and family. The disappointment of slow results and multiple surgical procedures along with pain in the postoperative period at this early stage of growing up means that many affected children become withdrawn or aggressive in nature and subsequently become labelled as having 'behavioural problems' (Visintainer and Wolfer, 1975). Hospitalization requires them to spend more time in the company of adults, such as parents and nursing and medical staff, and reduces their contact with healthy children, possibly affecting social skills through a lack of interaction with the same age group. This can result in isolation and a feeling of being different from other children, making adolescence a much more troubled time for themselves and those around them.

It is reported that the non-compliance rate among schoolchildren with long-term medical problems has been estimated to range between 17% and 64% (Friedman *et al.*, 1986).

Trends in illness

As child mortality decreases in westernized countries and life-threatening illnesses are better controlled, emphasis is shifted from acute infectious diseases to the care of chronically ill or handicapped children (Garrison and Mcquiston, 1989). Selekman (1991) noted that 10–20% of all American children have some form of chronic illness or disability and that the majority of these children are diagnosed during the first year of their life. The baby who is born with a chronic condition or genetic abnormality will alter the environment for the family, making it more difficult for them to cope. This in turn may influence the environment in which the child develops (Paton and Brown, 1991).

Children with congenital abnormalities face a lifetime of hospital appointments, diagnostic procedures and sometimes painful treatments. Their parents and siblings will be touched and changed by an unexpected diagnosis (Eiser, 1993). These children can experience social restrictions because of their disabilities. These restrictions could be as a result of the condition or of parental anxiety in discouraging children from taking up activities that are perceived to be dangerous and carry the risk of further injury which the parents feel would be wise to avoid.

What is adolescence?

Although teenagers have always been with us, their existence as a specific group with their unique psychological characteristics has only recently been recognized by Western society. Until the eighteenth century teenagers were regarded as either overgrown children or undergrown adults. In the Victorian era they were expected to be seen and not heard. Nowadays, however, adolescents have become identified as a separate social group, with a process of identifying themselves as a group and the development of their own music and dancing, hairstyles and make-up (Lowe, 1972). In Western society adolescence is defined simply as a period of transition between childhood and adult life. There is no limit on the age group but the onset of puberty is accepted as a starting point, and it can end with adopting the role of adult within a given culture (Paton and Brown, 1991). In many parts of the world adolescence as a separate stage of growing up does not exist. The transition is marked instead by some ritualistic ceremony. The person can wake up as a child and by the end of the day go to bed as an adult (Paton and Brown, 1991). The major developmental task in this period of life is to invoke a sense of identity.

The World Health Organization (1977) defined adolescents according to chronological age, stating that adolescence begins at the age of 10 years and ends at age 20 years. The legal definition of adolescence is not clear. Young people under the age of 18 years are considered legally to be minors. However, under Section 8 of the Family Law Reforms Act (1960) a minor aged 16–17 years can give consent to treatment (Dimond, 1990). Succeeding events such as 'Gillick competence' considered that children below the age of 16 years can also give consent to treatment under certain circumstances. The Children Act (Department of Health, 1989), in relation to giving consent, rules that 'parental responsibility itself diminishes as the child acquires sufficient understanding to make his or her own decisions'.

Identity

A major developmental task that confronts adolescents is that of acquiring a sense of identity, a sense of who they are as people. Until Erikson (1968) formulated his concept of identity, psychologists had found it extremely difficult to explain, or even to understand, the psychological preoccupations of adolescence.

Identity is a basic, general feature of our lives, apparent in one form or another at all developmental stages. During adolescence, identity becomes predominant and is disturbed by biological changes which are not only extreme and profound, but are in many ways inconsistent. Biological changes, whenever they occur, always have important psychological consequences. The mere fact that the muscles of boys become nearly twice as large between the ages of 12 and 16 years gives rise to a more energetic output which can in turn give them greater self-confidence when comparing and competing with older people. These changes will affect the adolescent's concept of who they are. They may find their physical strength equal, if not superior, to their father as their new body image is disturbed (Lowe, 1972).

According to Erikson (1977), the adolescent's sense of identity develops gradually out of various 'identifications' of childhood. A young child's values are largely taken from and moulded by those of their parents, and their self-esteem arises from the views their parents express about them directly or indirectly (Paton and Brown, 1991). In adolescence, the values of their peers become important. Adolescents clarify their identity by interacting with other people in groups and in constant conversation where it is possible to explore a variety of ideologies and beliefs (Paton and Brown, 1991). Adolescents are faced with the task of developing a value system and preparing to make decisions about their future. This may be in the form of continuing education or choosing a job or career. It is during this period that individuals prepare themselves for independence.

Crucial issues related to the adolescent developmental tasks of identity and independence are those of establishing an independence from parents and developing positive feelings regarding sexuality and body image (Dewis, 1989). Identity in adolescence is affected not only by biological changes within the individual but also by the social expectation and opportunities available (Lowe, 1972). In today's multicultural climate the importance of different cultural backgrounds must be taken into account if the adolescent's beliefs, attitudes and behaviour are to be understood (Paton and Brown, 1991).

Development of independence

Adolescence is a period in which young people usually become relatively independent from their parents. As adolescents grow up and become physically independent, their needs may change. Peer groups become a more important part of their life, family ties are weakened and replaced by peer group activities, new experiences and relationships (Taylor and Muller, 1995). Adolescents begin to question family values and require explanations and reasons. This demand for independence increases tension within the family structure. There are many factors that influence the extent to which independence is gained. Taylor and Muller (1995) pointed out that family structure, family regulation and parenting patterns are important in gaining independence, but other factors such as socioeconomic states of adolescence, culture and religion are important issues in today's society.

Children who were 'overprotected' owing to chronic illness may find it difficult as adolescents to cope with the demands of becoming independent, and in some cases parents will find it hard to let go and allow an adolescent the choice to make their own decision (Taylor and Muller, 1995). Adolescents with health problems may find independence from their family much more difficult to achieve, in part because of the restriction their condition puts on their lives and the security and importance the family relationship and interaction within it offer, although these qualities are an important issue in gaining independence from the family itself.

As to when adolescents should become responsible for their own self-care, Johnson et al. (1982) focused on young diabetic patients, pointing out that this group were poorly informed about many aspects of their self-care which had an effect on management of their disease, and that they could not realistically be expected to cope alone.

The nurse's understanding of family dynamics in our society is crucial. Careful intervention can assist adolescents in gaining independence from their families by, for example, being taught how to perform tasks for themselves or how to detect a urine infection by observations of colour, smell or texture. Encouragement to find out about self-help organizations can help in breaking dependence on family ties.

Cognitive development

Piaget (1952) argued that during adolescence cognitive abilities are characterized by an ability to think logically at a theoretical level (Table 16.1). Whereas 'concrete operational' thinkers (7–11 years) (see Figure 16.1) cannot separate themselves from the objective world and think about purely hypothetical propositions, the 'formal operational' thinker can. Whaley and Wong (1993) pointed out that in this period of life, adolescents are also concerned with the 'possible'. At this stage their thoughts can be influenced by logical principles rather than just their own perceptions and experiences. They now become capable of scientific reasoning and formal logic. It is during this period of life that adolescents may think about their future role as adults and of having children. It is at this time that the question of their fertility arises and they become aware of the risks involved in passing their genetic disorder to their children.

Sexual development

Puberty increases glandular changes in adolescents and produces new and turbulent sexual feelings which are often strange and disturbing when first experienced. They may indeed change drastically the adolescent's attitude towards the opposite sex. Sexual identity, sexual urges and sexual limits and boundaries constitute an important preoccupation among adolescents (Lowe, 1972).

Sexual development is an area that often causes concern to some young people with urological disorders. Delayed puberty, lack of or scattered pubic

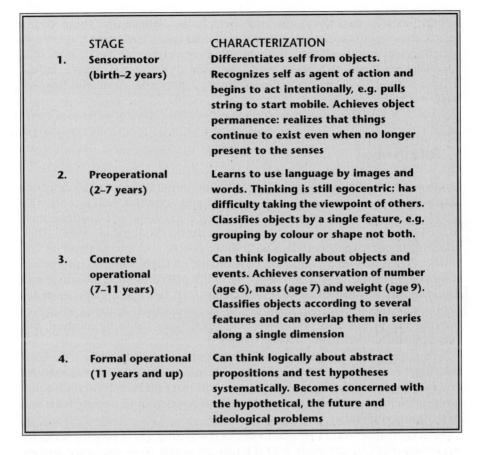

	STAGE	CHARACTERIZATION
1.	Sensorimotor (birth–2 years)	Differentiates self from objects. Recognizes self as agent of action and begins to act intentionally, e.g. pulls string to start mobile. Achieves object permanence: realizes that things continue to exist even when no longer present to the senses
2.	Preoperational (2–7 years)	Learns to use language by images and words. Thinking is still egocentric: has difficulty taking the viewpoint of others. Classifies objects by a single feature, e.g. grouping by colour or shape not both.
3.	Concrete operational (7–11 years)	Can think logically about objects and events. Achieves conservation of number (age 6), mass (age 7) and weight (age 9). Classifies objects according to several features and can overlap them in series along a single dimension
4.	Formal operational (11 years and up)	Can think logically about abstract propositions and test hypotheses systematically. Becomes concerned with the hypothetical, the future and ideological problems

Table 16.1   Piaget's stages of cognitive development

hair owing to surgical scars, and alternative voiding mechanisms such as in self-catheterization (urethral or continent diversion), may cause lack of confidence when seeking to form relationships, thus causing further isolation from peer groups. Mackenzie (1988) pointed out that during this stage the peer group becomes all-important, and in order to feel secure the adolescent must feel accepted in the group.

Taylor and Muller (1995) pointed out that the need to 'find oneself' is an important psychological driving force in this turbulent period of adolescent life. This is an important element in directing and enabling them to identify with peer groups. Adolescents who have urological abnormalities find themselves even more isolated from peer group activities, which may take the form of who can drink the most or who is able to 'pee' the furthest. This limitation in their lives keeps them from mixing with their own age group and therefore denies them the feeling of belonging.

The lack of confidence in overcoming their physical limitations is seen in outpatient departments and on the wards. The strong feelings of inferiority, anger, of not being like everybody else and particularly of not being 'fixed' yet is, as an 18-year-old young man said, the cause of extra stress for themselves and their families. Some will lose the desire to care for their appearance and hygiene, which may result in being avoided by friends. The desire to interact socially may disappear and there is the danger that these young people may stop mixing with others of a similar age. Others may not comply with medical treatment and their health may deteriorate because of this, necessitating frequent admissions to hospital and the consequent falling behind with schoolwork, as well as forming a dependency on the hospital staff.

Self-esteem

Developing a healthy sense of self-esteem is an important part of adolescence and involves evaluating one's own qualities and activities. Adolescents who are ill or disabled may find it difficult to develop a sense of self-worth because of the limitations placed upon them by their illness (Muller *et al.*, 1988). They continually compare themselves with other people and find themselves less worthy. Their deficiencies may become central to their thoughts and preoccupy them constantly (Gills, 1980). Basic life activities such as eating and drinking, which most of us take for granted, can become a major issue for people with incontinence in the necessity to restrict their drinking whenever they go out in order to stay dry. These restrictions cause resentment and eventual withdrawal from social activities.

Factors that can help people with long-term problems to deal with such situations are unique to the individual. People with different personalities and varying mental and physical abilities will react differently to their long-term problems. Family dynamics and support are crucial in dealing with and overcoming difficulties.

Nurses can help young people to develop a greater sense of self-esteem by involving them in decisions and discussions about their own care and by promoting self-care. Education plays an important role in the adolescent period. Gaining knowledge of their condition can be an area in which adolescents may be involved, thus increasing their understanding and empowering them to make an informed decision about their future. Support groups can be a way of learning about each other and interacting with each other. Belle (1989) in a study of young adolescents with cancer noted that the amount of support received by friends and peer groups increases during adolescence. In the UK, the Great Ormond Street Hospital for Sick Children runs a support group called the Bladder Exstrophy and Epispadias Society (BEES), which provides newsletters, organizes an annual meeting and presents lectures by paediatric urologists for parents and their children. This can be a useful area in educating patients and their families. The BEES organizers run a holiday camp once a year to bring together adolescents of different ages to socialize during the time together. The older ones usually take care of the younger ones with the organizer's supervision. This is an area which in an adolescent can develop self-esteem by helping younger children to overcome their limitations and feel they are not the only one with problems. An awakening of other values may occur, such as pride in oneself and mastery of tasks. Drench (1994) calls it 'promoting self-esteem'. Other strategies include promoting increased motivation, co-operation and achievement which can eventually be perceived as of greater personal value than the 'body beautiful' (Drench, 1994).

Body image

Price (1990) pointed out that 'body image' is the complex and sometimes an abstract way in which we picture our bodies. As discussed earlier in this chapter, the components necessary to form and maintain these images of ourselves are:

- ◆ body reality – the way in which our body is constructed
- ◆ body ideal – how we think and would like our body to look
- ◆ body presentation – how we present ourselves in terms of dress, pose, behaviour and actions

In the social world, body image plays a crucial part in our lives. Media, especially television, play an important part in telling us how we should look. How people feel about themselves is related to how they feel about their body. Adolescents in searching for identity have problems with body image and body changes due to puberty (Paton and Brown, 1991). Saylor (1990) suggested that because a great deal of value is placed on health and beauty in our culture, images of physical perfection – in contrast to their perceived 'body imperfection' – prevent the chronically ill from interacting effectively in society. Whenever we watch television or read magazines, the 'normal' successful person is projected as a healthy and attractive one. This media image places pressure on disabled or chronically ill people by high-lighting their imperfections. Diabetic teenagers may worry about what their friends will think about the fact that they have to inject themselves with insulin. This may reduce their willingness to interact with others through fear of the response, thus reducing the quality of their life (Paton and Brown, 1991).

Adolescents with urological abnormalities find it difficult to overcome their 'body reality' which may comprise surgical scars, strange genitals or an alternative voiding system. Their 'body ideal' from television and other media images, causes them to feel that they are not like their peer group, resulting in feelings of isolation and lowered self-esteem. The outcome of this is a failure to present themselves well, therefore losing out in social activities with peer groups. Reduced interaction with others results in poorer social skills, anger, frustration, lost trust in their abilities and a reduced sense of self-worth.

Another factor in dealing with the problem is the 'coping mechanism'. A 'coping mechanism' is defined by Folkman (1984) as 'efforts to manage demands, regardless of the success of those efforts'. Because as individuals we are unique, people react differently to their problems and demands, therefore the coping mechanisms used are different. Gills (1980) divided coping mechanisms into accepting the illness or disability and dealing with it, or reacting negatively to the problem (i.e. a denial mechanism), therefore dismissing it. In order for adolescent patients reacting in the latter way to adapt to their situation and overcome their limitations, they must receive psychological as well as clinical help. Nichols (1984) noted the importance of psychological care and its aims. He pointed out that 'the aim is to minimize the trauma of illness by giving instruction and information, providing supportive intervention to help with psychological reactions and social difficulties when they arise, and of course, standard medical procedures'. He based his psychological care on four aspects:

- ◆ emotional care
- ◆ information care, acting as an agent on behalf of the client
- ◆ counselling
- ◆ monitoring psychological states and referring when necessary (Nichols, 1984)

The role of the psychologist has in the past been one of intervention during crises. The urology nurse can provide emotional support to both parents and adolescents, dispense accurate information, and also act as advocate for the adolescents and their families. Nurses should be aware of the psychological problems this group of clients may encounter and facilitate prompt referral to a counsellor or psychologist whenever the situation demands. We often ask for too little help too late from psychologists and counsellors. In today's caring climate, it is common to see a psychologist attached to special units dealing with life-threatening conditions such as cancers, but it is rare for children with chronic diseases and their families to be offered routine 'non-crises orientated psychological help'. Eiser (1993) argued that this situation should be changed for two reasons. Firstly, by intervening earlier in the problem, escalation of the crisis into a major event can be reduced and routine psychologial input will be associated with earlier presentation of a problem and managed sooner rather than later. The second reason is that the children themselves may encounter problems that may not be disease-related. These problems may be interpersonal problems with siblings or relationships with others in school, anxiety about a relationship with someone of the opposite sex, or arguments with parents. These issues may seem trivial (and part of normal adolescent development) as healthy children may encounter the same problems, but 'trivial' problems may seem immense to an individual who already faces disease and its treatment as part of the daily stress load. A recent study by Olsen (1988, cited by Eiser, 1993), found that 42% of the psychologist's workload was accounted for by children with medically related problems. The most frequent problems were depression, suicide attempts, poor adjustment to the illness and behavioural problems.

The psychological care starts with talking to the client. This gives an insight into their experiences of growing up with a physical abnormality. While medical staff and parents may be satisfied with the adolescent's achievements in education, grateful for the child having fewer urinary infections, and happy that the surgical operations have helped, children may not share these views and may have other criteria for success. They may believe that social relationships within the school are more important to them, or they would like to be able to do what others do without restrictions. There has been very little research undertaken in regard to children and adolescents with long-term illnesses, and the consequences of spending so much time in the company of adults rather than their peer groups. With more children surviving childhood urological diseases and abnormalities, our aim should be to develop closer working relationships between paediatric and adolescent urologists and psychologists. Uniting physical and psychological care from the outset will ultimately provide the adolescents and their families with the tools to access their own support network, and will subsequently have a beneficial effect on their self-esteem.

REFERENCES

ANDREWS S (1988) Coping with the sexual health interview. *Journal of Nurse-Midwifery* **33**(6): 269–273.

ASHWORTH P D and Hagan M T (1993) The meaning of incontinence – a qualitative study of non-geriatric urinary incontinence sufferers. *Journal of Advanced Nursing* **18**(9): 1415–1423.

AUDIT COMMISSION (1993) Children First: A Study of Hospital Services. London: HMSO.

BATES P (1979) The standard of terminology of lower urinary tract function. *Journal of Urology* **121**: 551–554.

BELLE D (ed.) (1989) *Children's Social Networks and Social Supports*. Chichester: John Wiley and sons.

BOORE J R P (1978) *A Prescription for Recovery: The Effects of Pre-operative Preparation of Surgical Patients on Post-operative Stress, Recovery and Infection*. London: Royal College of Nursing.

BRINK P J (1987) Cultural aspects of sexuality. *Holistic Nursing Practice* **1**(4): 12–20.

CHEATER F (1991) Attitudes to urinary incontinence. *Nursing Standard, 20 March*, **5**(26): 23–27.

DAVIS K (1990) Impotence after surgery. *Nursing* **4**(18): 23–25.

DEVLIN H B (ed.) (1995) *Surgery on the Prostate*. London: Royal College of Surgeons of England.

DEPARTMENT OF HEALTH (1989) *The Children Act*. London: HMSO.

DEPARMENT OF HEALTH (1991) *The Welfare of Children and Young People in Hospital*. London: HMSO.

DIMOND B (1990) *Legal Aspects of Nursing*. New York: Prentice Hall.

DOUGLAS J W B (1975) *Early Hospital Admission and Later Disturbances of Behaviour*. Cited in: *Nursing Children, Psychology Research and Practice*, D Muller (ed.), 1988. Oxford: Harper & Row.

DRENCH M E (1994) Changes in body image secondary to disease and injury. *Rehabilitation Nursing* **19**(1): 31–36.

DEWIS M E (1989) Spinal cord injured adolescents and young adults: The meaning of body changes. *Journal of Advanced Nursing* **14**: 389–396.

EISER C (1993) *Growing up with Chronic Disease: The Impact on Children and their Families*. London: Kingsley Publishers Ltd.

ERIKSON E H (1968) *Identity: Youth and Crisis*. London: Faber and Faber.

ERIKSON E H (1977) *Childhood and Society*. Harmondsworth: Penguin Books.

FAUGIER J (1988) Incontinence: hidden for whom? *Senior Nurse* **8**(3): 19–20.

FOLKMAN C (1984) Personal control and stress and coping process: a theoretical analysis. *Journal of Personality and Social Psychology* **46**(4): 839–852.

FRADD E (1988) It's child's play. *Nursing Times* **3**(6): 6–8.

FRIEDMAN I, Litt I, Henson R, King D, Holtzman D, Halverson D and Kraemer H (1986) Compliance with anticonvulsant therapy by epileptic youth. In Pidgeon V (ed.). Compliance with Chronic Illness Regimens: school aged children and adolescents. *Journal of Pediatric Nursing* **4**(1): 36–47.

GARRISON W T and McQuiston S (1989) *Chronic Illness During Childhood and Adolescence. Psychological Aspect*. London: Sage Publications.

GILLS L (1980) Human Behaviour in Illness, 3rd edn. London: Faber and Faber.

HEYWOOD (1975) *Information – A Prescription Against Pain*. London: Royal College of Nursing.

JACOBSON L (1974) Illness and human sexuality. *Nursing Outlook* **22**(1): 50–63.

JOHNSON S B, Pollak T, Silverstein J H, Rosenbloom A L, Spillar R, McCallum M and Harkavy J (1982) Cognitive and behavioural knowledge about insulin–dependent diabetes among children and parents. *Pediatrics* **69**: 709–713.

KÜBLER-ROSS E (1973) *On Death and Dying*. London: Tavistock.

LIPETZ M J, Bussigel M N, Bannerman J and Risley B (1990) What is wrong with patient education programmes? *Nursing Outlook* **38**(4): 184–90.

LOWE G R (1972) *The Growth of Personality from Infancy to Old Age*. London: Cox & Wyman.

MacKENZIE H (1988) Teenagers in hospital. *Nursing Times 10 August* **84**(32): 58–61.

McKENZIE F (1988) Sexuality after total pelvic exenteration. *Nursing Times* **84**(20): 27–30.

McLEOD Clark J (1981) Communication in nursing. *Nursing Times* **77**(1): 12.

MITTENESS L S (1990) Knowledge and belief about urinary incontinence in adulthood and old age. *Society* **38**(3): 374–378.

MULLER D, Harris P and Wattley L (1988) *Nursing Children: Psychology Research and Practice*. London: Harper & Row.

NICHOLS K A (1984) *Psychological Care in Physical Illness*. Sydney: Croom Helm Ltd.

NORTON C S (1982) The effects of urinary incontinence in women. *International Rehabilitation Medicine* **4**(1): 9–14.

NORTON P A, MacDonald L D and Stanton S L (1987) Distress associated with female urinary complaints and delay in seeking treatment. *Neurological Urodynamics* **6**(3): 170.

PATON D and Brown R (1991) *Lifespan Health Psychology Nursing Problems and Interventions.* London: Harper Collins.

PETERSON G (1989) Let the children play. *Nursing* **3**(41): 22–25.

PIAGET J (1952) *The Origins of Intelligence in Children.* New York: International Universities Press.

PLATZER H (1987) Body image: Helping intensive care patients to cope with changes – a problem for nurses part 2. *Intensive Care Nursing* **3**(3): 125–132.

PRICE B (1986) Keeping up appearances. *Nursing Times* **82**(40): 58–61.

PRICE B (1990) *Body Image – Nursing Concepts and Care.* London: Prentice-Hall.

QUINTON D and Rutter M (1976) *Early Hospital Admissions and Later Disturbances of Behaviour.* Cited in Hazardous secrets and reluctantly taking charge: parenting a child with repeated hospitalizations, Ogden Burke et al., 1991, *IMAGE: Journal of Nursing Scholarship* **23** (1): 39–45.

RODIN J (1983) *Will It Hurt?* London: Royal College of Nursing.

ROPER N, Logan W and Tierney A (1985) *The Elements of Nursing.* Edinburgh: Churchill Livingstone.

ROY C (1976) *Introduction to Nursing: An Adaptation Model.* New Jersey: Prentice-Hall.

SALTER M (Ed.) (1988) *Altered Body Image – The Nurse's Role.* London: Scutari Press.

SALTER M (1996) Sexuality and the stoma patient. In: *Stoma Care Nursing – A Patient-centred Approach.* Arnold Publishing.

SAYLOR C R (1990) The management of stigma: redefinition and representation. *Holistic Nursing Practice*, October, pp. 45–52.

SELEKMAN J (1991) Pediatric rehabilitation: from concept to practice. *Pediatric Nursing* **17**(1): 11–14.

TAYLOR J and Muller D (1995) Nursing Adolescents: Research and Psychological Perspectives. Oxford: Blackwell Science.

VISINTAINER M A and Wolfer J A (1975) Pediatric surgical patients' and parents' stress responses and adjustment. *Nursing Research* **24**: 244–255.

WHALEY D and Wongs L (1993) *Essentials of Pediatric Nursing.* New York: Mosby.

WILSON-BARNETT J (1980) Prevention and alleviation of stress in patients. *Nursing* **1**(10): 432–436.

WORLD HEALTH ORGANIZATION (1977) *Health Needs of Adolescents.* WHO expert Committee Technical Report Series 609. Geneva: WHO.

WRIGHT L (1974) *Bowel Function in Hospital Patients.* Royal College of Nursing Research Project, series 1, no. 4. London: RCN.

DEVELOPMENTS IN UROLOGICAL NURSING

17

Contents

RESEARCH NURSING IN UROLOGY

What is research nursing?

Research nursing has long lacked a clear definition of its precise meaning. The great majority of posts are moulded to the requirements of the individual consultant clinician or academician (Jordan, 1990). Most involve the conduct of clinical trials in one form or another and for many this is the only type of work involved. Research is expensive for academic or National Health Service establishments to fund, and relatively few research nursing posts involve purely academic work. In the authors' unit, the research nurses have taken on most of the responsibility for the actual running of clinical trials, a role which used to be undertaken purely by doctors.

The word 'research' derives from the French '*recherche*', meaning to look or search again. It is a systematic approach used to discover previously unknown facts. In the European Community (EC) guidelines on good clinical practice (CPMP, 1990), a clinical trial is defined as a 'systematic study on medicinal products (and more recently, medical devices) in human subjects . . . in order to discover or verify the effects of and/or identify any adverse reactions to investigational products . . . in order to ascertain their efficacy and safety'. Traditionally scientific (academic) research is poorly funded and often reliant on donations, grants and charities to secure its development. The so-called 'soft money' generated from drug company sponsorship of clinical trials can be viewed as a good source of finance for the more academic work.

Although the attitude of many people in Britain towards clinical research has essentially been one of caution (Bishop, 1983), recent innovations such as the Patients' Charter, ethical concepts of informed consent and the relative ease of litigation have done much to reassure potential candidates for trials and research and dissipate many of the old fears. The legislation governing clinical trials is complex and voluminous. Very little is written on the subject, and many nurses entering research are left to learn the processes involved by trial and error. This chapter is intended to clarify the basic rules which, although not specific to urology, are nevertheless of paramount importance and to provide an informative resumé of the clinical research process.

Standards in research

All research involving human subjects must abide by certain international standards. Since the 1960s there has been a tremendous increase not only in clinical research, but also in the government regulations controlling it. The sudden sharp rise in the incidence of phocomelia in newborn babies following the ingestion of the antiemetic drug thalidomide by pregnant women for first-trimester nausea sparked a furore which has never been forgotten. This disaster fuelled such anger amongst both the public and members of the medical profession that a call for stricter controls led governments to concede to scientific and political pressures and examine the entire research procedure. These regulations started in developed countries and now apply virtually worldwide. Mostly they are based on the regulations of the Food and Drug Administration (FDA) in the USA. Modern legislation and procedures have substantially increased the volume of paperwork generated, but have been designed to

- prevent fraudulent practices
- protect the rights of the individual volunteer subject
- avoid recurrence of pharmaceutical disasters such as thalidomide
- set universally recognized standards for the conduct of clinical research and trials

Good clinical practice

The EC guidelines for good clinical practice (GCP) are the European 'gold standard' for the conduct of clinical trials. European GCP closely parallels the FDA laws from which it was developed and is accepted by the USA as conforming to its own standards. It has been defined as the term used to describe the package of procedures needed to ensure that clinical studies meet the required international standards (Rondel, 1995). The GCP guidelines define the obligations of three main groups:

1. The sponsor, i.e. the company developing the drug or device and funding the research.
2. The monitor, i.e. the person allocated to check and regulate the progress of the trial and assist in providing an advisory role and a liaison between the investigator and the sponsor.
3. The investigator, traditionally the qualified medical practitioner (usually a consultant) conducting the trial but more recently including the research doctors and nurses who are increasingly assuming most of the responsibility for the day-to-day running of clinical trials. The investigator, however, remains wholly accountable for the written data collected from the research.

Obligations of the investigator

The obligations of the investigator are to ensure that all ethical controls are adhered to, assure the safe custody of the investigational product, conduct the study and maintain the agreed standard of record-keeping.

The minimal ethical standards are those specified in the World Medical Association Declaration of Helsinki. This is a document that was first drawn up in 1964 as a consequence of the atrocities of Nazi human experimentation during the Second World War. The Declaration has undergone various amendments, the most recent (World Medical Association, 1989) being that to which clinical trials and research must conform. Although almost everyone involved in human research has heard of the Declaration of Helsinki, few are able to summarize its contents, although it is an exceedingly important document with regard to subject welfare and as such deserves every attention. The Declaration states that the purpose of biomedical research involving human subjects must be to improve diagnostic, therapeutic and prophylactic procedures and the understanding of aetiology and pathogenesis of disease (World Medical Association, 1989). It recognizes that human research involves certain hazards but concedes that experimentation on human subjects is ultimately inevitable. It outlines the rights of the individual subject, the main points being as follows:

- the research must conform to generally accepted scientific principles
- the research protocol must be submitted to an independent ethics committee for approval
- the responsibility for the trial must always rest with a medically qualified person
- the objectives must be in proportion to the risks to the subject
- the interests of the volunteer are more important than those of science and society
- the subject's confidentiality and anonymity must be preserved
- the potential hazards of the research should be predictable

- ◆ the published results must be accurate
- ◆ the subject must receive an information sheet outlining risks, benefits, aims and methods using language that is comprehensible to members of the public. The subject is free to withdraw consent at any time without jeopardizing future care and management.

Informed consent

The European guidelines for GCP base their advice on informed consent on the Declaration of Helsinki (Rondel, 1995). Participation of volunteers must be voluntary, and if possible oral as well as written information regarding the research study should be given. Patients should be given the opportunity to ask questions and should have ample time (i.e. a few days) to make a decision. It is always an important element of informed consent that patients should not feel pressurized or obliged to enter a trial and may withdraw their consent at any time without having to give a reason for doing so.

The information given to patients must contain clear indication of any risks involved, for example urodynamic investigation of the lower urinary tract carries a small risk of urinary tract infection. If such tests are required, the patients should be told of the risk but also informed that they will be given prophylactic antibiotic cover. Another example could be the potential hazard to an unborn fetus from hormone manipulation, e.g. 5-alpha reductase inhibitors used in benign prostatic hyperplasia. Men contemplating entering a trial involving these drugs must be warned of the dangers and given contraceptive advice. Should a man wish to father children during the treatment period then he should not participate in any trial of such drugs.

Patients generally appreciate receiving detailed information and once they feel that their feelings and rights are being respected, they are far more likely to commit themselves to a trial and remain compliant. Such co-operation is essential to ensure that the quality of the data collected is of a good standard. It is important that the patient is always encouraged to express any concerns and thus is given the feeling of being in control, not just a 'guinea-pig'.

Patients agree to participate in clinical trials for a variety of reasons but there are some strong recurrent themes. Some wish to avoid surgery; for example, the man who prefers to try alpha-blockers before resorting to prostatectomy. Many men prefer this option on the understanding that they will remain on the waiting list for surgery during the course of the trial so as not to prolong the amount of time they have to wait should they change their mind or should the medication not be effective. Some patients hope to gain some benefit that has so far eluded them, such as the patient who has tried every medication available to relieve the symptoms of an unstable bladder. Others feel that they have some debt to repay to the health service and enter trials for altruistic reasons. A commonly expressed view is that although the study drug may not be of use to that particular volunteer, the study results may benefit other people with similar problems in the future. Whatever the patient's reasons are, the rules of informed consent apply universally.

Selection criteria

Each clinical trial is designed to target a specific patient population. This is done by defining a set of inclusion and exclusion criteria which must be met in order for a patient to enter.

The inclusion criteria specify the limits of the variables as well as the definitive diganosis. An inclusion criterion for an anticholinergic drug trial could therefore be detrusor instability or hyperreflexia. Such a trial would usually require some objective proof of the diagnosis such as urodynamic evaluation and also subjective evidence such as symptomatology.

The exclusion criteria are those conditions that must not be present in the patient prior to entry into the trial. For the above example, the exclusion criteria would include significant bladder outflow obstruction, usually defined as a maximum flow rate of less than 15 ml s^{-1}. Administering an anticholinergic drug to such patients could send them into urinary retention.

There are some general criteria which apply to most urological clinical trials. Patients included are usually between the ages of 18 and 85 years. Exclusions include uncontrolled diabetes mellitus, significant cardiac disease such as unstable angina, congestive cardiac failure or serious arrhythmias, and concurrent malignancy (unless it is a cancer trial).

Approaching and recruiting volunteers

For a nurse working in clinical trials, a large proportion of the time is taken up by identifying and recruiting suitable volunteers. One needs to identify the patient group that will comply with the inclusion and exclusion criteria. Patients can only be entered with permission from a suitably experienced doctor, in this case a urologist.

Investigating consultants will enter their own patients when suitable, but as large numbers of patients with specific diagnoses may be required within a certain time limit, other sources of potential trial candidates may be needed. Other urologists can refer patients for trials, but the overall responsibility for their well-being during the trial must always rest with the named investigator. If nurses are performing the day-to-day running of the trial it is important that the referring doctor writes a letter confirming the referral or that a referral form is completed. Sometimes potential recruits can be identified from test results, e.g. video urodynamics or cystometrogram reports. This can be a useful source of patients with bladder instability or benign prostatic hyperplasia. In these cases it is essential that the patient is given the diagnosis by the doctor before being approached by research staff, and only after this may the patient be contacted by telephone or letter. It is useful if research nurses trawl outpatients clinics and check through patient records before they see a doctor. A memorandum can be placed on those who may be suitable and the clinic doctor can then discuss the idea of a trial with the patient. A patient who wishes to pursue the matter further can see the research nurse afterwards or arrange a mutually convenient time for a further appointment. The personal contact often makes this the easiest method of recruitment. In cases of external referrals, the consultant in charge of the patient's care must be fully aware of the details of the trial and the care of the patient is temporarily transferred to the investigating consultant for the duration of the trial.

Once a volunteer has been identified, a full explanation and discussion take place and the patient is given a printed information sheet. Telephone contact is made after a few days once the patient has had time to read the information and discuss it with family or general practitioner. Patients who are first contacted by telephone or by letter sometimes wish to pay a visit to the unit to meet staff and see the equipment that may be involved. Occasionally they request that the research staff discuss the trial with their general practitioner. The patients are always given as much information as possible and are reminded of their status as a volunteer. It is stressed that they may withdraw at any time without prejudice to their future care and management.

Some patients require a letter to their employer in order to be able to obtain time off. It is unethical and forbidden to offer remuneration for participation in a trial or for time off work, but the fares incurred for hospital visits and incidental expenses such as food and drink are refundable.

As mentioned above, male patients who wish to father children are prohibited from entering some trials. Women of childbearing potential may participate in most trials provided that they use adequate contraceptive precautions. The definition of this will be laid down in the trial protocol but generally refers to the contraceptive pill, intrauterine devices, cap and spermicide or condom and spermicide. Even if the patient states that she is celibate at the time, she must be given this advice. All protocols are designed for safety, thus, during the screening phase, the urine of women of childbearing potential is subjected to a pregnancy test. If this is positive, a serum sample is sent for testing. The result must be negative prior to dosing with the trial drug. The results of all tests taken during screening must be scrutinized by the research doctor. The patient can only start taking the trial compound in a drug trial when it is confirmed that all the tests are within normal limits.

When patients have been successfully screened and included, they are given a card stating this and listing emergency contact numbers. If there is a time lapse between a visit and starting medication it is helpful if the research nurse telephones the patient as a reminder the day before dosing is due. The benefits of this are threefold. Firstly, the patient is less likely to forget to start the tablets; secondly, the contact gives the nurse the opportunity to reiterate any specific instructions; and thirdly, it helps patients to feel valued and that they have not been abandoned.

The use of placebo in clinical trials

Placebo has been defined as a medicine given to humour, rather than cure, the patient (Sykes, 1983). In some trials the efficacy of the trial compound may be compared with a placebo or 'dummy' drug. The presentation of each is identical in colour, taste, weight and smell. When a placebo is used in a comparative study, the patient is made aware of the possibility of not receiving active treatment, or of receiving both active and passive treatment, without knowing which is the case. No trial will proceed without signed informed consent from the patient.

Sometimes a trial is designed to include a placebo run-in. For example, on screening a patient with benign prostatic hyperplasia for an alpha-blocker trial, the patient completes an international prostate symptom source (IPSS) sheet. He is then given a bottle of placebo tablets to take for 2 weeks, but in this instance he is not aware that the tablets he is taking are inactive. Following this he returns for a second visit and completes a further IPSS sheet. If there is an appreciable improvement in his symptoms he is said to have had a 'placebo effect' and is therefore withdrawn from the trial, as any subjective data he would provide cannot be regarded as valid.

New drugs and other innovations in urology

Clinical trials and research are important for the progress of treatment and there are many possibilities for the development of new products within urology. This section describes innovations in the treatment of benign disease, as well as providing a short explanation of how current urological drugs work.

As occurs in most groups of drugs, the first generation is usurped by newer (and usually more expensive) alternatives. The aim of any drug company developing a new compound is to find one that acts by a completely different mechanism and/or is safer, more effective and better tolerated than those already available.

Drugs act by three main mechanisms:

- ◆ at the cell membrane (e.g. alpha-blockers, anticholinergics)
- ◆ within the cell itself (e.g. chemotherapy, 5-alpha reductase inhibitors)
- ◆ outside the cell (local anaesthetic gel)

Most urological drugs fall into the first category, that is, they act at the cell membrane. These drugs target molecules, usually proteins, called receptors which are present at the cell membrane. Receptors recognize certain chemicals produced by the body and bind with them in competition with natural substances, so changing the response of the cell.

There are three types of drugs acting on receptors; agonists, antagonists and partial agonists. Current receptor-active urological drugs have antagonistic properties. Antagonists, also known as blockers, are drugs that are sufficiently similar to the endogenous substance to occupy the receptor, thereby deactivating it or blocking its action.

Oxybutynin and alpha-blockers both work in this way. Oxybutynin is a muscarinic receptor antagonist. When muscarinic receptors are activated, certain smooth muscle (e.g. detrusor) is caused to contract. Oxybutynin blocks this action, thereby reducing bladder contractions. Not surprisingly, alpha-blockers target alpha-receptors and reduce smooth muscle contraction at the bladder neck and in the prostate.

Muscarinic and alpha-receptors are not only present in the genitourinary tract but also in other parts of the body. For example, muscarinic receptors can be found in the bowel, the acinar cells of the salivary glands, the ciliary muscles controlling the curvature of the lens of the eye, and so forth. This explains oxybutynin's side-effects of constipation (reduced gut motility), dry mouth (reduced salivary secretion) and blurred vision (relaxation of the ciliary muscles). Alpha-receptors are also present in the small blood vessels, hence blockade can cause relaxation (dilation) of these vessels and therefore hypotension and dizziness.

Drug manufacturers are particularly interested in producing drugs with fewer side-effects and are therefore looking for more specific drugs or (perhaps more accurately) drugs that target more specific receptors. New compounds currently in development or on trial are aiming to block subtypes of receptors which are found in greatest quantities in the genitourinary tract and in only small numbers elsewhere in the body. Recent research has identified several subtypes, for example, alpha-1_A receptors (Lepor *et al.*, 1993) in the prostate, which were previously unknown. Targeting specific receptor subtypes will, it is hoped, have a greater therapeutic effect and reduce side-effects experienced by patients.

Intravesical therapy is a growing area of interest and the possibility of this as a route of administration for several new compounds is being explored. Its use in carcinoma in situ of the bladder is well established, and there are possible applications for its use in conditions such as primary bladder instability and sensory urgency.

Drug treatment for erectile impotence is an area undergoing many changes. Intracavernosal papaverine used to be the standard remedy for this condition, but owing to its severe alpha-blocker side-effects of hypotension and priapism it has now been replaced by alprostadil, a prostaglandin vasodilator, PGE_1. Although the incidence of priapism is considerably less, the hyperalgesic effects of prostaglandins can cause painful erections and pain at the site of injection. The drug is also unstable in solution, which necessitates the preparation of the injection by the patient just prior to its use. Other vasoactive compounds are being investigated for their potential use in impotence, the aim being to find a drug that is more easily administered and has minimal side-effects.

Not all clinical trials involve completely new drugs or devices. Different applications for established treatments may also be investigated. A good example of this is finasteride, an anti-androgen which prevents metabolism of testosterone to dihydrotestosterone by the enzyme 5-alpha reductase. Finasteride chemically resembles the enzyme sufficiently to compete with it and so inhibit testosterone metabolism. This leads to a reduction in prostatic tissue and therefore outflow obstruction in benign prostatic hypertrophy. The possible benefit derived from such hormone manipulation can unfortunately take months to become apparent, significantly limiting the use of this drug. Recent clinical trials aim to discover a potentially more effective alternative by using finasteride with alpha-blockers as a combination therapy. Preliminary results from a study in American veterans has suggested that monotherapy with alpha-blockers is as effective as combination therapy, but there are several other studies whose results may or may not confirm this.

The unsuitability of many patients as candidates for surgery, the unwillingness of others to undergo such intervention and current financial and managerial pressures related to reducing waiting lists and treatment costs are strong incentives for companies to search for alternatives.

Intraurethral devices for female stress incontinence are another area of particular interest and are being developed and tested. Trials with a disposable urethral 'plug' have already been conducted, and a more permanent intraurethral 'valve' is undergoing clinical studies. The long-term practicality, viability and safety of such devices remain to be seen. Although urethral stents for males are not a very new idea, the search is on to develop more effective designs with longer-lasting results.

Basic research

Basic research usually falls under the jurisdiction of scientists and doctors with students or higher surgical trainees taking on projects leading to a PhD or other higher degree. Much of the work can appear very remote from the patient whom it is supposed to benefit. This is partly because of the length of time, very often years, which it takes for the technology or discovery to reach a stage where it can safely be tested or used in human subjects. Nurses are not often involved in such research unless it is directly concerned with patients as subjects. The author has become involved with work on neuromodulation using healthy volunteers and patients. The nurses' role includes providing patients with information about the tests involved during the recruitment phase, patient care during the procedures including placement of filling and pressure catheters for urodynamics, and assisting the investigators with the actual experiments.

Neuromodulation in urology has its origins in the 1970s with work on pudendal nerve electrical stimulation to inhibit detrusor instability (Godec et al., 1975). Permanent electrical implants to stimulate S3 nerve roots are being used in spinal injury patients to suppress detrusor hyperreflexia and initiate bladder emptying. Prior to permanent implantation, temporary wires are left in place for a week to assess patient suitability for the device. A new non-invasive method with potential investigative and therapeutic benefits in the treatment of both detrusor instability and hyperreflexia is magnetic stimulation of the sacral nerve roots. Early work using this method has been successful in suppressing both hyperreflexia (Sheriff et al., 1996) and instability (McFarlane et al., 1996). By performing simultaneous urodynamic studies with magnetic stimulation, our understanding of bladder physiology and dysfunction is expanding.

As urology is a growing specialty and much is still not known about the causes of many urological disorders – and indeed their physiology – there is undoubtedly a wealth of knowledge to be discovered and explored. As science progresses, and the understanding of urology increases, the quest to provide better treatment will continue and clinical trials and research are unlikely to be in short supply.

EXPANDING NURSING ROLES IN UROLOGY

The provision and delivery of health care in the UK is currently undergoing a period of rapid change (Leathard, 1990). The purchaser-provider split, new technology and increasingly high public expectations have transformed the structure and philosophy of care for everyone. The nursing profession has needed to respond to these changes as well as to specific professional issues.

Since clinical grading was introduced in the late 1980s there has been a recognition that nurses need a career structure that supports and rewards clinical expertise and experience (Wade and Moyer, 1989). Nursing initiatives from the Department of Health have discussed strategies for the development of nursing including the concept of specialist and advanced practice (Department of Health, 1993). The nurses' own regulatory body has issued guidelines for expanding traditional nursing roles (UKCC, 1992b) which emphasize personal accountability rather than formal certification.

In addition to these issues, junior doctors are also facing changes in working hours and training (Calman, 1993). The working practices and availability of junior doctors inevitably have an impact on the patient, the nurse and the nursing role. Nurses are finding themselves faced with a multifactorial problem. They need to reconcile the needs and demands of the patient, the service and their own professional development, while ensuring that the nursing profession is also advanced in the process. This is an awesome task which in many areas is being tackled with enthusiasm and commitment.

A prime example is in the area of urological nursing. In many centres, urological nurses are expanding and extending their practice in response to the patient and the service. Some of these initiatives are discussed below within the context of the nurse's role. Many of these innovative roles are local ideas which have succeeded because of the vision and commitment of individuals. This chapter aims to draw together some themes and ideas and identify any recurring problems, and by doing so provide advice for nurses who are interested in developing their role in this way.

The role of the nurse

Role expansion is not a modern concept. The nursing profession has been evolving and changing since the Middle Ages. Nursing has progressed from being a simple extension of a woman's role, through to the influences of Florence Nightingale and onwards towards the search for professional status (Wainwright, 1994). Yet a common argument used when looking at aspects of role expansion is the question, 'Is it nursing?'. Often we have a personal instinctive idea about what nursing is, but this is not always articulated or defined. The move away from the pre-1960s idea of the nurse as the doctor's handmaiden is reflected in the definition of the role of the nurse by Virginia Henderson:

> 'The unique function of the nurse is to assist the individual, sick or well, in the performance of those activities contributing to health or its recovery (or to a peaceful death) that he would perform unaided if he had the necessary strength, will, or knowledge. And to do this in such a way as to help him gain independence as rapidly as possible. This aspect of her work, this part of her function, she initiates and controls; of this she is master.' (Henderson, 1966)

What is clear is that nursing cannot be defined by the tasks that nurses do. Perhaps that is why it has been unhelpful to look at role expansion as the process whereby the nurse acquires extra skills, usually skills that were previously the domain of another professional group. Maguire (1980) suggested that the term *expanded practice* should be reserved for roles that require nurse education and in which nursing skills are used, and that *extended practice* should describe roles where tasks are basically medical and nurse training is not essential. True role expansion is a response to the holistic needs of the patient and reflects the nurse's ability to see and meet a range of needs. This may involve the acquisition of new skills which have traditionally been the province of another profession such as medicine. The important issue is that the art and science of nursing is being augmented by the new skills rather than being undermined (Mitchinson and Goodlad, 1996). This may be the most powerful argument for ensuring that any changes in the nurse's role in individual areas should be a nurse-led initiative.

Making changes

A review of the role of a nurse may be initiated for many reasons, e.g. by nurses themselves, or may be instigated because of management issues or for political or financial reasons. Whatever the precipitating factor, the nurse will need to take a leading part in redefining the boundaries of her practice. The nurse may like to consider three issues:

1. What is the objective of change?
2. What limitations does the nurse face?
3. How do we maintain standards and ensure the safety of the patient and ourselves?

Alongside these issues also runs the ongoing question of whether the change benefits nursing as a profession.

The objective of the change

A major criterion for the instigation of change, according to the UK Central Council for Nursing, Midwifery and Health Visiting (UKCC, 1992b), is that 'each aspect of practice is directed to meeting the needs and serving the interests of the patient'. Therefore, for example, the fact that a nurse's role adjustment results in a reduction in the hours worked by a junior doctor is not in itself a sufficient reason for change. The UKCC is clear that the nursing role remains patient-centred and any role expansion should seek to improve patient care.

Limitations on practice

We do face some limitations in our practice and it is vital that we are confident where these limitations lie. This may be expressed in terms of our duties and obligations, i.e. to the employer, the profession, the patient and the public.

The employer

The relationship with the employer involves an employment contract with the health authority or trust. Nurses undertake to provide a service, but the employer must be aware of any change in duties from those performed by someone working in what would generally be considered to be a traditional nursing role. Therefore the job description or contract should include details of the expanded role. Then, in the event of complaint or litigation, providing we have not acted in a negligent fashion, the employer accepts vicarious liability. It is also wise to belong to a professional organization providing indemnity insurance for its members.

The profession

The UKCC provides registration to practice. By this process the public can expect a certain level of competence. The nurse is bound to adhere to its code of conduct (UKCC, 1992a), which with its subsequent publications provides principles and guidelines by which to judge practice.

The patient

Each individual patient has a range of rights protected by civil law. An abuse of these rights may result in litigation. Dowling et al. (1996) highlighted some particular problems that may occur with the emergence of new breeds of practitioners. They particularly stress the areas of negligence and battery. They remind us that in the event of an accusation of negligence against a nurse undertaking a traditionally medical task, the nurse will be judged against the standard of any competent practitioner, i.e. in this case a doctor.

A battery is committed if a patient is touched without consent. Dowling et al (1996) argued that the patient may assume the nurse to be a doctor because of the nature of the contact or the lack of uniform. If nurses do not properly identify themselves the consent to treatment may not be valid and a battery may be committed.

The public

There are specific Acts of Parliament which protect the public in hospital. These include the Nurses, Midwives and Health Visitors Act 1979, the National Health Service Act of 1977 and the Medicines Act of 1968. Within these Acts are definite legal parameters which limit the practice of a non-medical practitioner. These include such issues as the prescription of drugs and certification of death.

Maintaining standards and ensuring safety

The UKCC's publication *The Scope of Professional Practice* (UKCC, 1992b) gives nurses guidelines for change rather than the more restrictive system of requiring certification for individual tasks. This was also a recognition that the boundaries of any profession are not fixed. Any professional group needs to be able to respond to changes including advancing technology and new techniques. The UKCC guidelines state that when expanding the scope of practice the nurse must:

> 'endeavour always to achieve, maintain and develop knowledge, skill and competence to respond to the [needs and interests of the patient] . . . and acknowledge any limits of personal knowledge and skill and take steps to remedy any relevant deficits.' (UKCC, 1992b)

This ongoing learning and identification of educational needs may include formal courses and skill acquisition, but equally may consist of private study, reflection and one-to-one learning opportunities. It is important that the nurse keeps a record of this personal education and development, both as a tool for reflective practice and as evidence towards proof of competency. The nurse should also maintain a record of assessments and reviews for the same reasons.

The nature of role expansion means that nurses may need to gain skills traditionally performed by other professions to complement their nursing practice. Some professional groups may have a different cultural approach to teaching and supervision. The nursing profession has never been a great advocate of the 'see one, do one, teach one' method, and in practice some nurses have expressed worries that they may be expected to perform tasks that they do not feel able to do. The UKCC guidelines indicate that the nurse should be responsible for ensuring that this does not happen.

Professionally, therefore, the UKCC provides clear guidelines about the nurse's continuing responsibility to identify educational needs and deficits and take appropriate action to remedy these. However, we may also need to take a wider look at hospital policy and the nurse's status as employee. In the event of any investigation, complaint or litigation, the nurse must be able to show that he or she was working within the recognized boundaries of the role of the nurse. If the nurse has moved away from what would generally be considered the traditional role, the employer may refuse support. Therefore in order to be protected by vicarious liability nurses must ensure that the role and duties they perform are formally recognized. In many centres the use of protocols are favoured. These are defined by Lanara (1994) as:

> 'a written plan specifying the procedures to be followed in a given particular examination, in conducting research or in providing care for a particular condition.'

These protocols should be written or agreed in collaboration with medical staff and management. The sanctioned protocol then has the joint purpose of proposing an agreed level of care for the patient and giving the nurse the documented support or consent of management, medical staff and the hospital administration. Following this theme, Scott (1995) defined the protocol as:

> 'a framework for additional responsibilities we have not previously held, and is the contract between ourselves, our medical colleagues and the employer.'

As mentioned previously, the nurse's job description should clearly define the specific nature of the post. Subsequent protocols will provide guidelines in individual areas of practice.

The expanded role in practice

There are a number of areas in urology where key duties are traditionally undertaken by junior doctors on short-term rotations, occasionally with little experience or even interest in urology. In some of these areas motivated and experienced nurses are making a vast difference to the quality of care delivered to the patient. These include services for men with erectile dysfunction, continence and stoma care, and prostate assessment.

In some centres a nurse is incorporated into the medical team, often replacing a junior doctor. In terms of professional issues this is probably one of the more controversial models of role expansion. Some nurses have argued that this is so removed from the traditional role of the nurse that it is not a true nursing role at all. This may be true if the nurse is assisting the care and treatment of the patient by performing extended skills only. The nurse may have no input into the role definition and may in effect be taking over a hotchpotch of jobs that no one else wants. In these cases the nurse is likely to feel poorly used and undervalued. It is also a waste of resources and talent, as a technician could equally perform many routine tasks. The nursing role in this case is being extended to incorporate aspects of a junior doctor's job, but without really being expanded or advancing the profession of nursing.

However, the incorporation of the nurse into the consultant team may work in a different way. It can create a cohesive team where the nurse has a direct influence on the management of the patient and a unique chance to see the whole care experience of the patient from a different angle, while retaining and using the unique nursing insight. The role can provide an effective means of communication between medical and nursing staff and encourage a holistic approach to the patient.

The nurse may be able to gain an in-depth knowledge of a client group throughout their inpatient and outpatient episodes and be in a position to identify client groups who may benefit from a 'medico-nursing' approach to the assessment of their needs, the diagnosis and treatment of their condition and the ongoing support of themselves and their family.

The second analysis of the role requires a team who understand the value of nursing and who are willing to both teach and be prepared to stand back and allow some of their traditional territory to be changed. Also needed is a strong and supportive nurse manager or advisor who is willing to act as a guide in professional issues. Without these the nurse is likely to feel isolated and unsupported. The good communication which is the linchpin of the model will not be present and the initiative is likely to fail.

Nurse-led clinics

In addition to the above role, or as a separate initiative, nurses have set up assessment and treatment services for patients presenting with a defined range of urological problems. These include men with bladder outflow obstruction, men with erectile dysfunction, adults and children with continence problems and individuals with haematuria. Again, there are wide variations in provision for patients. We can look at an outflow obstruction assessment service or prostate clinic as an example which highlights the difference between extended and expanded roles.

The following are descriptions of two imaginary prostate clinics run by nurses. We may wish to consider the benefits and drawbacks to the patient and the nurse.

Clinic 1

Nurse Smith runs a prostate assessment clinic one day a week, where she sees men presenting with lower urinary tract symptoms. She has a pro-forma written by her consultant with which she is able to take a history from the patient. She orders some blood tests following the guidelines for investigating prostates. She similarly obtains a flow rate and the patient is then ready to see the doctor in order to be examined, assessed and treated with either medication or surgery. The patient is followed up by whichever doctor is present at the clinic on the day he returns.

Clinic 2

Nurse Jones runs a prostate assessment clinic one day a week, where she sees men presenting with lower urinary tract symptoms. She sees men in a dedicated clinic and works to a protocol devised by herself and a group of clinicians. The protocol has been approved by the clinical director, her line manager and the Health Trust. She has received training and education in the relevant clinical skills and is competent to perform these. She has a recognized source of support should an unfamiliar situation occur which she feels unqualified to deal with. She introduces herself as the nurse to the patient and explains her role, although the patient has already received this information with his appointment.

Nurse Jones is able to take a full medical history with clinical examination including flow rate, ultrasound estimation of residual volume of urine and digital rectal examination. After listening to the patient's account of the problem and his perception of the effect of this on his health and well-being, she uses her clinical judgement as to the possible cause and effect of the presenting symptoms. She is able to assess the medical, nursing and individual social and emotional needs of the patient to augment her clinical judgement. She is able to provide information, education (written and verbal) and advice as to subsequent treatment including preventive measures, and either refer the patient on for surgical intervention or advise the general practitioner about medical or non-interventional options according to what the patient has chosen. Follow-up or ongoing support may be also at the nurse clinic. If the patient needs surgical intervention, according to the structure of the nursing role she may go on to care for the patient during his inpatient stay including his admission clerking, where she will be able to effectively reinforce the information already given and build on the therapeutic relationship already initiated on first presentation.

The patient's perspective

For the patient there may be an initial worry or anxiety about seeing a nurse instead of a 'proper doctor'. In practice, anecdotal reports suggest that most nurses have found that as long as the patient is given the relevant information very few actually mind. For most people, a knowledgeable practitioner with a courteous, respectful approach, honesty and competence are the ingredients for a successful hospital visit. Often, what the nursing approach actually means for a number of patients is more time, more empathy and more understanding with no associated loss of competence or confidence.

However, some patients still wish to see a medical practitioner and this should be respected.

The patient is one of the reasons for the role change so the nurse should be able to identify areas of care for possible improvement. In the case of the prostate clinic these may include:

◆ provision of a consistently high standard of care in an area where there may be a high turnover of medical staff
◆ improved advice for men with lower urinary tract symptoms
◆ early preoperative education for men about to undergo prostate surgery
◆ provision of continuity of care for a vulnerable group of patients

In Clinic 1 there is little evidence of any nursing intervention. The clinic is used as a clearing house for patients so that the technical 'legwork' is done before the patient sees the doctor. As the patient is not actually assessed there is little scope for advice or health education. There may be a chance for the nurse to begin to form a relationship with the patient, but the benefits are negated when the continuity of care is disrupted as the patient is moved on to an unfamiliar person for the potentially embarrassing and unpleasant part of the consultation, the examination.

In Clinic 2 the patient is the focus of the episode. Hopefully there is more scope for the building of a trusting and therapeutic relationship where the patient's needs and fears are allowed to be expressed and taken into account. Hence his needs are not only recognized but addressed at that point. In incorporating the technical tasks needed for a full assessment of the patient's physical status in the nurse's remit, she is able to provide for the patient a truly holistic service.

The nurse's perspective

The role of the nurse in Clinic 1 is that of a technician. There is no scope for autonomy or clinical judgement. It can be easy to get stuck at this point without professional and clinical support. There may be a lack of confidence in the acquisition of the necessary clinical skills such as rectal examination, or it may be a reluctance on the part of the medical staff to relinquish the role to a nurse. There has been considerable debate by urologists as to who is the appropriate person to perform and interpret digital rectal examination and the themes of the argument are as discussed before. Peer support and the sharing of experiences are the key at this time.

Clinic 2, in contrast, is truly nurse-led. With support and ongoing review for this nurse she can continue to develop herself and the service for the benefit of the patient. Ongoing audit and review is an essential part of the clinic and encourages optimum evidence-based practice and the early identification of resource or education needs.

The problems of the expanded role

There are inevitably problems associated with any new initiative. Each area will experience some that are common to all. It is hoped that as more nurses share their experiences we may begin to learn from each other.

Education

Some centres are considering or have just finalized Master's degree level courses in advanced practice as discussed by the UKCC (1994). These should provide a core curriculum including professional issues and health assessment. The course will not provide a step-by-step educational programme consisting of all a urology nurse practitioner would need to know, but will rather nurture the ideals of therapeutic nursing care and expand on the framework for role expansion.

Career structure

Currently there is little scope for advancement or progress clinically past the level of nurse practitioner or nurse specialist. It is a source of frustration to many nurses who want to continue to care for patients, but may reach the top of their earning potential in their mid-20s. This is an area which is currently being addressed by the profession.

What of the bedside nurse?

We are in a time of great change and advancement in nursing and we have concentrated on some of the ground-breaking initiatives that are taking place. However, most urology nursing takes place at the bedside and we should not ignore the equally important work being done there. One danger when discussing expanded practice is that despite talking about patient-centred care we can forget that for the patient, high-quality nursing care is not about the profession or academic arguments, but is about receiving what is needed, when it is needed, in a compassionate, competent and caring manner.

The object of role expansion is not to create a breed of super-nurses who are superior to the traditional nurse in status and pay, but rather to allow all nurses to examine their role and adapt their practice to the specific need of the patient if it is needed. It involves the appreciation of all aspects of care and the flexibility and discernment to adapt to given situations. It is hoped that neither ward nurses nor nurse practitioners will become threatened or deskilled in the process.

The way forward

As a profession and as a speciality, urology nurses need to continue to take a lead in fighting for and delivering high-quality nursing care to the patient. The formation of the British Association of Urological Nurses has united more than 650 nurses in the common goal of improving the standard of care for the urological patient. Within this there is the scope to look at many expanded roles and evaluate the contribution to the patient and the profession. The expansion of the nurse's role must be a nurse-led initiative if it is to benefit the patient, the nurse and advance the profession. We need educational opportunities, appropriate supervision and the ongoing support of our medical colleagues to achieve this. For the immediate future we must look urgently at uniting education and a career structure in order to support and ultimately improve the individual pockets of excellent work going on. These are exciting times and urology nurses must be congratulated for responding to so many diverse needs in such innovative ways. The ultimate beneficiary is the patient.

REFERENCES

BISHOP V (1983) Anxiety and the volunteer. *Nursing Mirror* **156**(3): 62.

CALMAN K (1993) *Hospital Doctors: Training For The Future*. Report of the Working Group on Specialist Medical Training. London: DHSS.

CPMP WORKING PARTY ON EFFICACY OF MEDICINAL PRODUCTS (1990) *Good Clinical Practice for Trials on Medicinal Products*. EEC Note For Guidance, pp. 361–372.

DEPARTMENT OF HEALTH (1993) *A Vision of the Future. The Nursing, Midwifery and Health Visiting Contribution to Health and Health Care*. London: DOH.

DOWLING S, Martin R, Skidmore P, Doyal L, Cameron A and Lloyd S (1996) Nurses taking on junior doctors' work: a confusion of accountability. *British Medical Journal* **312**: 1211–1214.

GODEC C, Cass A S and Ayala G F (1975) Bladder inhibition with functional electrical stimulation. *Urology* **6**: 663–666.

HENDERSON V (1996) *The Nature of Nursing*. London: Collier-Macmillan.

JORDAN S (1990) Look before you leap. *Nursing Times* **86**(11): 42.

LANARA V (1994) Protocol matters. *Nursing Standard* **8**(24): 14.

LEATHARD A (1990) *Health Care Provision: Past, Present and Future*. London: Chapman & Hall.

LEPOR H, Tang R, Meretyk S and Shapiro E (1993) Alpha$_1$ adrenoceptor subtypes in the human prostate. *Journal of Urology* **149**: 640–642.

McFARLANE J P, Foley S J, de Winter P, Shah P J R and Craggs M D (1996) Suppression of detrusor instability in man by magnetic stimulation of the sacral nerve roots. *Journal of Physiology* **497**: 16.

MAGUIRE J (1980) *The Expanded Role of the Nurse*. London: Kings Fund.

MITCHINSON S and Goodlad S (1996) Changes in the roles and responsibilities of nurses. *Professional Nurse* **11**(11): 734–736.

RONDEL R K (1995) *Syllabus for GCP Workshop for Research Nurses*. Oxford Workshops.

SCOTT G (1995) Challenging conventional roles in palliative care. *Nursing Times* **91**(3): 38–39.

SHERIFF M K M, Shah P J R, Fowler C, Mundy A R and Craggs M D (1996) Neuromodulation of detrusor hyperreflexia by functional magnetic stimulation of the sacral roots. *British Journal of Urology* **78**: 39–46.

SYKES J B (ed.) (1983) *Concise Oxford Dictionary* 7th edn. Oxford University Press.

[UKCC] United Kingdom Central Council for Nursing, Midwifery and Health Visiting (1992a) *Code of Professional Conduct*. London: UKCC.

[UKCC] United Kingdom Central Council for Nursing, Midwifery and Health Visiting (1992b) *The Scope of Professional Practice*. London: UKCC.

[UKCC] United Kingdom Central Council for Nursing, Midwifery and Health Visiting (1994) *The Council's Standards for Education and Practice Following Registration*. London: UKCC.

WADE B and Moyer A (1989) An evaluation of clinical nurse specialists: implications for education and the organisation of care. *Senior Nurse* **9**(9): 11–15.

WAINWRIGHT P (1994) Professionalism and the concept of role extension. In: Hunt G and Wainwright P (eds) *Expanding the Role of the Nurse*. Oxford: Blackwell Scientific.

WORLD MEDICAL ASSOCIATION (1989) Declaration of Helsinki. *41st World Medical Assembly, Hong Kong*. Ferney-Voltaire: World Medical Association.

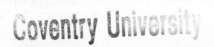

INDEX

Note – Page references in **bold** indicate major references, those in *italic* indicate illustrations and tables.